Alpha Development Team

Publisher
Kathy Nebenhaus

Editorial Director
Gary M. Krebs

Managing Editor
Bob Shuman

Marketing Brand Manager
Felice Primeau

Editor
Jessica Faust

Development Editors
Phil Kitchel
Amy Zavatto

Production Team

Development Editor
John Jones

Production Editor
Stephanie Mohler

Copy Editor
Krista Hansing

Cover Designer
Mike Freeland

Photo Editor
Richard Fox

Cartoonist
Bryan Hendrix

Designers
Scott Cook and Amy Adams of DesignLab

Indexer
Tim Tate

Layout/Proofreading
Angela Calvert
Gina Rexrode
Julie Trippetti

Contents at a Glance

Part 1: The Fountain of Youth   **1**

1 So, You Want to Live to Be 100?   3
Why living to 100 may not be so far-fetched.

2 The Physical Exam   13
Things to keep in mind when consulting your doctor.

3 The Dietary Balancing Act   25
How not to fall short of your minimum dietary requirements.

4 Isn't Carrot Cake a Vegetable?   37
How to choose what your body needs to use.

5 Super Foods to the Rescue   51
Learn which foods contain powerful antioxidants and phytochemicals.

Part 2: Supplements Made Simple   **65**

6 Nutrients Knocking at Your Door   67
Why you really do need to take your supplements.

7 The ABCs of Vitamins   79
Using vitamins to prevent and reverse the dreaded diseases of aging.

8 Minding Your Minerals   95
Sifting and sorting through the benefits of marvelous minerals.

9 Nutrients in the News   105
Advanced research: going beyond vitamins and minerals for peak performance.

10 An Introduction to Botanicals   115
Weeding out the facts about medicinal herbs.

Part 3: Combating the Diseases of Aging   **127**

11 Strengthening Your Immune System   129
Just the facts you need to know to bolster your immune system.

12 Healing Your Heart   139
Cleaning up coronary heart disease with super supplements.

13 Cancer: The Danger Zone   153
    Breaking with tradition: Seeking out alternatives to
    chemotherapy and radiation.

14 Osteoporosis   167
    Laying the foundation for building better bones.

15 Menopause: Get Out of the Heat   177
    Natural options every woman needs to know about for
    optimum health.

16 An Arsenal Against Arthritis   187
    Using nutrients and diet to eliminate those achy, breaky
    joints.

17 Solving Prostate Symptoms   199
    Learning new ways to help you sleep through the night
    again.

18 Depression Is Not a Prozac Deficiency   209
    Discover dietary recommendations, vitamins, and herbs to
    heighten your spirit.

19 Alzheimer's Disease   223
    Promising therapies to boost your memory.

20 Seeing Eye to Eye   231
    Cutting cataracts and macular degeneration to a
    minimum.

Part 4: Whole Body Fitness   **241**

21 Adding Life to Your Years   243
    Stress: choices for relief and rejuvenation.

22 It's Your Bod, Baby!   255
    Jogging, jumping, and pumping for couch potatoes.

23 Oh, Those Raging Hormones   265
    The latest scoop on natural hormones and how they can
    add flavor to your life.

24 So, Is There Really a Fountain of Youth?   283
    Making the most of everyday by putting yourself first.

Appendices

A Additional Nutritional Information   289
B Organizations   295
   Index   301

Contents

Part 1: The Fountain of Youth   **1**

1 So, You Want to Live to Be 100?   **3**

The Inevitability of Aging 4
Reversing the Process 4
Are You Sick of Feeling Sick? 6
The Aging Process of Cheese 6
   Defining the "Normal" Range 7
   Horizontal Versus Vertical Disease 8
The Great Human Experiment 9
Expanding Your Horizons 10

2 The Physical Exam   **13**

Passing Inspection 13
   Eyes, Ears, Mouth, and Nose 15
   Head, Shoulders, Knees, and Toes 16
Understand Your Lab Results 18
   Cholesterol: The Good and the Bad 19
   Blood Basics 20
Listen to Your Body 21
Digestion and Assimilation 22
   Gas, Gas Go Away 22

3 The Dietary Balancing Act   **25**

Our Infamous Food Pyramid 26
The SAD Diet 27
   Avoiding Anti-Nutrients 29
   Sugar and Spice and Everything Nice 31
   Faux Finishes: Additives and Preservatives 32
   To Spray or Not to Spray 32
Are the RDAs Adequate? 33
To Market, To Market 35

4 Isn't Carrot Cake a Vegetable?   **37**

It's a Matter of Taste 38
   The Vegetarian Diet 38
   The Macrobiotic Diet 38

The Ornish or Pritikin Diet *39*
The Atkins Diet *39*
The Zone Diet *39*
Cutting Calories 40
Trimming the Fat 41
All Carbs Are Not Created Equal 43
Fabulous Fiber 44
Conscientious About Cholesterol 45
The Power of Protein 46
What's Left for Dinner? 47

5 Super Foods to the Rescue   51

Soy What? 52
The Soy Shield *52*
The Bone-Bean Connection *53*
What About Flavonoids? 54
Fabulous Phytochemicals 55
How to Make Every Meal a Phyto-Feast *55*
Red Wine Wonders *56*
The Broccoli Connection *57*
Berry, Berry Best *58*
The Roots of Relief *58*
Potent Remedies *59*
Green Tea for Two *60*
Tomatoes: The Lycopene Link *61*
Beans, Beans, They're Good for Your Heart *62*

Part 2: Supplements Made Simple   65

6 Nutrients Knocking at Your Door   67

Who Needs Supplements? 67
Deficiency Versus Dependency 72
Are All Supplements Created Equal? 73
Are Your Medicines Making You Mad? 74
What About Antioxidants? 76
Assessing Your Nutrient Status 77

7 The ABCs of Vitamins   79

Beginning with A and Beta Carotene 80
The Benefits of the B's 82

Vitamin B1 (Thiamin) 82
Vitamin B2 (Riboflavin) 83
Vitamin B3 (Niacin and Niacinamide) 83
Vitamin B6 (Pyridoxine) 84
Vitamin B12 (Cobalamin) 86
Folic Acid 87
So What's Left? 88
C Is for Citrus 89
Don't Forget D 91
E Is for Everyone—Almost 92
And Tag-Along K 94

8 Minding Your Minerals   **95**

Assessing Your Mineral Status 95
Does Your Diet Do You Right? 96
Bone Up on Boron 97
Calcium: More Than Just Milk 97
Chromium in Control 98
Pumping Iron 99
Magnesium the Magnificent 100
Don't Sell Selenium Short 101
Think Zinc 102

9 Nutrients in the News   **105**

Alpha-Lipoic Acid 105
CoQ Who? 106
Essential Fatty Acids Are Essential 107
Omega-6 Fatty Acids 107
Omega-3 Fatty Acids 108
Glutathione Goes After Free Radicals 108
The Arthritic Answer: Glucosamine Sulfate 109
Relaxing with 5-HTP 109
Medicinal Mushrooms 109
NADH 110
Quercetin: The Allergic Response 110
Pycnogenol and Grape Seed Extract 111
P.S. Don't Forget the PhosphatidylSerine 111
What's on the Horizon? 112

10 An Introduction to Botanicals   115

The Healing Power of Herbs 115
Selecting and Shopping for Herbs 117
Bilberry: The Eyes Have It 118
Echinacea: Nature's Antibiotic 118
Feverfew: Migraine Medicine 119
Ginkgo Biloba: Memory Booster 119
Ginseng: For the Weary and Stressed 120
Hawthorn: Helping Healthy Hearts 120
Kava: Controlling Anxiety and Stress 121
Milk Thistle: Liver Cleanser 122
Peppermint Oil: Irritable Bowel Be Gone 122
Saw Palmetto: Prostate Protection 123
St. John's Wort: Diminishing Depression 123
Stinging Nettle: Nothing to Sneeze at 124
The Case of Doris and Her UTI 124

Part 3: Combating the Diseases of Aging   127

11 Strengthening Your Immune System   129

How the Immune System Works 129
Causes of Immune Dysfunction 130
The Sugar Connection 130
Food Allergy Facts 131
Toxins in the Environment 132
Is Your Immune System Weak? 133
How to Enhance Your Immune Response 133
Nutrients Necessary for Immune Support 133
Helpful Herbs 135
Behaviors Affecting Immunity 136

12 Healing Your Heart   139

Let's Get to the Heart of the Matter 139
Is Heart Disease Inevitable? 140
Cardio Treatment 141
Heart Healthy Hints 142
Zero in on Exercise 142
Relaxing from Stress 143

Controlling Cholesterol 143
   Medications: The Only Answer? 144
   Foods and Nutrients That Work 145
High Blood Pressure: The Silent Killer 145
Agonizing over Angina 147
Homocysteine and B Vitamins 148
Super Supplements for Super Hearts 149
Chelation Therapy: The Controversy Continues 150
   The Case of Irv 151

13 Cancer: The Danger Zone   153

Cancer in a Nutshell 153
Assessing Your Cancer Risk 154
Breast Cancer 155
Maintaining Lifestyle Modification 157
Dietary Decisions 159
   Macrobiotics in Micro 160
   Phytochemicals and Antioxidants 161
What Should You Do? 163
   Tradition, Tradition 164
   Over the Border of Mexico 164

14 Osteoporosis   167

Where Has Your Height Gone? 167
Preventing Osteoporosis in the First Place 169
More than Calcium 170
   Calcium Sources 170
   The Vitamin D Dilemma 171
   Mineral Metabolism 172
   Don't Forget the K 173
   Dietary Delights 173
   Exercise Essentials 174
Drug Therapy 175

15 Menopause: Get Out of the Heat   177

Are Hot Flashes Inevitable? 178
Menopausal Symptoms 178
Hormone Replacement Therapy: Help or Hindrance? 179

My Doctor Never Told Me I Had Options 181
   Dietary Decisions During Menopause 182
   Soy to the Rescue 183
   Vital Vitamins for Menopause 184
   Exercise for Everyone 185
   Herbal Remedies 185

16 An Arsenal Against Arthritis   **187**

Oh, Those Aching Joints 187
Are Anti-Inflammatories the Answer? 189
Diet and Arthritis 190
Supplements You Should Reach For 192
   The Glucosamine Sulfate Secret 194
   Funky Fish Oils 194
Arthritis and Exercise 195

17 Solving Prostate Symptoms   **199**

Where Is That Thing Anyway? 199
Is Prostate Enlargement Inevitable? 200
   Symptoms of Enlargement 201
   Diagnosing BPH 201
   What Causes BPH? 202
Is Proscar Your Only Option? 202
Avoiding Surgery 203
   Food Factors for Prostate Power 204
   Botanical Solutions 205
   Nutrients Not to Be Missed 206

18 Depression Is Not a Prozac Deficiency   **209**

Singing the Blues 210
It's Not All in Your Head 210
Overcoming Depression 213
   Sugar Snacks 214
   Dietary Decisions for Depression 214
   Boost Your Energy with Exercise 215
   Turning SAD into Glad 216
I Never Really Did Drugs 216
   St. John's Wort: Nature's Antidepressant 217
   5-HTP: The Mood Enhancer 218

Inositol: The Forgotten B Vitamin 219
NADH for Brain Energy 219
Alternative Aminos 220
A Freudian Slip 220
It's Never Too Late to Make a Friend 221
Busy as a Bee 221

19 Alzheimer's Disease   223

Was I Always Like This? 224
Alzheimer's Disease 224
The Dreaded Diagnosis 224
Signs of Concern 225
Tell Me Again About Diet 226
B Wise 227
Grab the Ginkgo 228
E and Me 228
Promising Possibilities 229
Helpful Hormones 229

20 Seeing Eye to Eye   231

20/20 on Prevention 232
Ophthalmology Options 232
Antioxidants and the Cataract Connection 233
Seeing with C 234
Eyeing Vitamin E 235
Macular Degeneration: The Mac Attack 236
Nutrients.NET 238
A Host of Herbs 239
Getting Some Shut Eye 239

Part 4: Whole Body Fitness   241

21 Adding Life to Your Years   243

Aging Gracefully 243
Keeping Your Mind Sharp 244
The Eight-Year Plan 245
Smart Drugs 246
Getting in Touch with Your Spiritual Side 246
Yoga: Practice Makes Perfect 247

Meditation Matters 250
Biofeedback 251
Planned Parenting 251
Live, Laugh, and Love 252

22 It's Your Bod, Baby! 255

Who Said You Can't Teach an Old Dog a New Trick? 256
Calculating Your Target Heart Rate 258
Warming Up 260
You Gotta Walk the Walk 260
Shake, Rattle, and Roll 261
Pump It Up 261
Setting Up a Personal Program 262

23 Oh, Those Raging Hormones 265

Feeling 20 Again 266
Natural Versus Synthetic Hormones 266
Making Way for Melatonin 268
DHEA Does It All 269
Well, Sex Is Still Good 271
The Answer to Your Prayers 272
Beyond Viagra 273
Getting Your Hormones in Balance 274
Estrogen for Everyone 275
The Power of Progesterone 276
Touting Testosterone 277
Hormones on the Horizon 279
Pregnenolone Prowess 279
Homering with Androstenedione 279
Growing Younger with HGH 280

24 So, Is There Really a Fountain of Youth? 283

There's Always Cosmetic Surgery 284
The $6 Million Man 285
The Bionic Woman 285
Preserving Your Most Visible Asset 286
Helping Your Body Heal Itself 287
Finding a Like-Minded Health Care Practitioner 287
You Are What You Think 288

Appendices

A Additional Nutritional Information   **289**

B Organizations   **295**

Index   **301**

Foreword

People are confused about nutrition. A recent magazine cartoon entitled "Random Health News" depicted a satirical TV news broadcast à la *Wheel of Fortune*. The newscaster sits amid three wheels offering a multitude of health news permutations: (selection of foods) causes (selection of diseases) in (selection of animals). Consumers are left to take their pick of fast-changing and often contradictory health headlines. Small wonder that the average citizen feels like a "complete idiot!"

But the public remains undaunted. Sales of herbs and vitamins are soaring to unprecedented levels. The health food and supplement industries are showing major economic clout and a majority of Americans are seeing one or another type of alternative practitioner. Even the fledgling Office of Alternative Medicine of the National Institute of Health was recently elevated to the status of a "Center" with an annual research budget of 50 million dollars.

But with such a bewildering array of choices, how does the average consumer select wisely from among the options? To the uninitiated, buying products willy-nilly in a health food store is a little like a novice investor shopping stocks via the Internet: a perilous adventure!

To the rescue comes my esteemed colleague Dr. Allan Magaziner. Using a concise, easy-to-understand approach, **Dr. Magaziner brings to the readers of this book the same cutting-edge information that he provides his patients on a daily basis.** The beauty of this book is that Dr. Magaziner takes nothing for granted: No prior nutritional sophistication is required to access state-of-the-art, relevant information. To the oft-repeated questions "What should I eat?" and "What nutritional supplements would work best for me?" Dr. Magaziner provides simple, direct answers. The clever format of this book enables readers to rapidly glean the information they seek.

Inevitably, many of you will complain, "Why can't I ask my doctor these questions?" Repeatedly frustrated, some of you have just given up. Fortunately, the woeful knowledge gap among health professionals is narrowing. New courses in nutrition and complementary medicine are rapidly pushing their way into medical school curricula—a response to intense demand from a new crop of student doctors who deplore the lack of training opportunities that have existed until now. Doctors like Dr. Magaziner and myself are increasingly being pressed into action to teach such courses—a changing of the guard if there ever was one!

So, if you're feeling like a "complete idiot" about nutrition, don't despair. By reading this book, you're embarking on a sure path to nutritional sophistication. And while you're at it, you want to pick up an extra copy. Send it to your doctor, and make sure it arrives before your next appointment. Bon Voyage.

—Ronald L. Hoffman, MD

Ronald L. Hoffman, MD has been the Medical Director of the Hoffman Center in New York City for more than 15 years. He is a licensed acupuncturist. Dr. Hoffman has a nationally syndicated radio program. He is also a contributing editor of *New Life* and *Conscious Choice* magazines, and the author of several books, including *Intelligent Medicine: A Guide to Optimizing Health and Preventing Illness for the Baby Boomer Generation.*

Introduction

We are all looking for a magic remedy to ensure a long and healthy life. Explorers in the New World once searched for the Fountain of Youth, in hopes of achieving eternal youth and immortality. While that fountain is only mythical, it really is possible to achieve some of the benefits the miraculous waters were thought to provide. By following the ideas suggested in this book, we can slow down the aging process and add more quality years to our lives.

Keeping the Heart and Mind Young, and the Body Youthful

As you read this book chapter by chapter, you will unlock more and more doors to renewed vitality. You will learn about the necessary nutrients and supplements that enhance your health, and the vitamins, minerals, and herbs that protect against the most common diseases associated with aging. You'll learn how to fit fitness into your life forever. You'll discover diet and nutritional advice to keep you young from the inside out, and mind strategies for defying the aging process.

Virtually anyone can benefit from this book, regardless of your current age, health status, or medical sophistication. That's why we call it a *Complete Idiot's Guide*: It's written for everyone, not just for those who are experts in medical lingo and scientific jargon. By integrating the comprehensive programs, therapies, and modalities suggested in this guide, you can enjoy living longer and healthier.

How to Use This Book

This book is divided into four parts to make it easy to use. Part 1, "The Fountain of Youth," covers the basics in longevity strategies, from understanding the process of aging, to getting a physical examination, to helping you make the right food choices for healthy living. Part 2, "Supplements Made Simple," provides comprehensive information on the vitamins and minerals, nutrients, and botanicals that can make healthier living a reality. Part 3, "Combating the Diseases of Aging," begins with a program to strengthen your immune system. Chapters 12 through 20 focus on specific ailments, including heart disease, cancer, Alzheimer's disease, prostate problems, menopause, and arthritis. Part 4, "Whole Body Fitness," provides an exploration of mind and body techniques and lifestyle modifications to ensure longevity. Topics in this section range from yoga and meditation, to setting up an exercise program, to an analysis of hormones on the horizon of anti-aging medicine.

To get the most from this book, I suggest reading the first two parts to determine where you should begin your anti-aging program. This will get you in tune with your body and help you determine what your body needs to achieve optimum health. Then go shopping for heart-healthy foods and body-balancing supplements. Next, read Part 4 for tips on additional healthy changes you can incorporate into your life to help add more life to your years. Part 3 is disease-specific. Everyone should read about bolstering the immune system; it's our body's first line of defense in fighting disease and infection. Then pick and choose from the rest of the chapters on diseases, according to your own needs and interests. You will learn some of the latest techniques to help prevent the most common conditions associated with aging. Hopefully, the information and healthy tips will provide the foundation to keep you healthy or to help someone you know and love.

Throughout the book, you will find sidebars filled with additional useful information and tips. Make sure you read them for added insight into the subject.

Note from Your Doctor

These sidebars are longer discussions of themes that are of special importance or that are too often ignored. These include information about recent scientific studies and insights into the origins of many medicines.

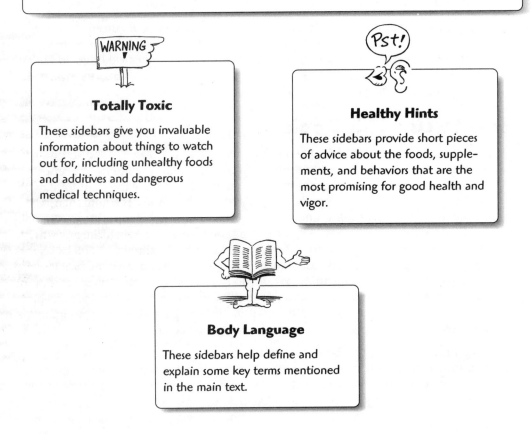

Totally Toxic

These sidebars give you invaluable information about things to watch out for, including unhealthy foods and additives and dangerous medical techniques.

Healthy Hints

These sidebars provide short pieces of advice about the foods, supplements, and behaviors that are the most promising for good health and vigor.

Body Language

These sidebars help define and explain some key terms mentioned in the main text.

Special Thanks from the Publisher to the Technical Reviewer

Our thanks to Michael Janson, M.D. Dr. Janson is president of the American College for Advancement in Medicine, past president of the American Preventive Medical Association, and a charter member of the American Holistic Medical Association. He received his M.D. from Boston University in 1970. He lectures internationally on nutrition, holistic health, vitamin supplements, and natural medicine. He is the author of *The Vitamin Revolution in Health Care, Chelation Therapy and Your Health,* and *All About Saw Palmetto and The Prostate.* He is also the director of the Center for Preventive Medicine in Barnstable, Massachusetts, and can be reached via e-mail at janson@healthy.net.

Dedication

To my beautiful children, who remind me every day of the miracles of life and inspire my quest for a long and healthy life.

Acknowledgements

Special thanks to my staff and patients at the Magaziner Center for Wellness and Anti-Aging Medicine, who support a nutritionally oriented philosophy of health care and possess a wisdom to heal themselves from within first. Much thanks for the inspiration from my predecessors and colleagues in the field of nutritional medicine who continue to carry the torch of good health. In particular, my thanks to Michael Janson, M.D., for his technical editing of this manuscript.

Much gratitude goes to all those who helped get the words to print—the team at Macmillan, including John Jones, Krista Hansing, Stephanie Mohler, Jessica Faust, Bob Shuman, and all others who have helped along the way. My personal thanks to the tireless efforts of Gayle Cohen and Linda and Bill Bonvie for their timely help and assistance.

And these thanks would not be complete without expressing my gratitude and love for my wife, Suzanne, whose writing, editing, and reviewing helped pull this entire project together. Thanks always for all your hard work and constant support.

Trademarks

All terms mentioned in this book that are known to be or are suspected of being trademarks or service marks have been appropriately capitalized. Alpha Books and Macmillan General Reference cannot attest to the accuracy of this information. Use of a term in this book should not be regarded as affecting the validity of any trademark or service mark.

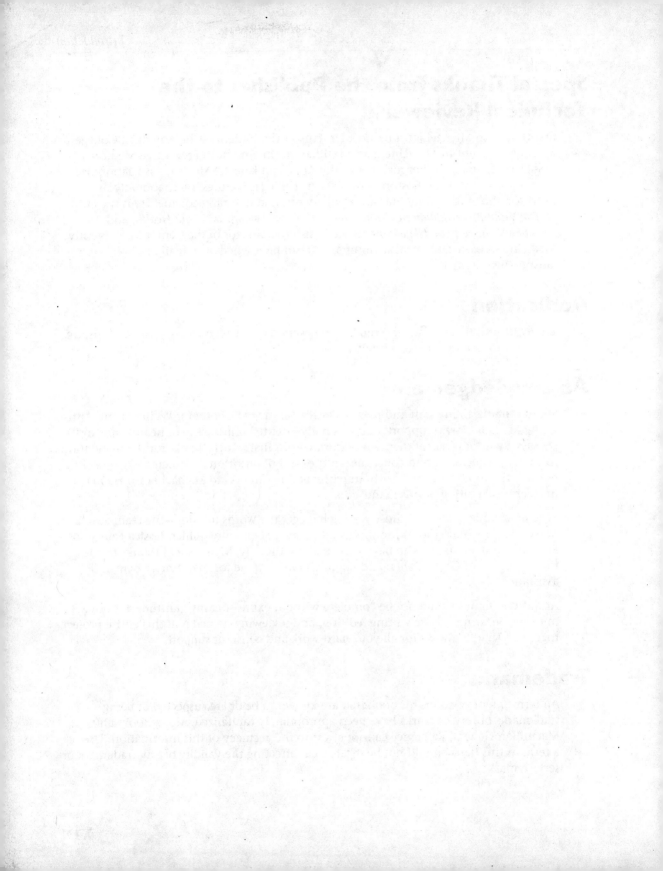

Part 1
The Fountain of Youth

We are all explorers still looking for the magical waters that promise immortality on earth. While our geographic search has yielded little, recent scientific advances have improved our odds of living a long and healthy life. Our quest for longevity should not be directed at immortality, but at living longer with quality. In this book, there is no magical spell for eternity. There are, however, pages filled with the latest medical advances and strategies for dramatically increasing your lifespan.

Always keep your health and longevity goals in mind. What are you living for and how can you live better to help ensure meeting your objectives? Read on for simple and painless lifestyle modifications that can increase your odds of survival and get you to your goal.

Let's cut through the fog of often confusing and conflicting medical messages we receive from the media, from our friends and family, and even from our healthcare practitioners. We're getting right to the point. We want to start living today with tomorrow in mind.

Chapter 1

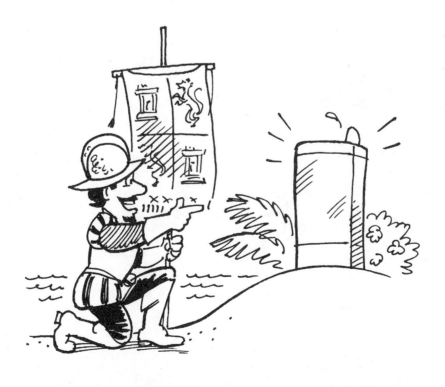

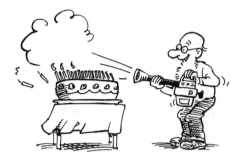

So, You Want to Live to Be 100?

In This Chapter

➤ How getting older differs from aging

➤ The diseases associated with aging

➤ The natural changes that occur with aging

➤ Why being in the "normal" range is not so normal

Like Ponce de Leon in search of the Fountain of Youth, it seems we're always chasing after dreams of renewed longevity. Why is it that so many of us want to live to be 100 or more? Some days I do, too—especially when I'm on vacation, or when I watch my kids reaching for the stars, or when I'm feeling like a kid myself or pretending to be a star. Then there are those other days when living longer doesn't sound like such a great idea. You know the ones I mean: your achy, breaky back days, your "I'm too sick to move" days, and your overwhelmed and stressed-out days.

For the purposes of this book, let's assume that we all have a finite number of days on planet Earth. What can we do to extend them and make the most of them? How can we be healthier and hopefully live a little bit longer with our full range of capacities? Is there a way we can increase the number of healthy years we have and add quality to those years? Let's find out.

The Inevitability of Aging

People say they want to have a long life, but is it enough just to survive for 100 years? I don't just want a big birthday cake with 101 candles—I want to be healthy enough to blow out all the candles. Life should be about quality—pleasure, satisfaction, independence, and achievement, not just quantity. I want a long life worth living. I know the risks, and I'm willing to put in a little bit of effort now in return for the future payoff. Aren't you?

While all of us are getting numerically older, it doesn't necessarily mean that we are aging. And when we do finally age, we can do it with grace. You can make wise decisions to slow the aging process—or at least delay its onset.

As it turns out, your dream of living to 100 may not be so far out. More Americans than ever are centenarians—an estimated 70,000. By the year 2004, that number may go as high as 140,000. Better yet, by the year 2050, there may be well over a million centenarians. Maybe the waters from that mythical fountain are finally trickling toward us. Here's some more water to splash in.

During the last century:

➤ the number of Americans who are 65 years or older has tripled, from 4 percent to 12.5 percent.

➤ the total world population of people older than 65 has increased from 3 million to 31 million.

➤ the number of people ages 65 to 74 has increased eightfold, and the survival of people ages 75 to 84 has increased more than 25 percent.

The average American now lives to be 76, but we all know people in their 80s and even 90s who are still vibrant and sharp. We also know that it is statistically quite possible to make it to 100. So how can we increase our chance of survival? Darwin's Survival of the Fittest theory applies to us, too.

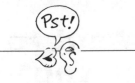

Healthy Hints

There's one way to ensure eternal life and prosperity: Be like an Egyptian and get mummified. The ancient Egyptian Pharaohs and all their worldly belongings have been remarkably well preserved. If the Egyptians could do that 5,000 years ago, imagine what we should be able to do today. But where are you going to park your pyramid?

Body Language

The word *centenarian* is derived from the Latin word *centum*, meaning 100. A centenarian is any person at least 100 years old.

Reversing the Process

Oh, to be 75 and feel like 29 again: Wouldn't that be great? In fact, it may be entirely possible. Cutting-edge medical research is discovering possible ways to prevent or even reverse some of the maladies most commonly associated with aging. This list includes Alzheimer's disease, cancer, heart disease, diabetes, osteoporosis, strokes, arthritis, and Parkinson's disease.

While we wait for mainstream medicine to catch up to us, we can look toward the vast array of alternative treatments and anecdotal remedies that already exist. Much of this information is readily available, but it might not have caught the eye or interest of your doctor. It's up to you to put in the work, energy, and effort to seek out the information that will help prolong your life and vitality—you have to become your own Director of Prevention.

You might have developed unhealthy habits along the way, such as a poor diet, cigarette smoking, excessive drinking, or inappropriate use of medications. Or perhaps you have become overweight, sedentary, or super stressed-out. Each of these factors contributes to premature aging and the early onset of chronic diseases.

Eating a wholesome diet consisting largely of fresh fruit and vegetables, on the other hand, provides antioxidants and phytochemicals that can help protect you from the ravages of aging. Specific antioxidants, such as vitamin C, vitamin E, and beta carotene, also can protect you from premature aging. Incorporating other nutrients, hormones, and herbs into your diet, as well as starting a regular exercise program and having a great attitude, go a long way toward keeping you young in mind, body, and spirit.

Staying young can also help us stay out of debt. If we could slow the onset of aging and eliminate many degenerative diseases, we could cut our nation's total health-care expenditure significantly. And think how much we could accomplish with all the money we'd save. We could provide needed immunizations for children of welfare recipients, clean toxic waste and pollution from our oceans, maybe even buy another set of china for the White House. The bottom line is: A healthier population means a healthier economy.

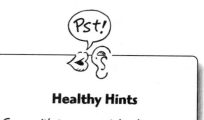

Healthy Hints

Genes, it's true, certainly play an important role in determining longevity. But we can still make the most of our inheritance, whatever it is, and perhaps even turn a modest endowment into something much longer lasting.

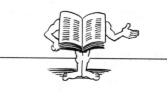

Body Language

Phytochemicals, also called phytonutrients, are components of fruit and vegetables that medical researchers believe can actually ward off disease. It is thought that phytochemicals may prevent heart disease and even reverse some cancers, including melanoma and breast and prostate cancer.

Are You Sick of Feeling Sick?

Are you the kind of person who never feels quite right, who is always complaining of some low-grade, nagging ache of some sort? Maybe you have chronic back pain, loose bowels or constipation, headaches, fatigue, intestinal gas, bloating, or some other embarrassing ailment you don't even want to talk about. If so, you're probably like most of the other people reading this book and the majority of patients I see in my office every day. And you've probably had this condition for so long now that, unfortunately, you have forgotten how it feels not to have the problem. In other words, you can't remember what feeling good really feels like.

Hardly a week goes by when a patient doesn't tell me that they're "just sick and tired of feeling so sick and tired." But just as aging can be avoided, feeling sick can be avoided, too, provided you're doing your job as Director of Prevention. It really is possible to feel good again. The changes along the road to achieving optimal health are so subtle that, one day, you'll suddenly realize you no longer feel the way you used to. You're okay now. No more incontinence, no more headache, no more arthritic pain, no more congestion. That moment of realization is pretty amazing: Maybe your lifestyle didn't change that much, but your life sure did.

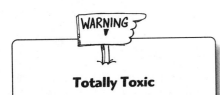

Totally Toxic

On any given day in America, an alarming 22 percent of the population eat no vegetables at all and 45 percent have no fruit, even though these are considered fundamental to good health and disease prevention.

The Aging Process of Cheese

Yup, we're cheese. We start out fresh, we have a fairly long shelf life, and then we get moldy fast. During that shelf life, many changes actually occur as we go about our daily routine. For example, in your 20s and 30s you may begin to feel less flexible and limber. Your metabolic rate starts to slow down. You start tweezing a few gray hairs. Your skin loses its elasticity, and you may begin to develop those dreaded wrinkles.

In your 40s, you can't see as well. You can no longer pluck your gray hairs because you can barely make them out, and even if you could, you'd have too many to pull. Along with the decline in your visual acuity comes the decline in your hearing. (Maybe that's why so many husbands can't hear their wives most of the time.) And the worst of it is, your waistline is gone and your stomach and hips begin to bulge. Your hormones decline, frequently taking your libido down with them. You have started sliding down the other side of the bell curve.

In your 50s you usually undergo further deterioration. You develop even more wrinkles. While this won't make you happy, it will be a source of delight to your plastic surgeon. Your metabolic rate becomes even slower and your hormones almost disappear. Just when you thought you were reaching the golden years, your gold will have turned to bronze.

Defining the "Normal" Range

Let's set the stage. You have just presented your doctor with a list of every ongoing, nagging complaint you have ever had. Your doctor taps his fingers on his desk and looks you straight in the eyes. The script reads something like this:

> **Doctor:** "Well, you're in the normal range."

> **Patient:** "But Doctor, I don't want to be normal if it means being sick all the time."

You may have performed in this role so often that you should be nominated for an Academy Award by now. Who wants to be normal when normal feels so lousy?

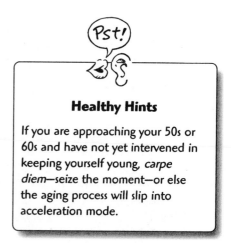

Healthy Hints

If you are approaching your 50s or 60s and have not yet intervened in keeping yourself young, *carpe diem*—seize the moment—or else the aging process will slip into acceleration mode.

If you have been clinically diagnosed as "normal," that tells me that you are probably prone to all the health problems you are trying to avoid or overcome by reading this book. The average "normal" person usually feels lousy—and sometimes even looks lousy.

Let's rewrite the script. Suppose the doctor used a more precise way of speaking: "There was nothing that I could find wrong with you that I wouldn't expect to find in people in your age group." Your doctor is telling you that according to the textbooks he studied in medical school, it is statistically not surprising—"normal"—for you to develop poor eyesight, heart disease, poor memory, osteoporosis, obesity, and so forth. Now you have an opportunity to consult with someone else or request another study.

Because normal in this sense is not enough. You aren't interested in being on the curve: You want to be on a different curve. You want better than "normal," or you wouldn't have invested in this book. You want optimum. And the key to achieving optimum health is going beyond the normal range to find the sources of what is bugging you and fix them at a cellular level.

To give you an example, let's talk about B_{12}, the vitamin responsible for keeping your red blood cells healthy and preventing heart disease. The normal range for your serum B_{12} level runs approximately 200 to 900 pg/ml. Now, if you're suffering from numbness and tingling in your legs and you have poor memory, poor concentration, and difficulty with your balance, it is probably worthwhile to have your B_{12} status assessed.

Note from Your Doctor

Most doctors check your level of vitamin B12 with a simple B12 blood test. But there are probably more effective ways to assess your functional level—that is, how well your B12 is working. Have your doctor check your methylmalonic acid level or homocysteine level.

If your blood tests indicate that your B12 level is 220, chances are your doctor will tell you that "you're in the normal range" and so no further therapy is needed. I would disagree. Why? Because you're very close to below normal. You're so close, in fact, that even if I gave you B12 supplements and was able to double your B12 level to 440, you'd still be in the lower half of the normal range. Your symptoms might subside, however, if we could move your serum level higher. The moral of this story is: Don't accept what's "normal" if you don't feel normal.

Horizontal Versus Vertical Disease

How sick do you have to be before someone will really listen to you? Do you have to be flat on your back with a water bottle, watching *I Love Lucy* reruns to get attention? So many of us are "just making it" through the workday, the school day, or the day at home. We wake up every morning still tired, some days with a headache or nasal mucous and congestion. Then we get dressed and pretend a cup of coffee is going to help get us through the day. Sounds familiar, doesn't it? Perhaps you're just getting by. You're still walking, you're upright—but you're barely functioning. I call this vertical disease, and vertical disease usually precedes horizontal disease, when you are so sick you're flat on your back.

Millions of Americans suffer from low-grade, chronic, annoying symptoms that prevent them from feeling vibrant and full of zest. Don't wait for help until you're stricken with horizontal disease. You need to be empowered to take responsibility for your own health, to take an active role in your own well-being—your primary responsibility in your new role as Director of Prevention. This may mean lifestyle modifications: quitting smoking, changing your diet, reducing stress, and starting on an individualized wellness program. These will help keep you upright and outta sight—the doctor's sight, that is!

Note from Your Doctor

As the classic diseases of nutritional deficiency (such as scurvy and beriberi) have diminished, they have unfortunately been replaced by diseases associated with overconsumption and dietary excess, such as obesity, heart disease, and alcoholism.

Hopefully by now you have made a promise to yourself that you are going to begin your rejuvenation process. You'll be looking younger, feeling healthier, and glowing in no time. But remember not to expect results overnight—it took you a lifetime to get to where you are now.

The Great Human Experiment

Perhaps you've resolved that tomorrow, you'll start walking, reducing stress, and eating well-balanced meals. In the meantime, however, watch out for the food you already have in your refrigerator and cupboards.

We are guinea pigs in a very large food experiment—we are the first generation of humans to be ingesting food that is devitalized of nutrients, refined, depleted, transported, colored, preserved, and sprayed with millions of pounds of pesticides every year.

It wasn't until about 100 years ago that our food supply was drastically changed with the advent of "modern" farming techniques. Luckily, we also have "modern" medicine to try to keep up with the damage our food supply is causing.

Unless you are extremely conscientious, your dietary intake is probably deficient in many of the trace minerals, vitamins, and antioxidants. The lack of available wholesome foods is likely a significant contributing factor to many of the diseases of aging. We know that diet is a major factor in many of these diseases. I ask many of my patients why they seem to feed their dogs and cats better than they feed themselves!

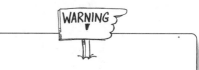

Totally Toxic

The world market for pesticides has seen continued steady growth, despite the fact that the number of harvested acres continues to decline. Total pesticides purchased by farmers increased from $184 million in 1955 to $1 billion in 1968, while harvested acres decreased from 335 million to 294 million.

Expanding Your Horizons

As more of us become interested in healthier lifestyles and longevity, we will see continued growth in the areas of preventative medicine. Nutrition and the impact of the environment on our health are already making headlines. This invigorating patient-driven approach to health care will ultimately influence our medical delivery system. There is an increasing interest in the areas of vitamin and mineral therapies, enzymes, amino acids and essential fatty acids, herbs, massage therapy, acupuncture, exercise, yoga, and Tai Chi.

Yet, with all the medical advances we've made in this century, we ultimately must resort to the ways of our ancestors to find good health. This growing trend is forcing the mainstream medical establishment to re-evaluate its methods of diagnosis and treatment so that it can respond to your needs and wants. Instead of treating the symptoms and covering up the disease, we need to prevent the disease from occurring in the first place. We are beginning to realize that there is no such thing as a magic pill to make all our diseases go away. Lifestyle changes and prevention will go much further toward ensuring our ability to live longer and healthier lives.

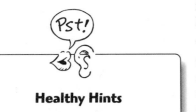

Healthy Hints

At latest estimate, nearly 50 percent of our population is participating in some form of alternative medicine in any given year. Most of the costs are out-of-pocket, but the satisfaction level remains high.

When I was in medical school, I thought I received a thorough education. I studied biochemistry and anatomy, pharmacology, and pathology. I learned how to look for and treat illness with diagnostic tools, medications, and surgery. But using only these methods is shortsighted. We need to look beyond the circle of mainstream medicine to understand the cause of the illness if we want to find the most effective treatment. If mainstream medicine had all the answers, we should really feel normal all the time.

We need to integrate new ideas—ideas that are intended not to replace but to complement conventional health care.

The insufficiency of traditional approaches has led to the emergence of an entirely new field of medicine known by several different names, including alternative medicine, holistic medicine, complementary medicine, functional medicine, or integrative medicine.

Note from Your Doctor

In 400 B.C., Hippocrates, considered by many to be the Father of Medicine, said "Let food be thy medicine, and medicine be thy food." Some 2,400 years later, these words still have resounding influence as medical scientists rediscover the value of food and nutrition to our health and well-being.

This new approach to medicine utilizes many different methods of health-care assessment and treatment. Complementary medicine incorporates all the best methods available, not just traditional medicine and surgery. While this is a relatively recent area of medicine, many of the ideas are centuries old. Alternative and complementary practices focus on nontoxic, effective treatments that can include the use of vitamins, minerals, herbs, acupressure, acupuncture, yoga, biofeedback, guided imagery, exercise, massage, music, and art therapy to help you live longer and healthier.

The Fountain of Youth you seek may be as close as your refrigerator. It is time to expand your horizons and make some simple changes. If you can succeed in your new capacity of Director of Prevention by preventing the disease before it attacks you, then true longevity may be yours.

The Least You Need to Know

➤ The number of people living past the age of 100 is significantly increasing.

➤ As you get older, it becomes more difficult to reverse the effects of aging.

➤ If you don't feel well most of the time, then you are not "well."

➤ Eating healthy and wholesome foods can slow the aging process.

➤ Numerous time-tested methods can help you achieve longevity and optimum health.

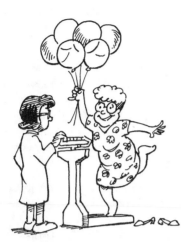

Chapter 2

The Physical Exam

In This Chapter

➤ What to expect during a physical exam

➤ The normal vital signs

➤ Body signs of a poor diet

➤ What laboratory studies your doctor might order

When is the last time you've had a physical exam? If you're over the age of 40, you might want to consider a thorough examination on a yearly basis. One way you can remember to schedule your exam is to call your doctor on your birthday each year. That way you won't forget (or will you then intentionally forget?), and hopefully you will be treating yourself to another year of good health. With advancing age, it becomes more important to get a good check-up on a regular basis.

The physical examination can identify any potential problems. It also gives you the opportunity to discuss new or lingering problems with your doctor, or explore preventive measures. She may suggest that you undergo other diagnostic studies—such as blood work, a cardiogram (EKG), a Pap smear, or a prostate exam, for example—to best keep you healthy.

Passing Inspection

If you're like me, you take your car in for inspection every year. (Actually, my wife sometimes does me the favor and takes my car in instead.) Your headlights are inspected, your brakes are evaluated, your horn and windshield wipers are checked, and hopefully your car is found to be "healthy" for at least another year. You replace a spark plug, tune up the engine, change the oil, and add brake fluid. Some of you probably take better care of your car than you take care of yourselves.

But you've been given only one body, one heart, one stomach, one spleen, one liver, and one nose. Fortunately, for some parts of your body you were actually given two:

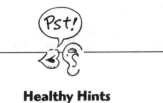

Healthy Hints

Just like you make out a grocery list when you go to the supermarket, take a list of your complaints with you so you won't forget any of the major points you want to review.

two eyes, two ears, two lungs, and two kidneys. Do your best to preserve these parts, because replacing them is a lot more difficult than replacing the parts on your car. As I tell my patients, "You've been given one body, you get one chance, so take good care of it."

Although some of you probably avoid getting a check-up, your doctor's visit does not have to be a terrifying experience. In fact, if you choose the right doctor it can actually be pleasurable. Hopefully your doctor will take a thorough history and not only discuss your complaints, but also inquire about your habits, your lifestyle, your medications, your supplements, your family history, your diet, your stress factors, and your exercise activity.

From there you should have a thorough physical examination. This usually starts out with a check of your vital signs, which include your height, weight, blood pressure, pulse rate, and number of respirations per minute. The normal blood pressure range for a healthy adult is 110 to 120 mmHg for your systolic blood pressure (the top number) over 70 to 80 mmHg for your diastolic blood pressure (the bottom number). If your pressure is significantly higher than 140/90, your doctor may want to discuss the possibility that you have high blood pressure, or hypertension. (This condition is discussed further in Chapter 12.)

Note from Your Doctor

About 10 percent of people with high blood pressure may experience "white coat syndrome." This means that their blood pressure goes up abnormally in the doctor's office. It's a good idea to buy a home blood pressure monitor to track your BP during real-life conditions.

Your pulse rate may vary depending on recent behavior and diet: for instance, whether you feel relaxed and comfortable or stressed or nervous, and whether you just drank two cups of coffee or ate a chocolate bar. The average pulse rate usually falls between 60 and 100, but keep in mind that a well-conditioned and well-trained athlete may have a pulse rate as low as 45 to 60 beats per minute. Certain medications can also affect your pulse rate. Relaxation techniques (discussed in Chapter 21) can also reduce stress and lower your pulse rate.

Your respiratory rate—that is, the number of breaths that you take per minute—is usually between 12 and 15. Obviously, if you just came in after running a 10k race, your respiratory rate will be much greater. Let's take a further look at what the remainder of your physical exam might entail.

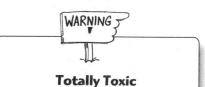

Totally Toxic

Two cups of brewed coffee may contain 300 mg of caffeine. This is enough to raise your blood pressure and pulse rate significantly and alter your reading.

Eyes, Ears, Mouth, and Nose

Your doctor will take a thorough look at your mouth and make sure that your teeth are in good condition. If you're drinking too much coffee or smoking cigarettes, the enamel on your teeth may be stained. (Hopefully you're also seeing your dentist at least once per year. We have to give him some business, too.) Cracks around the corners of your mouth may indicate that you are deficient in B vitamins, especially riboflavin (vitamin B_2). If so, try to eat more rice, green peas, tuna, avocado, collard greens, fish, or chicken. If you suffer from bleeding gums or periodontal disease, consider increasing your intake of vitamin C, bioflavonoids, and CoQ_{10}. (We will discuss more of these nutrients in Chapter 7, Chapter 8, and Chapter 9.)

Your tongue, too, can give clues about B-vitamin deficiencies. If your tongue is rough with peaks and valleys and looks like a topographical map of the Rocky Mountains, you might be deficient in vitamin B. In particular, consider extra B_{12} and folic acid. If your tongue and eyelids are pale, you might be anemic; your blood count will help diagnose anemia. The most common form of anemia is due to a lack of iron, but B_{12} or folic acid can also play a role.

Your scalp can also be a sign that you're following the "high Twinkie diet." If hair is thinning or has lots of dandruff, you may need more B vitamins and essential fatty acids. Make sure that you're getting enough protein to maintain a healthy scalp. If you're running into premature graying, you may be prematurely aging as well. And if your hair is dry, thin, and lacks luster, your diet may be too low in oils and essential fatty acids.

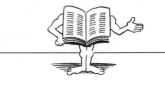

Body Language

Salicylates are food chemicals naturally occurring in apricots, berries, plums, tomatoes, cucumbers, and other foods. Salicylates also are used as a food additive, a food dye (such as tartrazine or yellow dyes) and in flavoring, including root beer, strawberry, and mint. Some people are allergic to salicylates and should monitor their intake.

If you're frequently taking your finger and pushing up on the bottom of your nose, you may have allergies— this is known as the allergic salute! And if your ears turn red after eating, think about food allergies. Red ears are commonly seen in allergic children, especially after eating dairy products, sugar, and sometimes wheat. If you are troubled by constant and excessive ear wax, you may be a candidate for more essential fatty acids in your diet. Think about fresh fish such as salmon, cod, tuna, mackerel, or halibut. You don't like fish? Then consider using more cold-pressed oils such as olive oil, canola oil, sunflower, or safflower oil. You can usually find these in a health food store. Add these to your salads, and they help make the skin silky and moist as well.

Let's move down the body a little bit and take a look at what's left. The doctor will probably check your nose. If he finds polyps inside, you may have allergies or perhaps be sensitive to salicylates. Be careful of taking aspirin or eating foods that contain artificial food colorings, since both of these may contain salicylates.

Head, Shoulders, Knees, and Toes

If you've been worshipping the sun for most of your life, you're probably developing premature sun-damaged skin and wrinkles. The best advice is exactly what you don't want to hear: Get out of the sun! Because you didn't prevent this in the first place, start wearing a hat, minimize your sun exposure, and use sunscreen. While you can't undo the damage already done, prevention can still help protect you from further sun-damaged skin—and from looking like a California raisin. If your skin bruises easily, consider upping your intake of vitamins C and K and bioflavonoids. Eating more peppers, spinach, cantaloupe, watermelon, grapefruit, oranges, broccoli, and lemon are all helpful. But at times you may need supplements to really do the trick. If your skin is dry and flaky, looks like sandpaper, or cracks easily, think zinc. You may not be able to get enough from your diet, and supplements may be necessary. Once again, essential fatty acids may be part of the rescue team here.

If your nails split, chip, crack, and won't grow, consider deficiencies in calcium or zinc, a problem with your metabolism, a deficiency of protein or essential fatty acids, or maybe even malabsorption. (We'll talk about malabsorption later in this chapter.) Frequently children and teenagers have small white spots on their fingernails; once again, think zinc. It's very difficult to eat enough zinc-containing foods—such as lean meats, beans, almonds, or oysters—to bring your zinc level up enough to get rid of those spots, so zinc supplements are necessary.

Note from Your Doctor

In the book *The Common Form of Joint Dysfunction: Its Incidence and Treatment* (1949), William Kaufman wrote that niacinamide can improve mobility, increase range of motion, and reduce pain associated with osteoarthritis.

What about those nodules or knots at the joints at the end of your fingers? You frequently see these on people as they get older. This is usually a sign of the aging process and the onset of arthritis. Once again, vitamin B comes to the rescue. In particular, niacinamide and vitamin B_6 may help keep the joints from becoming too swollen, tender, or puffy. You may respond positively to a "no nightshade" diet, whereby you avoid tomatoes, potatoes, eggplant, peppers, and tobacco. Although this doesn't help everybody, it may be useful for some. If you try this diet, give it at least a three-month trial.

Let's summarize some of the things to think about if your body shows signs of the following ailments:

Body Sign	Think About
Stained teeth	Too much coffee or cigarettes
Cracks in corners of mouth	B vitamins
Bleeding gums	Vitamin C, COQ_{10}, bioflavonoids
Periodontal disease	Vitamin C, COQ_{10}, bioflavonoids
Tongue grooves and cracks	B vitamins
Pale tongue	Anemia
Dry and flaky hair	B vitamins, essential fatty acids
Red ears after eating	Food allergies
Excessive ear wax	Essential fatty acids
Nasal polyps	Allergies, aspirin, salicylates
Skin bruising	Vitamin C, K and bioflavonoids
Dry and flaky skin	Zinc, essential fatty acids
Nails splitting and cracking	Calcium, zinc, protein, fatty acids
White spots on nails	Zinc
Finger nodules	B_6, niacinamide
Irregular/rapid heart beat	Caffeine, magnesium, COQ_{10}

During your exam, your doctor will also use a stethoscope and listen to your heart, your lungs, and your abdomen. Your heart rate should be regular, at approximately 60 to 100 beats per minute. Your lungs should be without rattles or gurgling sounds, and you should be breathing freely. Your abdomen should be soft and without tenderness to probing hands. Your doctor will usually proceed by checking your reflexes with that funny-looking reflex hammer and will probably check for swelling or fluid retention in your legs, ankles and feet. She also may check your strength, your coordination, and your balance.

Then comes that dreaded part for men. If you're over the age of 40, your doctor may ask you to drop your drawers to check your prostate and to check your rectum for nodules or for blood in your stool. She may also ask you to cough as she checks for a hernia.

If you're a female, you should have a regular gynecologic exam and Pap smear performed on a yearly basis. You, too, need a rectal exam to check for lumps or blood. A self–breast examination is also important; you should discuss this technique with your physician so that you can check yourself on a monthly basis. You may be able to detect a lump or breast cancer sooner than your physician and thereby prevent a potential catastrophe. After your full physical is completed, your doctor might feel that certain laboratory tests are appropriate.

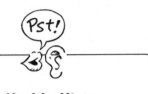

Healthy Hints

Most authorities recommend that women have a mammogram every other year from age 40 to 50, and then yearly thereafter.

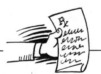

Note from Your Doctor

If your prostate is enlarged, your doctor may recommend a blood test called prostate specific antigen (PSA). If test results come back greater than 4.0, she may suggest further studies. The elevation may be caused by a benign or cancerous growth, prostate enlargement, or infection.

Understand Your Lab Results

After your physical exam, you may find yourself visiting the lab in your doctor's office for blood work. The following lists the most common laboratory tests that your doctor may order:

➤ Complete blood count (CBC)

➤ Cholesterol profile (including total cholesterol, HDL, and LDL)

➤ Blood glucose

➤ Liver profile

➤ Thyroid profile

➤ BUN and creatinine

➤ Electrolytes

Cholesterol: The Good and the Bad

By now you probably have some idea what your cholesterol level is. If it's over 200 mg/dl (milligrams per deciliter), it's too high. The ideal range is probably between 140 mg/dl and 180 mg/dl. When cholesterol builds up in the arteries, it begins to block blood flow and leads to arterial disease. When cholesterol circulates in the bloodstream, it attaches to other substances (known as lipoproteins) to be transported. Actually, two different types of lipoproteins exist: good cholesterol, known as HDL cholesterol, and bad cholesterol, known as LDL cholesterol. HDL, or high-density lipoprotein, helps take cholesterol to the liver, where it can be metabolized, broken down, and eliminated by the body. On the other hand, LDL, or low-density lipoprotein, carries the cholesterol and causes it to stick to the walls of your arteries and obstruct blood flow. This increases your risk of heart disease and high blood pressure. A third type of lipoprotein, called VLDL (or very low-density lipoprotein), primarily carries triglycerides, another blood fat that can wreak havoc.

Cholesterol is actually a fatty, waxy substance that is both produced by the human body and found in animal foods. Cholesterol is not found in plant foods at all. For example, chicken, beef, turkey, ham, pork, cheese, and eggs contain cholesterol, but apples, oranges, grapes, carrots, celery, corn, potatoes, and even nuts do not.

The more cholesterol you eat in your diet, the greater the chance that your bad cholesterol will increase.

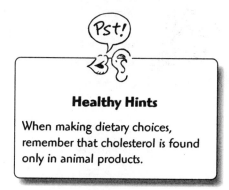

Healthy Hints

When making dietary choices, remember that cholesterol is found only in animal products.

The higher your level of HDL cholesterol, the lower your risk of heart disease. Conversely, the higher your LDL level, the greater your risk of heart disease. It is important to look at the ratio of your total cholesterol to HDL. If your ratio is 5:1 or lower, this is a favorable indicator.

For every 1 percent drop in LDL cholesterol, your risk of heart disease drops by 2 percent. For every 1 percent increase in HDL cholesterol, your risk of heart disease drops by 3 to 4 percent. Obviously, it is important to know not only your total cholesterol but your HDL and LDL levels as well. Your desirable levels of cholesterol and triglycerides should fall in this range:

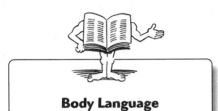

Body Language

A *CBC* is a complete blood count. It measures levels of white and red blood cells and platelets.

➤ Total cholesterol→Less than 200 mg/dl

➤ LDL cholesterol→Less than 130 mg/dl

➤ HDL cholesterol→Greater than 35 mg/dl

➤ Triglycerides→Less than 150 mg/dl

➤ Ratio of total cholesterol: HDL→Less than 5.0

➤ Ratio of LDL cholesterol: HDL→Less than 3.0

Even though you might have heard that cholesterol is bad, keep in mind that it is necessary for the development of your sex hormones, such as estrogen, progesterone, testosterone, and DHEA. For this reason, you don't want your cholesterol level to drop too low. And remember that cholesterol is only one risk factor associated with heart attack and stroke; other risk factors for vascular disease are discussed in Chapter 12.

Blood Basics

In addition to cholesterol, your doctor may order a complete blood count (CBC) to take a look at your white cells, red cells, and platelet count. All are important parameters to make sure you do not have anemia, a common cause of fatigue. Your white count is an indicator of infections and other illnesses. Platelets help prevent you from bleeding inappropriately so that, if you cut yourself, you clot appropriately and don't bleed excessively. The normal range for the main cells tested in the CBC are listed here:

➤ WBC: 4,000–10,500

➤ RBC: 4.5–5.5

➤ Hemoglobin: 12.5–16

➤ Hematocrit: 38–45

➤ Platelets: 150,000–415,000

If you're concerned about diabetes, you should have your blood sugar checked. This is also known as your fasting glucose level, and the normal range is approximately 70 to 120. Most adult-onset diabetics have levels greater than 120 and have to be very cautious with their diet, exercise, and weight loss.

Note from Your Doctor

A variety of nutrients—such as chromium, magnesium, zinc, vitamin C, and B-complex—may also help bring down abnormal glucose levels. A low-sugar, high-fiber diet and regular exercise is also advised.

If you're fatigued, depressed, and worn out all the time, and if you have mood swings and constipation, your doctor might want to check your thyroid to determine your T4 (thyroxine) and TSH (thyroid-stimulating hormone) levels. This helps tell whether you might be revved up as a result of hyperthyroidism, or suffering from a sluggish and underactive thyroid, a condition known as hypothyroidism.

A liver profile helps detect liver inflammation or hepatitis. This test commonly includes several different blood parameters of funny abbreviations such as SGPT, SGOT, GGT, alkaline phosphatase, and total bilirubin.

If you've been on different blood pressure medications or water pills, your doctor might want to check your electrolytes. No, he won't have to go into your home to check the electric meter, but instead will have some blood drawn to examine your levels of sodium, potassium, and calcium. A low level of calcium, potassium, or magnesium might contribute to high blood pressure, an irregular heart beat, or other heart problems.

Two blood tests help assess your kidney function: the BUN (blood urea nitrogen) and creatinine. A urinalysis may be part of a complete physical exam to see whether you're spilling sugar, protein, or blood into the urine, or whether you have bacteria that can indicate an infection. Certainly, your doctor might order many other blood tests if he feels that they are indicated for your particular problems; but don't let him get too carried away with drawing blood. If too much blood is drawn, you might feel dizzy; if excessive amounts are drawn continuously, anemia can occur.

Listen to Your Body

Each day the patients who come into my office teach me a lot. I learn a lot about myself from them, and there's no reason you can't learn a lot from yourself, either. You probably know your body better than anyone else. And a 15- or 30-minute examination may not be sufficient for your doctor to learn as much about you as you need him to know. For example, if you notice that eating peanuts causes headaches, then perhaps you should avoid peanuts. If you become tired, drowsy, or foggy-headed after eating wheat products, perhaps you should avoid wheat. If taking the latest blood pressure pill seems to make you feel depressed and moody, inform your doctor. This doesn't necessitate $2,600 worth of laboratory studies and diagnostic tests, and you don't have to be a rocket scientist to make the appropriate changes. Simply listen to your body. Most of the time it's telling you the truth.

Healthy Hints

Take your time when eating; don't rush it. Chew your food well—30 times per bite, if you can. That's the very beginning of the digestion process. Your saliva produces digestive enzymes that begin to break down carbohydrates and protein so that they can be better absorbed and assimilated. The more time your food is in contact with saliva, the more efficient your digestion may be.

Digestion and Assimilation

When I was growing up, I was always told, "You are what you eat." But are we really? I certainly don't look like the barbecue potato chip I'm snacking on while writing this book. After seeing patients on a regular basis for more than 15 years, I began to realize that perhaps you aren't what you eat but rather you are what you absorb, assimilate, and utilize. Just because you eat a food doesn't mean that you're getting the proper vitamins, minerals, and nourishment from that food. The food must be broken down in the digestive tract, and then the nutrients must be transported to the different organs to be utilized. If you are experiencing a lot of bloating, gas, indigestion, heartburn, diarrhea, or loose bowels, you may not be absorbing and utilizing your nutrients as effectively as you might think. So just because you eat it doesn't mean you utilize it.

Gas, Gas Go Away

Gas, that embarrassing stuff! Millions of Americans are troubled by excessive amounts of intestinal gas and resort to taking antacids or other acid-inhibiting drugs. If you are troubled by excessive amounts of gas and bloating, chances are you're not assimilating or digesting your food effectively. Some people find that peas, beans, greens such as broccoli, and citrus fruits are gas-forming. Others experience gas and bloating from dairy products.

You also might be lacking digestive enzymes, bile acids, or hydrochloric acid and pepsin produced by the cells of the stomach. Frequently, the standard diagnostic tests such as an upper or lower GI, or those tubes your doctor may want to put down your throat or into your rectum, may not be able to fully diagnose the problem. These tests primarily look at the anatomy of your gastrointestinal tract and do very little to evaluate the function of your gut. Unfortunately, excessive amounts of gas and bloating are often caused by a problem with the function of your bowel and not usually the anatomy. Additionally, if you don't have adequate enzymes to break down your food, these incompletely metabolized foods are more likely to provoke intestinal gas. Frequent ingestion of antibiotics can have a similar effect.

Another problem that may be triggering your intestinal gas is eating poor quality foods, ingesting too many sweets, too many refined foods, or foods that might trigger allergies or sensitivities in your body. If you notice that a particular food (and not only beans!) is causing intestinal gas, listen to your body once again. It usually tells you the truth.

Totally Toxic

Be cautious not to use antacids too frequently. Some contain aluminum, a metal that many believe may contribute to poor memory and Alzheimer's Disease.

Note from Your Doctor

Antibiotics may destroy the normal, friendly bacteria in your gut. The lack of good bacteria can contribute to intestinal gas, bloating, and irregular bowel movements. Supplements called probiotics (which contain acidophilus and bfidobacteria) can help relieve your symptoms.

The Least You Need to Know

➤ As an adult, you should have a physical exam on a regular basis.

➤ Normal blood pressure is approximately 120/80.

➤ Cracks in the corner of your mouth can be a sign of B–vitamin deficiency.

➤ A desirable cholesterol level is less than 200 mg/dl.

➤ HDL cholesterol is considered the good cholesterol, while LDL is referred to as the bad cholesterol.

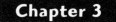

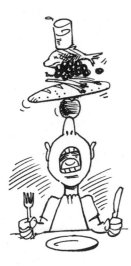

Chapter 3

The Dietary Balancing Act

In This Chapter

➤ Why the food pyramid may not cut the mustard

➤ What to include in your daily diet

➤ What's wrong with the standard American diet

➤ Foods to avoid

➤ Why the RDAs and RDIs may not be adequate.

So you think your diet is terrific. You rise and shine with a bowl of Wheaties with skim milk, a cup of coffee, and, of course, orange juice. Lunch—on the run—is a peanut-butter-and-jelly sandwich, a bag of chips (or pretzels, if you're trying to cut some fat from your diet), and a can of soda, either diet or regular. For dinner, you actually sit down and take more than 10 minutes to enjoy your meal. Dinner is your big meal: chicken or beef, lasagna or something Parmagiana; bread, potato, or rice; and a lovely salad: a bowl with iceberg lettuce in it and maybe a diced tomato or cucumber. An hour later, you have a few cookies, perhaps some ice cream, and fall asleep watching TV. Then you finally muster enough energy to walk upstairs and go back to sleep. If you're like most of us, you repeat that cycle—or a variation on that theme—the next day and the next day after that until the weekend, when you go out to dinner and eat twice as much.

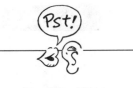

Healthy Hints

It turns out that we eat a very repetitious diet. The average American ingests 80 percent of his nutrients from only 20 different foods. Try to add new food into your diet. You might surprise yourself and enjoy it. By eating a greater variety, we'll get a better balance of the different amino acids needed to build protein, different types of fiber, and a wider variety of trace minerals and essential vitamins.

Let's examine this diet. You did not indulge in any fresh fruit. You certainly didn't get enough healthy fiber in your diet. And what about those dark-green leafy or yellow-orange vegetables that you probably left on your grocer's shelf for the next guy to enjoy? You missed out on a whole world of healthy and nutritious whole grains and beans. But what you did get was the minimum requirements to keep you going for just one more day. In fact, if you keep on eating like this you'll probably have trouble even making it through the day. You may be lucky just to make it through the morning, let alone the afternoon.

So what should you fix in this picture? Remember that immortal mummy in his pyramid? Somehow our government thought that if it could recreate a pyramid for our diet, then we could all live forever, too.

Our Infamous Food Pyramid

You're probably tired of hearing it. When I was growing up, I heard about those four major food groups over and over again: meat, dairy products, fresh produce, and cereal grains. As it turned out, the four food group plan was far from perfect. The plan allowed for excessive amounts of some nutrients and was terribly short on others.

In 1992, after much debate, the U.S. Government changed the direction of a balanced diet from the four basic food groups to the now infamous food pyramid. Though an improvement, this plan is still far from perfect:

➤ It doesn't differentiate between unhealthy hydrogenated oils or saturated fats found in animal meat and the more healthful unsaturated fats found in plants and vegetable oils.

➤ It doesn't differentiate between whole grains and white flour products.

➤ It makes no distinction between beneficial oils such as canola or olive oil and the rancid oils used to cook French fries or other fast-cooking delicacies, especially those used in fast-food restaurants.

➤ It doesn't take into account the difference in nutritive value between fresh fruit and vegetables and canned carrots or vegetables that have had all their nutrients boiled, stewed, and cooked right out of them.

But the new food pyramid is certainly a step in the right direction. What does it tell us? It tells us that we should be eating the following on a daily basis:

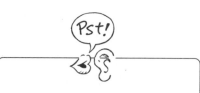

➤ At least 6–11 servings of bread, cereal, rice, or pasta

➤ At least 2–4 servings of fruit

➤ At least 3–5 servings of vegetables

➤ At least 2–3 servings of meat, poultry, fish, dried beans, eggs, or nuts

➤ At least 2–3 servings of milk, yogurt, or cheese

➤ Fats, oils, and sweets used sparingly

Healthy Hints

Eat brown rice, not white rice. I know you really like the white rice you get in Chinese restaurants, but brown rice contains much more fiber, vitamins, and essential trace minerals.

It's fairly safe to assume that most of us passed the fourth grade many years ago, so here is a new diagram of our revised food pyramid to replace the chart that you once studied diligently.

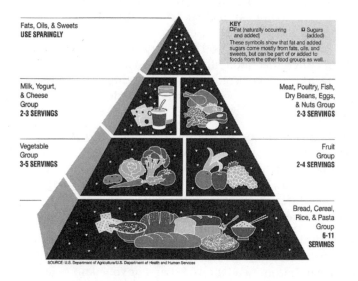

The new food pyramid.

But are we really getting what we need from this new pyramid? It seems to me that this pyramid has plenty of room left for renovation and modernization.

The SAD Diet

Would you believe that even though 90 percent of our population thinks that they're eating a healthy diet, only 1 percent actually meets the dietary guidelines outlined in the food guide pyramid? Consider these dietary faux-pas performed by the typical American on any given day:

➤ The average person eats only one and a half servings of vegetables and less than one serving of fruit.

➤ Forty-five percent have no fruit at all, and 22 percent eat no vegetables at all.

➤ Only 27 percent eat three or more servings of vegetables, and only 29 percent consume two or more servings of fruit.

➤ Overall, only 9 percent meet the U.S. Department of Agriculture's minimum recommendations of eating at least five servings of fruit and vegetables.

So even with all the bureaucratic rhetoric regarding what we should eat, we still haven't cut the mustard. Our Standard American Diet is just that, SAD. Not only are we not getting enough fruit, vegetables and wholesome grains, but we're eating far too much refined and processed white food like white bread, enriched pasta, French-fried potatoes, and instant rice.

Totally Toxic

The average American ingests approximately 43 teaspoons of table sugar per day. One can of Coca-Cola or Pepsi contains 10 teaspoons of sugar. It's not surprising that so many children turn into sugarholics.

What else is wrong with our diet? For starters, we eat too many calories. And then we eat too many saturated fats and too much total fat, contributing to excess cholesterol in our diet. We also consume large amounts of quick and easy food. This is packaged, processed, and often fried food filled with food additives, preservatives, and artificial colorings and flavorings. We also eat too much sugar, too much salt, too little fiber, and not enough variety of foods.

The bottom line is we simply don't eat a balanced or wholesome diet. Even though the National Research Council recommends that our diet consist of 20 percent of calories from protein, 30 percent from fat, and 50 percent from carbohydrates, we simply aren't doing that. And on top of that, all of us have different needs. For example, a clerk in a department store has different dietary requirements from a professional athlete. One size doesn't fit all when it comes to our diet.

Even if you try to comply with the food pyramid diet, who really has the time, energy, or interest to tally up and consciously pay close attention to their daily food intake? And even if you meet the dietary recommendations, I doubt anyone knows how much of the macro nutrients (such as carbohydrates, fats and proteins) or micronutrients (such as vitamins and minerals) she is really getting on any given day.

Note from Your Doctor

Do you realize that we get 20 percent of our total calories from sweets and sugars, and 40 percent from fat and food chemicals? That means 60 percent of our diet is of very low quality and barely provides any of the essential vitamins and minerals or fiber required for great health. It's no wonder that we see so much poor health in our society.

So what do we need to ensure that our diet isn't so SAD? We need to improve the quality of the foods we're eating. We need to eat a variety of foods that are fresh and non-processed or refined. We should snack more on fruits and vegetables instead of ice cream, pies, cakes, and donuts. Introduce new, unfamiliar foods that you may not be used to eating. Eat more kiwi, mangoes, yellow or red peppers, spinach, melon, or perhaps grains (such as millet, barley, oats, couscous, and quinoa), and beans (such as navy, azuki, garbanzo, lima or soy). Be creative, take chances, go to a vegetarian or even macrobiotic cooking class. You might even like it. Turn that SAD diet into a healthy, nutrient-dense, fiber-packed, wholesome, delicious, health-enhancing diet.

Avoiding Anti-Nutrients

Not only do we need to optimize our intake of foods rich in vitamins, minerals, amino acids, essential fatty acids, antioxidants, and phytonutrients (all of which are discussed in later chapters), but we really need to reduce our intake of foods that stress our body. These are the anti-nutrients.

Limit your intake of fried foods. The frying process generally heats oils at high temperatures, which promotes the formation of dangerous free radicals. It's much better if you can bake or broil, because you require less oil and little chance of any oils

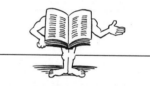

Body Language

To convert a liquid vegetable oil into a solid or creamy margarine, hydrogen atoms are rapidly added to the oil. This process is called *hydrogenation*, and in doing so the structure of the fat is altered to an unnatural and abnormal atomic configuration. Do your best to avoid products with hydrogenated fats. The trans-fats produced by hydrogenation can raise your cholesterol level, clog your arteries, and contribute to heart disease.

becoming rancid from continual reheating. Also try to avoid trans-fatty acids, commonly found in margarine, shortening, cake, pie, cookies, crackers, and other baked products or any hydrogenated vegetable oils; these are unhealthy. Trans-fatty acids found in hydrogenated vegetable oils act like saturated fats and can raise your cholesterol level, increase your blood pressure, and perhaps make you more susceptible to cancer.

Trans-fats account for up to 60 percent of the fat in many processed foods. The average American's intake is between 10 and 20 grams of trans-fat per day. Try to keep your intake as close to zero as possible, since there is no safe dose and no known benefits to eating trans-fatty acids. It's been estimated that these fats may contribute to 30,000 deaths each year as a result of heart disease.

So, is margarine, which is loaded with trans-fats, your best bet? Absolutely not—unless you're an undertaker. According to the Nurses Health Study conducted at the Harvard School of Public Health, women who had the highest intake of margarine were at twice the risk for heart disease, compared to women who ate very few hydrogenated fats. Women who ate 4 teaspoons per day were 66 percent more likely to suffer from heart disease compared to those who ate less then 1 teaspoon each month. The message is clear: Avoid hydrogenated oils and trans-fatty acids. The following list reveals some insightful information about those not-so-transparent trans-fatty acids.

Food	Trans-fatty acids (grams)
French fries, large order	4.0–7.9
Packaged doughnut (1)	5.0–6.0
Chocolate cake roll (1)	2.0
Vegetable shortening (1 Tbsp)	3.0
Hard stick margarine (1 Tbsp)	2.0–4.6
Crackers (1)	2.4
Cheese danish (1)	2.2–5.2
Sugar cookies (2)	1.33
Pound cake (1 oz)	1–2.1
Dinner roll (1)	.85
Mayonnaise (1 Tbsp)	.55
Butter (1 Tbsp)	.40

Limit your intake of caffeine, since it has a diuretic effect and may wash out key nutrients. Caffeine is found not only in coffee but also in tea, soft drinks, and chocolate. One or two cups of coffee per day might be okay, but drinking more than three cups per day is not advisable.

Go easy on alcohol. Excessive alcohol intake can stress your liver and increase your risk of certain cancers, including esophageal, pancreatic, colon, and liver cancer. Alcohol also depletes B vitamins, vitamin C, and numerous trace minerals, not to mention the extra unnecessary calories.

Taste your food before deciding whether you need salt. Most of the time, food has enough naturally occurring salt to make it palatable. Try adding spices, seasonings, and herbs to your food in place of table salt. If you're concerned about your blood pressure, you might want to try potassium salt as opposed to the more common sodium salt.

Don't be a chimney and continue smoking. Smoking accelerates aging and increases your risks for heart disease, stroke, high blood pressure, diabetes, and cancer. Plus, if you successfully quit, you'll have extra money to buy organic food and enjoy a night out at the movies.

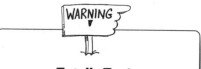

Totally Toxic

The average American consumes 15 lbs. of salt per year—the weight of an average bowling ball! Although the association between salt and high blood pressure is still somewhat controversial, most authorities agree that salt should be limited and that it may play a role in cases of hypertension. Some people also find that salt causes swelling, fluid retention, and weight gain. If that occurs, shake your booty instead of your salt shaker.

Sugar and Spice and Everything Nice

As previously mentioned, approximately 20 percent of our calories comes from sugar alone. White sugar, in particular—the type that you generally add to your cup of coffee in the morning or that you use when baking a pie—is virtually devoid of any key vitamins and minerals. Sugar contains 16 calories per teaspoon and has no B vitamins, chromium, magnesium, zinc, or other trace elements necessary to metabolize it. As a result, the sugar in your sugar jar essentially robs your body of beneficial nutrients from healthy foods that you might be eating. To fully metabolize sugar, your body has to take B vitamins and other trace minerals from healthy grains, beans, fruits, and vegetables instead of being utilized for more efficient and important purposes such as fighting infections, warding off allergies, and preventing cancer or heart disease.

Be sure to read labels. Sugar is everywhere: in sodas, cake, pie, ice cream, donuts, candy, chocolate, breakfast cereals, breads, ketchup, and even salad dressings. And it may be disguised with an alias such as corn syrup, cornstarch, or high fructose corn syrup.

Note from Your Doctor

If you're looking for alternatives to plain table sugar, consider using stevia, pure unfiltered honey, pure maple syrup, or date sugar. These are equally sweet, are generally well tolerated, and have greater nutritional value than refined sugar. But be cautious when using artificial sweeteners. Many of these contain aspartame, found in NutraSweet or Equal, which has been associated with dizziness, headaches, heart palpitations, flushed feelings, seizures, blurred vision, and depression.

Faux Finishes: Additives and Preservatives

While food additives and preservatives have their benefits, I recommend that you do your best to limit your intake of them. These chemicals are generally used in an effort to preserve and prevent food spoilage and to retard mold growth. However, some people experience symptoms such as headaches, asthma, wheezing, dizziness, fatigue, or hives from some of these added ingredients. How to avoid them? It's quite simple. Buy fresh food that's not packaged or prepared, and read food labels. A little bit won't hurt you, but the less you eat, the better off you'll be.

This caution applies not only to food, but to your prescription medication as well. Drug manufacturers add food coloring and dye to their medications. Why? Do you really care whether your antibiotic is white or pink? Some pharmacies compound prescription medications so that they are completely free of artificial colorings, flavorings, dyes, and preservatives. If you're concerned, ask your pharmacist to compound your medication without these unnecessary chemicals.

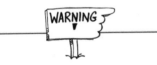

Totally Toxic

More than 10,000 different food additives are actually used in our food supply. If you have asthma or other forms of breathing problems, avoid sulfites, which are frequently added to alcoholic beverages, dried fruit, frozen fish, soup mixes, and a variety of other foods. Read labels! Sulfites may be disguised as sodium bisulfate, metabisulfite, or sulfur dioxide, all of which can trigger severe allergic reactions.

To Spray or Not to Spray

If you have ever tasted the difference between organically grown produce and conventionally grown produce, you know why organically grown fruits and vegetables are gaining in popularity. Organic foods have not been sprayed with chemical insecticides or pesticides. More natural forms of insect repellents and fertilizers are used to keep these products nutrient-rich and delicious.

Although some are skeptical of the merits of organic food, I am in favor of a toxin-free diet. Besides tasting better, organically grown fruits and vegetables also contain greater amounts of trace minerals. A recent study indicated that the amounts of calcium, magnesium, potassium, sodium, manganese, iron, and copper in five different vegetables were higher in those that were organically grown—in fact, as much as 50 percent to 390 percent greater!

A debate also rages about the potential health risks associated with pesticides, herbicides, and fungicides. These chemicals are stored in your fatty tissue and stay there for many years. They can accumulate in your brain, liver, and in virtually all the cells in your body. Do we really need them? Of course not. If possible, try to find a local grocer or farmer who is promoting fruits and vegetables as well as grains and beans that are not sprayed with chemical pesticides. The produce generally costs a bit more (sometimes 10 to 30 percent more, depending on the food), but you'll taste the difference.

Of particular concern is the fact that pesticide exposure may contribute to weakening your immune system and making you prone to colds or infections. Pesticides have also been linked to headaches, fatigue, skin rashes, muscle aches and pain, and possibly even some cancers.

Totally Toxic

Are you using pesticides in your home? In the United States, 91 percent of all households use pesticides in their gardens or homes. This adds up to 80 million pounds of toxic chemicals used by you and your neighbors per year. Many pesticide residues stay active for days and even months. Chlordane, used to kill termites, can remain active for up to 20 years.

Are the RDAs Adequate?

The RDAs may be adequate, but for whom? For you? For me? For pregnant women? For the children who avoid fruit and vegetables like the plague? For the elderly who barely keep track of all the medications they take daily? How is it that we can all have the same requirements?

We are all built differently. I like to think I'm 6 feet tall with the same physique I had in college. Truthfully, I'm about 5 feet 10 inches and 175 pounds now, up a few pounds from my college days and down a few muscles. You might be 5 feet 2 inches and 200 pounds, or 6 feet 3 inches and 150 pounds. So how can the recommended daily allowances (RDAs) be adequate for everybody? In my opinion, they're not.

Actually, the RDAs—which represent the minimum amounts of nutrients that you need each day to prevent obvious deficiency symptoms—have now been replaced by the RDIs (Reference Daily Intake). This newer term has been used since January 1997

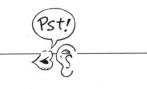

Healthy Hints

According to a recent survey, most adult women do not ingest the RDA minimum requirements for vitamin B6, E, calcium, magnesium, iron, or zinc; the average man falls short on zinc and magnesium.

and represents an average need for each individual. The newer RDIs, however, are quite similar in value to the RDAs and so fall short of what might be necessary for feeling your best.

The original RDAs for vitamins and minerals were established in 1941 and have since been revised several times. However, their original goal was to provide guidelines to prevent diseases that were linked to severe deficiencies. For example, it was recognized that vitamin C would prevent scurvy, that niacin could prevent pellagra, that vitamin D helped prevent rickets, and that thiamin (vitamin B_1) prevented beriberi. These RDAs were designed for groups of people instead of for individuals.

Consequently, the RDAs did not address the special nutritional needs of many individuals, including those listed here:

➤ Cigarette smokers

➤ Alcoholics

➤ Pregnant or lactating woman

➤ Teenagers going through a growth spurt

➤ People exposed to toxic fumes and chemicals

➤ People under tremendous stress

➤ Individuals taking diuretics, antacids, or birth control pills

➤ People with malabsorption

➤ People performing heavy strenuous exercise

➤ Any others with diseases or conditions that can increase their specific nutritional needs

Sounds like most of us, doesn't it? Of course, the RDAs do not take into account the fact that most of us do not eat adequately or that the vitamins and minerals we do get around to eating are often destroyed with the refining, bleaching, and milling of our flour, grains, and other foods.

The RDAs are simply inadequate. They don't give us guidelines for the intake of nutrients for optimal health and enhanced longevity. For these reasons, nutritional supplements are becoming increasingly important for most if not all of our population. (More about this is addressed in Chapter 6.)

To Market, To Market

"To market, to market to buy a fat pig." Oops, wrong book! Let me try that again. To market, to market to buy some fresh fish, lean meat, apples, grapes, carrots, and peppers. That sounds a lot better. If you're really adventurous, maybe you'll even pick up some tofu or seitan (protein derived from wheat).

When cruising up and down the aisles of your local grocery store, try to spend most of your time around the outer perimeter. These areas generally have the fresher, more wholesome foods that are usually lower in fat and less processed. This is where you would generally find fresh vegetables, fruit, cheese, fish, chicken, eggs, and maybe even freshly baked whole-grain breads. Minimize your time in the inner aisles, as they generally contain more of the processed and packaged foods such as cookies, cakes, mixes, potato chips, and carbonated beverages. These foods are usually higher in the anti-nutrients discussed earlier in this chapter. And if you walk around the perimeter enough times, you'll get a whole lot more exercise than if you only walk up and down the center aisles.

The Least You Need to Know

➤ Most Americans fall exceedingly short on their minimum dietary requirements.

➤ Avoid hydrogenated vegetable oils and trans-fatty acids.

➤ Limit your intake of sugar, saturated fat, salt, and alcohol.

➤ Try to avoid artificial colorings, dyes, preservatives, food additives, and processed food.

➤ Increase your consumption of fresh fruit, vegetables, whole grains, beans, and lean meats and fish.

Chapter 4

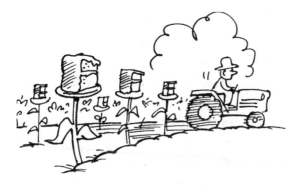

Isn't Carrot Cake a Vegetable?

In This Chapter

➤ Is there one diet for everyone?

➤ Calories from carbohydrates, fats, and proteins

➤ Are all fats the same?

➤ Simple and complex carbs

➤ Finding fiber to put into your diet

➤ Sources of protein

Carrot cake: It sort of sounds like a vegetable. So what is it—just carrots, raisins, and some flour, right? Sort of like a fruit and vegetable sandwich. Great, I'll eat three servings a day and get my recommended daily three to five servings of vegetables. It's easy, right? No need to worry about a trip to the produce department and all that washing, peeling, and steaming. The only problem is that my weight keeps going up, and I don't seem to have all the vigor of those people in cereal commercials who can go from dawn to dusk with the energy of a two-year-old running through the mall.

So, since I don't seem to be getting any healthier, what else is in this carrot cake?

Let me take a look. Oh my gosh, 275 calories per serving—and I just ate three servings. And what is all this? Hydrogenated vegetable oils, high fructose corn syrup, leavening, sodium acid pyrophosphate, monocalcium phosphate, calcium sulfate, glycerin, soy lecithin as an emulsifier, sodium stearyl lactylate, whey, and yellow #6. What happened to the carrots? Is it any surprise that I'm gaining weight and not feeling well? Let's get back to the basics.

It's a Matter of Taste

Many diet specialists and nutritionists suggest the same diet for everybody. But does that make sense? What may be good for one of us may not be good for another. Furthermore, several different diets are all good for you rather than just one. Eating the right nutritious foods can certainly go a long way toward keeping you healthy, slowing the aging process, and perhaps even extending your life span.

Let's touch on some of the more common diets that are currently popular in our society.

The Vegetarian Diet

Basically, this diet requires you to cut out any foods derived from animal sources. This includes veal, chicken, beef, ham, pork, steak, and fish—and anything else that was once part of a creature with two eyes. Vegetarian diets primarily focus on whole grains, beans, legumes, fruit, vegetables, and sea vegetables.

If you're a vegan—that is, a more orthodox vegetarian—you'll also have to cut out cheese, milk, ice cream, yogurt, eggs, and anything else that may have come from that same animal with two eyes. So if you're taking the vegan route, it is especially important to learn how to combine your foods effectively to get adequate protein. You'll probably also want to eat plenty of tofu, tempeh, and seitan as a substitute for meat, chicken, and fish. Combining beans, grains, nuts, and seeds can also provide complete protein.

Vegetarians generally have a lower incidence of high blood pressure, osteoporosis, cancer, diabetes, arthritis, and obesity.

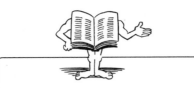

Body Language

Tofu, tempeh, and *seitan* are all vegetarian meat substitutes. The two T's—*tofu* and *tempeh*—are both textured plant proteins made from soybeans, and *seitan* is derived from protein-yielding wheat gluten. These products are becoming increasingly available in our markets due to their popularity and meat-like taste and texture. These products are all low in fat and calories and are cholesterol-free.

The Macrobiotic Diet

This diet is based on the principle of balancing yin and yang, the forces of energy controlling the world we live in. Many believe that balancing these forces in our diet as well as in every aspect of our lives has a great impact on whether we are healthy or sick.

The macrobiotic diet consists of 50 to 60 percent whole grains, 20 to 25 percent vegetables, 5 to 10 percent seaweed and beans, and 5 to 10 percent soups. Some fish and fruit is also permitted. Medicinally, macrobiotics is somewhat controversial, but this diet has been popular among individuals seeking holistic therapies for cancer, diabetes, and heart disease, as well as with those seeking a healthier alternative lifestyle.

The macrobiotic diet excludes all meat, eggs, dairy products, caffeine, sugar, alcohol, and processed foods. It is fairly complicated in terms of food preparation and in obtaining some staple ingredients. Many classes are offered on how to do "macro" right; check with your local health food store for class information and ingredient assistance, or read up on the topic in books or on the Internet.

The Ornish or Pritikin Diet

Both of these diets are very similar, although they're technically considered separate by staunch supporters. They promote very low-fat vegetarian cuisine and are beneficial in lowering cholesterol and blood pressure, as well as in controlling diabetes. They call for the elimination of all meat, poultry, nuts, and whole eggs. Egg whites and non-fat dairy products are generally acceptable, but butter, margarine, and oils should usually be avoided. Instead of giving you 30 percent of your calories from fat, these diets are generally restrictive to 10 percent fat. Regular exercise and stress reduction are also part of these health-conscious regimens.

The Atkins Diet

This controversial diet focuses on the restriction of most carbohydrates and suggests that you eat high quantities of fat and protein. It's based on the fact that your body secretes excessive amounts of insulin when you eat simple carbohydrates, fruit, or sugars, which wreaks havoc on your cholesterol, triglycerides, blood sugar, and weight. Initially, the carbohydrate intake is restricted to less than 6 percent of your total calories, and virtually all fruit, bread, cereals, and pasta—along with starchy vegetables such as corn, peas, and potatoes—are avoided. Eventually, the intake of carbohydrates is gradually added back.

The Zone Diet

This diet is a little more lenient on the carbohydrate intake, compared to the Atkins diet. It derives 40 percent of its calories from carbohydrates, 30 percent from fat, and 30 percent from protein. In addition, the type of fats, whether saturated or unsaturated, is a major focus because fats can regulate prostaglandin secretion. This diet is helpful in regulating inflammatory pathways in your body that play a role in high blood pressure, diabetes, obesity, and possibly cancer.

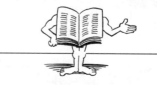

Body Language

Prostaglandins are hormone-like substances produced by your body. They control many bodily processes, influence inflammation, provide moisture to your skin, and control constriction or dilation of your blood vessels.

Cutting Calories

Do calories count? Of course they count. If you're eating 4,000 calories per day and hoping to lose weight . . . well, there's no way, José. Calories certainly are important. They are a unit of energy, indicating the amount of heat produced by metabolizing food. For example, if one medium-size apple contains 100 calories, then metabolites in that apple produce 100 units of heat energy that your body can then use for work.

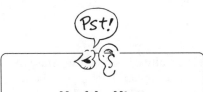

Healthy Hints

Calories count. If you take in more calories than your body burns, you'll gain weight. On the other hand, if you take in fewer calories than you use up, you can lose weight most of the time.

Not all the food that you eat contains the same number of calories. That's why when you eat a lot of fat, it may end up on your hips. Carbohydrates and protein generally contain half as many calories as does fat:

➤ One gram of carbohydrate has 4 calories.

➤ One gram of protein has 4 calories.

➤ One gram of fat has 9 calories.

One of the biggest dietary problems we face is that not only are we eating a lot of calories, but we're simply eating too many *empty* calories. These come from foods that provide very little nutrition, vitamins, minerals, or fiber—but they still give you extra calories. At the top of the list are table sugar and alcohol, which give you calories but have almost no nutritional value.

To determine whether you weigh too much or not, use this method. (You may need to get out your calculator.) Called your BMI (body mass index), this index measures the relationship between your height and weight. Here's what you need to do:

1. Multiply your weight (in pounds) by 703.

2. Multiply your height (in inches) by itself.

3. Divide the total in step #1 by the total in step 2.

For example, to calculate your BMI if you weighed 145 pounds and were 5 feet 2 inches tall, you would do the following calculations:

1. 145 pounds x 703 = 101,935

2. 62 inches x 62 inches = 3845

3. 101,935/3,845 = 26.5

The ideal BMI is less than 25. If your BMI is 26 to 30, you face a higher risk for weight-related diseases. If your BMI is greater than 30, you are at a much higher risk for illnesses such as heart disease, stroke, hypertension, diabetes, and cancer. If your BMI is above 30, you're considered unfit and unhealthy.

Trimming the Fat

Somehow fat seems to creep into most of the foods that we like. Fats are everywhere: in beef, chicken, pork, fish, nuts, seeds, milk, cheese, and vegetable oils. The good news is there's hardly any fat in most fruits and vegetables. As previously mentioned, fats contain almost twice as many calories per gram as do carbohydrates and protein. But not all fat is bad. The problem is that we simply eat too much of the wrong types.

Fats play an important role in synthesizing hormones and helping you absorb fat-soluble vitamins such as A, D, E, and K. They help to conserve body heat and are a major source of energy. They also line every cell membrane in your body so that your cells hold together. Fat is a component of myelin, which provides the insulation around your nerves. And while you may not want to believe it, your brain and liver are primarily composed of fat.

Too much fat—and especially saturated fat—has been associated with a variety of common medical diseases. These include heart disease, cancer, obesity, and diabetes. Too little fat, too, may cause a host of medical problems.

Most authorities recommend that you get no more than 30 percent of your total calories from fat, with no more than 10 percent coming from saturated fat. I generally suggest that you limit your fat intake to no more than 20 to 25 percent of your total calories if you're really hoping to stay healthy and prevent disease.

Generally, three types of fat or fatty acids exist in your diet: saturated, polyunsaturated, and monounsaturated. All three types of fatty acids are found in virtually all food. As a rule, saturated fats (found predominantly in butter, whole milk, beef, and cold cuts) carry a high risk of future health problems. The monounsaturated fats (found mostly in olive and canola oil) are liquid at room temperature and may have beneficial effects on your cardiovascular system. Polyunsaturated fats (found in safflower, sunflower, or corn oil) are also liquid at room temperature, but you should be cautious in heating these oils to high temperatures for long periods of time, as they oxidize and form free radicals. (We'll discuss free radicals in Chapter 11.)

When choosing oils, favor the monosaturated and polysaturated fats. To help with your selection, here's an overview of the most common oils and their fat content.

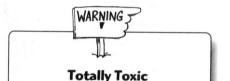

Totally Toxic

Don't go overboard in reducing your intake of fat. Eating too little fat can cause you to lose your menstrual period and may make it difficult to become pregnant. An inadequate fat intake may also make it difficult for you to assimilate and absorb your fat-soluble vitamins.

Fat or Oil	% Monounsaturated	% Polyunsaturated	% Saturated
Almond	73	18	9
Butter	30	4	65
Canola	62	31	7
Coconut	6	2	92
Corn	25	62	13
Margarine	46	33	21
Olive	77	9	14
Palm kernel	12	2	86
Peanut	48	34	18
Safflower	13	78	9
Shortening	45	27	28
Soybean	24	61	15
Sunflower	20	69	11

As a general rule, most fruits and vegetables are low in fat, ranging from 0 to 3 percent fat. Avocados are an exception, with 80 percent of their calories in the form of fat, but this is a very healthy fat and should be incorporated in your diet in reasonable quantities. As with avocados, nuts and seeds are also high in healthy fat, at more than 75 percent. Whole milk derives 49 percent of its calories from fat, while low-fat milk is much lower, at 31 percent. Hot dogs, hamburgers, bacon, spare ribs, and steak are generally all high-fat foods, with at least 66 percent of their calories from fat. Fish varies quite a bit but also is apt to contain healthy fat. Next time you're at the grocery store, check out the labels on the canned tuna. Typically, tuna, whether packed in water or oil, gets 4 percent of its calories from fat, but that can vary from can to can, even within the same brand. Salmon derives 35 percent of its calories from fat.

Note from Your Doctor

If you're reading labels and they tell you only the number of grams of fat your food contains, you might also want to know what percentage of calories are derived from fat. Here's a simple formula to calculate the percentage of fat calories from your food:

1. One gram of fat = 9 calories

2. If one serving has 7 grams of fat, then 7 x 9 = 63 calories from fat for the serving.

3. If the total calories of a serving are 110, then divide 63 by 110 = 57 percent of calories from fat. Don't eat too much of this food. It's simply too high in fat. Try to maintain your fat intake at no greater than 30 percent of your total calories; keeping in the 20 to 25 percent range is even better.

All Carbs Are Not Created Equal

While carbohydrates should probably be the mainstay of your diet, they are not all created equal. Two major forms of carbs exist: simple carbohydrates and complex carbohydrates. All are composed of a chain of sugar molecules linked together to give us energy. Simple carbohydrates generally contain only one or two sugar units. When more of them get together, they form a complex carbohydrate. Simple carbs are generally broken down by your body very rapidly, triggering your pancreas to release too much insulin. Examples of simple sugars are listed here:

➤ Molasses, corn syrup, glucose, fruit juice

➤ Fructose, maple sugar, dextrose, white sugar, brown sugar

➤ Honey, white rice

➤ White flour, sucrose

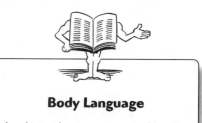

Body Language

Insulin is a hormone secreted by the pancreas to help regulate and control your blood-sugar level. Insulin is like an oil rig transporting glucose to your cells to be used as fuel by your body.

On the other hand, complex carbohydrates are generally much healthier for you. They break down much more slowly than simple carbohydrates and are higher in vitamins, minerals, and fiber. Complex carbohydrates are an excellent source of energy because they can be stored in your body and are converted to sugar to be utilized for energy when needed. Complex carbs won't send an insulin shock to your body. Examples of these favored complex carbohydrates or complex sugars include the following:

➤ Whole fruit

➤ Fresh vegetables, especially starchy ones

➤ Whole grains, including barley, millet, and oats

➤ Legumes, such as peas, beans, and lentils

➤ Whole-grain breads and cereals

You should certainly try to minimize your intake of simple carbohydrates and lean toward the more complex ones. It's generally recommended that in any given day you try to eat these amounts, at minimum:

➤ 6–11 servings of grains, including breads, pasta, rice, or cereals

➤ 2–4 servings of fresh fruit

➤ 3–5 servings of fresh vegetables

Fabulous Fiber

Fiber isn't just the stuff your socks or sweaters are made out of. It's also a quite edible complex carbohydrate that's a very valuable part of your diet. Fiber's fabulous benefits include the following:

➤ Preventing and helping to treat diverticulitis and colitis

➤ Improving bowel function and helping alleviate constipation

➤ Protecting you against colon cancer

➤ Helping to reduce your cholesterol level

➤ Reducing your risk of developing hemorrhoids or varicose veins

So where do you find this fiber without eating the shirt off your back? Fiber is found primarily in fresh fruit, vegetables, grains, beans, and legumes. You will not find any fiber in animal foods, including beef, chicken, pork, veal, lamb, or fish.

Two major types of fiber exist: insoluble and soluble. Both are important, and you should try to eat a variety of soluble and insoluble fiber. Insoluble fiber absorbs water and functions as a natural laxative by stimulating your gastrointestinal tract to keep moving waste out of your body. Good sources of insoluble fiber can be found in these foods:

➤ Starchy vegetables, including broccoli, carrots, peas, and potatoes

➤ Wheat bran and whole grains

➤ Popcorn, something you probably like that's good for you, too

Soluble fiber dissolves quickly and helps regulate the absorption of carbohydrates and fats into your bloodstream. Soluble fiber is largely responsible for lowering cholesterol and helping control diabetes. So start enjoying more of these foods:

➤ Fruit, especially apples and oranges

➤ Legumes (think of soups with lentils and beans)

➤ Oat bran, whether for breakfast, lunch, or dinner

Unfortunately, the average American eats only 12 to 17 grams of fiber per day. It's recommended that you try to eat at least 25 grams per day to reap the benefits of fiber. Make sure you drink more water when increasing the fiber intake in your diet. This will help decrease any intestinal gas, bloating, or cramping that some people may feel when eating a lot of fiber.

Conscientious About Cholesterol

Of all the different components in the foods in your diet that stir fear in our minds, cholesterol wins the prize. Virtually everybody is concerned about how much cholesterol their diet contains—and perhaps for good reason.

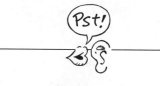

Healthy Hints

Carrots, sweet potatoes, corn on the cob, and cooked dried beans are great sources of both insoluble and soluble fiber. See, carrot cake and sweet potato pie can have some healthy benefits—if you can find carrot cake with healthy ingredients.

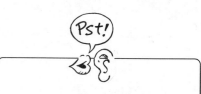

Healthy Hints

If you're concerned about an elevated cholesterol level, try eating oatmeal—or even better, oat bran—three to four times per week. You can either cook the oat bran or purchase it as a cold breakfast cereal. To help flavor it, try using raisins, bananas, or sliced fruit to add some sweetness and even more fiber. But avoid adding table sugar: It will drive your cholesterol level right back up.

As it turns out, elevated cholesterol levels play a role in increasing your risk of heart disease, cancer, and stroke. These are the three major causes of death in the United States, and the amount of cholesterol in your diet may contribute to your susceptibility. But eating cholesterol-rich foods is not the only way you increase your risk of disease. Eating saturated fat can also raise your cholesterol level.

As discussed earlier, dietary cholesterol is found only in foods of animal origin. There is no dietary cholesterol in plant foods. To avoid cholesterol, stick with the goodness of fruits, vegetables, and grains.

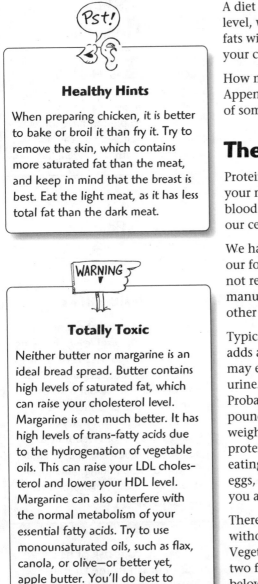

Healthy Hints

When preparing chicken, it is better to bake or broil it than fry it. Try to remove the skin, which contains more saturated fat than the meat, and keep in mind that the breast is best. Eat the light meat, as it has less total fat than the dark meat.

Totally Toxic

Neither butter nor margarine is an ideal bread spread. Butter contains high levels of saturated fat, which can raise your cholesterol level. Margarine is not much better. It has high levels of trans-fatty acids due to the hydrogenation of vegetable oils. This can raise your LDL cholesterol and lower your HDL level. Margarine can also interfere with the normal metabolism of your essential fatty acids. Try to use monounsaturated oils, such as flax, canola, or olive—or better yet, apple butter. You'll do best to restrict your intake of both butter and margarine.

A diet high in saturated fat will raise your cholesterol level, whereas monounsaturated and polyunsaturated fats will have no effect—or may even slightly reduce your cholesterol level.

How much cholesterol and fat are you eating? Refer to Appendix A for a look at the cholesterol and fat content of some commonly eaten foods.

The Power of Protein

Proteins are a part of your hair, your nails, your skin, your muscles, your bones, your DNA, and even your blood cells. They are one of the main building blocks of our cells and are made up of chains of amino acids.

We have to obtain nine essential amino acids through our food. Any other amino acids that our cells need are not referred to as "essential" because our body can manufacture them from other amino acids and from other normal metabolic activity.

Typically, most Americans eat too much protein, which adds additional stress to the kidneys and the liver, and may even contribute to the loss of calcium through the urine. So, how much protein do you really need? Probably about 1 gram of protein per kilogram (2.2 pounds) of body weight per day suffices. So, if you weigh 150 pounds, you'll need about 68 grams of protein a day. Unfortunately, many of us are probably eating two to three times that amount. If you are having eggs, chicken, and meat for breakfast, lunch and dinner, you are on protein overload.

There are also various ways of getting enough protein without eating meat and taxing your internal organs. Vegetarians do it all the time. Simply combine any two foods from two out of the three categories below to form a complete protein. For example, mixing a legume (such as chickpeas) with a whole grain (such as couscous) provides a nutritious, delicious, and protein-packed meal.

➤ Legumes: peas; kidney, navy, and lima beans; garbanzo beans or chickpeas; lentils; soy, or tofu

➤ Whole grains: millet, wheat germ, rye, quinoa, spelt, barley, couscous, brown rice, amaranth, buckwheat, barley, or oatmeal

➤ Nuts and seeds: sunflower, pumpkin, sesame, walnuts, pecans, almonds, peanuts, cashews, or filberts

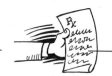

Note from Your Doctor

If you've been told that your kidneys are not working efficiently, or if you have a history of uric acid kidney stones or high uric acid levels in your blood, stick to a low-protein diet. Excess proteins often can't be metabolized efficiently in these cases.

Wondering what foods are packed with protein? Take a look in the appendix for a good overview.

What's Left for Dinner?

By now, you must be wondering: What the heck can I still eat to help ensure a longer and healthier life? Well, you may be pleasantly surprised.

Eat a variety of foods. If you're in the habit of eating the same food for breakfast or lunch every day, break it. Have some fun experimenting with new foods.

Change your fruits with the day of the week—or at least vary your bouquet seasonally. And if lunch is a bologna sandwich every day, try tuna or turkey between your bread, or go crazy and have a great salad. For dinner, experiment with different grains in place of rice or potatoes. Before you know it, you may be espousing a whole new vocabulary of foods you had never even heard of. Impress your friends with your new polenta and wild mushroom ragout dish.

Try a new vegetable every other day. Remember to eat at least three to five servings of your favorite vegetables on a daily basis, but also try different kinds of squash: acorn, butternut, and spaghetti squash. Make your mom proud, and eat a variety of cruciferous vegetables, such as broccoli, cabbage, and Brussels sprouts. All are high in antioxidants and help detoxify your body of hazardous chemicals and heavy metals. Try other vegetables such as beets, dandelion and mustard greens, artichoke, collards, parsnips, fennel, spinach, or endive. I promise, they won't bite back.

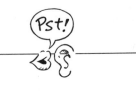

Healthy Hints

Here's a great healthy dish—and it's easy, too. Bake or steam a spaghetti squash. Scrape the skin off the squash with a fork. Top with tomato sauce and a sprinkle of Parmesan cheese. Mama mia—you've got pasta! Add a Caesar salad to make the meal complete.

Use a variety of different herbs and spices to season and flavor your food. Work your way through the alphabet and try a different seasoning each night, starting with A for anise, B for basil, and C for cinnamon. Most herbs and seasonings have the added benefit of containing important disease-fighting antioxidants and rejuvenating properties. Pay particular attention to garlic, onion, turmeric, oregano, and parsley, to name just a few.

Incorporate beans into your diet on a regular basis, perhaps four or five times each week. Take a class and learn how to cook, season, and flavor these high-fiber foods. Some of my favorites include garbanzo, kidney, navy, pinto, and soybeans. Extra time on your hands? Learn how to sprout beans such as alfalfa, mung, broccoli, and lentil. Or do it the easy way and pick them up at the grocery store, as they are more widely available now than ever. Add them to all your grains and greens. These are chock-full of nutrients and vitamins and will multiply the health benefits you are getting from your food.

Earlier in this book, I mentioned that the average American gets 80 percent of his or her calories and vitamins and minerals from only 20 different foods. Count up how many foods you really eat, and try to expand your diet to maybe 50 different foods on a regular basis. Try a new food every day or two. Each food has different vitamins, minerals, enzymes, amino acids, and fiber content that can benefit you in a variety of ways.

Choose a diet that is high in whole grains, vegetables, and fruit, and low in saturated fats and dietary cholesterol. Pick up a cookbook that grabs your eye at the library or bookstore. Take a vegetarian cooking class, or get competitive with a friend to see who can be more creative with a new vegetable or legume. Have a tasting party with everyone bringing a tofu, seitan, or tempeh dish. Mix grains and beans with a smattering of seeds such as pumpkin or sesame seeds for a non–animal-based complete protein meal. Try to have meatless meals several times throughout the week.

Food should be as fresh as possible. Avoid processed foods. Try to limit your intake of frozen foods, and try to avoid canned foods as much as possible, as they've lost some of their original nutrients. If you insist on having animal products for dinner, make it a side dish, maybe no more than 3 ounces. There's nothing wrong with having a meal made up of several side dishes of fruits, vegetables, rice, potatoes, or beans. Be a little concerned about appearances; arrange your food beautifully on your plate. This is a trick all chefs learn; if it looks good, it must somehow taste better.

Try to minimize your intake of salt and refined sugar. Avoid empty calories. And taste your food before deciding to add salt.

Water, water, water. Your body is more than 50 percent water, and you naturally lose 2 or 3 quarts per day, so you need to replenish water. Try to drink at least a gallon per day of either spring or filtered water. (I keep a 1-gallon jug next to my desk at work, and I try to make sure it's emptied each day.) If you're drinking alcohol, keep it to a minimum. Red wine? A glass or two a day may actually be beneficial, as we'll discuss in the next chapter, but don't drink a whole bottle. A beer or two during a football game is probably okay—as long as you're not watching football games all day long. (If you are watching that much football, read Chapter 22, and begin an exercise program.) The key, of course, is moderation, unless it's water—then drink like a fish.

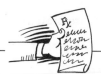

Note from Your Doctor

Do you know what the top 10 items purchased from grocery stores are? In a recent survey ranked by number of dollars spent, it wasn't milk, bread, eggs, chicken, or beef. Give up? Here's the very surprising list.

1. Marlboro cigarettes
2. Coca-Cola Classic
3. Pepsi-Cola
4. Kraft processed cheese
5. Diet Coke
6. Campbell's soup
7. Budweiser beer
8. Tide detergent
9. Folger's coffee
10. Winston cigarettes

Out of the top 10, four are carbonated beverages, two are cigarettes, two are not really food (processed cheese and detergent), and one is caffeine, which is as addictive as the cigarettes.

It's no wonder we're so sick!

The Least You Need to Know

➤ Eating too many calories can cause weight gain.

➤ Saturated fats and dietary cholesterol are associated with increasing your risk of obesity, heart disease, stroke, diabetes, and cancer.

➤ Simple sugars should be limited. Enjoy more complex carbohydrates.

➤ Animal-based foods contain cholesterol, while plant-based foods do not.

➤ It is possible to get adequate protein without eating meat.

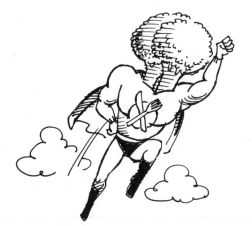

Chapter 5

Super Foods to the Rescue

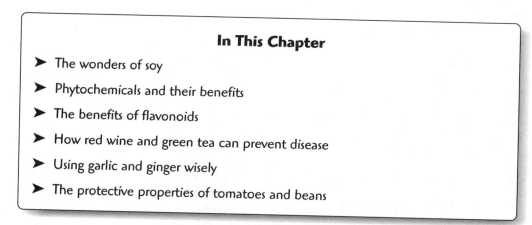

In This Chapter

➤ The wonders of soy

➤ Phytochemicals and their benefits

➤ The benefits of flavonoids

➤ How red wine and green tea can prevent disease

➤ Using garlic and ginger wisely

➤ The protective properties of tomatoes and beans

When penicillin was first introduced, it was referred to as the new miracle drug—as were discoveries that followed, such as cortisone and ibuprofen. Over the last 50 years, in fact, so many so-called miracle drugs have made their appearance that it's been nearly impossible to keep track of them. And now we have Viagra, the latest miracle drug, a pharmaceutical interpretation of the song "Never Too Late for Love."

Not that all these miracle drugs have proven to be so divine. For instance, that miracle Phen-Fen diet drug was popular for a few months before it became clear that its risks outweighed its weight-loss benefits and it was taken off the market. Then, too, a lot of antibiotic miracle drugs were so overused that they began to lose their healing powers.

By now you probably get my drift. We have seen miracle drugs come and go. Miracle foods, by contrast, have been around for centuries. They're not new and will probably be around long after you and I are around to derive any benefit from them.

What kinds of foods am I talking about, exactly? These are foods that can help detoxify your body, prevent cancer, prevent heart disease, and maybe even ward off headaches. These super foods may lower your cholesterol, stimulate your immune system, stop stomachaches, and even halt hot flashes. And, unlike fads that appear and disappear from year to year, they're a permanent part of the earth's bounty. They're also quite delicious—and a lot less expensive than miracle drugs. In this chapter, we'll examine the roles of some of these extraordinary edibles—foods that you definitely need to make use of, now that you've appointed yourself Director of Prevention.

Soy What?

If we all picked up and moved to Japan, soy would be a component of nearly every meal we'd eat. Foods that are high in soy are particularly important in protecting women against breast cancer and osteoporosis. For men, they're not so bad, either, helping to keep the prostate gland cancer-free. Soy can also lower cholesterol levels in both men and women.

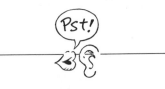

Healthy Hints

Try to drink a bowl of miso soup (soybean paste) each day. This could reduce your risk of stomach cancer by 66 percent. In addition to soy, celery, parsley, and fennel are also high in phytoestrogen and have estrogenic activity.

The Soy Shield

Soy can be found in soybeans, soy milk, soy cheese, soy flour, soy hot dogs, tofu, tempeh, miso, and textured soy protein. What makes soy so special? It contains estrogen-like compounds known as phytoestrogen, which provide protective benefits. Two phytoestrogens in particular—genistein and daidzein, both isoflavones—have been associated with the ability to inhibit cancers of the breast, the ovary, and the uterus. A third phytoestrogen, saponins (also found in soybeans), can help reduce the spread of cancer cells in the colon and reduce your cholesterol level. All three phytoestrogens can also help alleviate symptoms of menopause.

In fact, while about 75 percent of American women experience hot flashes, night sweats, and other menopausal symptoms, Japanese women rarely experience such problems or sleep disturbances at all in their menopausal years. Eating just two-thirds of a cup of cooked soybeans per day is sufficient to provide you with most of these benefits, providing a sort of "soy shield" against a whole host of problems ranging from merely annoying to life-threatening.

In fact, it's now believed that the phytoestrogen in soybeans can actually counteract cancer-promoting

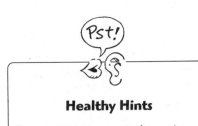

Healthy Hints

Try using soy as a meat alternative. Experiment or take a class, and learn how to use tofu, tempeh, or TSP (textured soy protein). All are healthy, inexpensive, versatile, and can provide great protein substitutes for meat.

estrogen in much the same way that the drug tamoxifen does. In Asian countries, those women who eat twice as much soy protein as their compatriots seem to have about 50 percent less chance of breast cancer.

The Bone-Bean Connection

Eating just 40 grams of soy protein per day can greatly increase the bone density in the lower spine in post-menopausal women. Soy helps you retain more calcium and build stronger bones. Soy isoflavones, known as genistein and daidzein, also help to reduce the risk of osteoporosis by preventing bone loss and bone breakdown—something you might think of as the "bone-bean connection."

Genistein has also been reported to directly lower blood cholesterol levels. Eating 25 to 50 grams of soy protein per day should generally be enough to accomplish that. To get an idea of how much is enough, about two servings (1 cup) of tofu will provide you with 40 grams of soy protein.

The following chart tells how much total isoflavones exist in different soy-based foods:

Soy Food	Total Isoflavones (mg)
Soy milk (1/2 cup)	40
Tofu (1/2 cup)	40
Tempeh (1/2 cup)	40
Miso (1/2 cup)	40
TSP (cooked, 1/2 cup)	35
Soy flour (1/2 cup)	50
Soybeans (cooked, 1/2 cup)	35
Soy nuts (1 ounce)	40

The next time someone offers you soy or soy products, don't think "soy what?" Think about soy's many benefits and possibilities instead.

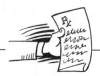

Note from Your Doctor

Soybeans are legumes, just like beans, peas, and lentils. However, soybeans are lower in carbohydrate content and are very high in dietary fiber and protein. In fact, their protein quality is equivalent to that which you would find in meat, milk, or egg protein. Soybeans are the only vegetable food that contains large quantities of complete protein.

What About Flavonoids?

Ever wonder how a blueberry became blue or how an apple became red or how an orange became orange? I hope you didn't really answer yes, because if you did, you need to get a life. I myself never wondered until I had to write this book.

As it turns out, most fruits and vegetables obtain their color and flavor from substances known as flavonoids or bioflavonoids. These terms are basically interchangeable, so for the purpose of brevity, I will refer to them as flavonoids.

Flavonoids are also members of a family of plant substances known as phytochemicals. These are strong antioxidants that protect your cells from free radicals—a kind of internal antiterrorism network, which should be essential to you as Director of Prevention. Flavonoids appear to act as deterrents to viruses, allergies, carcinogens, and inflammation. They may also help lower your total cholesterol level and prevent the oxidation of LDL cholesterol. Just as isoflavones act as phytoestrogen, flavonoids do, too. They help balance estrogen metabolism and encourage the body to convert estradiol to estriol, a safer, more protective form of estrogen.

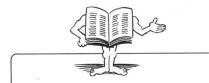

Body Language

Flavonoids are antioxidants belonging to the phytochemical family. They were actually discovered in 1936 by the Nobel Prize–winning scientist Albert Szent-Gyorgyi. He originally called them vitamin P because of their impact on vascular permeability. Flavonoids can actually strengthen the walls of small blood vessels known as capillaries.

Flavonoids can be found in most fruits and vegetables, as well as nuts, seeds, grains, and soy products. They are especially high in citrus fruit, tomatoes, berries, peppers, carrots, onions, kale, and grapes. You can also drink your flavonoids, which are present in tea, coffee, or red wine.

Flavonoids may also have other benefits. They may prevent swelling in the legs due to fluid retention and may help treat varicose veins, leg cramps, diabetic neuropathy, and high blood pressure. A recent study showed that men who consumed high amounts of flavonoids were 33 percent less likely to die from a heart attack.

Most of the studies performed on flavonoids have demonstrated their effectiveness in the prevention and treatment of various cancers. Some of the compounds that display antitumor effects are Quercetin, Hesperidin, Genistein, Rutin, Naringin, Catechin, and Pycnogenol.

Fabulous Phytochemicals

By now you've actually heard about two major groups of phytochemicals: flavonoids and isoflavones. Phytochemicals are naturally occurring substances in plants that have strong antioxidant activity. They're found in both fruits and vegetables and are associated with reductions in cancer rates and heart disease. Here are some of the most important phytochemical-containing foods that you should be aware of as Director of Prevention:

Phytochemical	Found In
Genistein	Soybeans, peas, lentils, cabbage
Indoles	Cabbage, broccoli, kale, Brussels sprouts
Carotenoids	Tomatoes, watermelon, grapefruit
Quercetin	Citrus fruits
Phytosterols	Alfalfa sprouts, yams
Isoflavones	Soy products
Lycopene	Tomatoes, red grapefruit, watermelon, strawberries
Capsaicin	Hot peppers
Allium	Garlic, leeks, onions
Sulforaphane	Broccoli, cabbage, mustard
Flavonoids	Citrus, tomatoes, berries, carrots, peppers, onions, kale, grapes, and red wine

How to Make Every Meal a Phyto-Feast

Consider these tips to make increasing the phytochemical content of your diet a little easier:

➤ Increase your intake and serving sizes of vegetables.

➤ Snack on fresh or dried fruit instead of candy.

➤ Include beans in your stews, soups, and pasta.

➤ Flavor your foods with herbs and spices, such as ginger, rosemary, thyme, garlic, parsley, basil, and chives.

➤ Add vegetables such as mushrooms, peppers, tomatoes, and onions, along with herbs when making an omelet.

➤ Eat meatless dinners three or more times per week.

➤ Drink 100 percent fruit or vegetable juice instead of soda.

➤ Add sautéed onions, mushrooms, and peppers to whole-grain dishes such as rice, barley, millet, couscous, or buckwheat.

➤ Use baby carrots for snacks between meals.

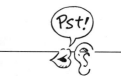

Healthy Hints

Even though you may see phytochemical supplements in your local health food store, it is still best to obtain your phytonutrients from plant-based foods such as fresh fruits and vegetables.

➤ Try hummus as a healthy vegetable dip.

➤ When preparing raw vegetable salads, try to include asparagus, red peppers, zucchini, broccoli, sweet potato sticks, cauliflower, carrots, and celery.

Red Wine Wonders

Health experts have found increasing evidence that drinking red wine in moderation—with emphasis on the word *moderation*—may be one of the secrets of a healthy heart and longer life. Numerous studies have indicated that moderate consumption of red wine has a beneficial effect on people with coronary artery disease.

Note from Your Doctor

For more than 6,000 years, while civilizations and empires rose and fell, wine has managed to retain its value as a prized beverage. In fact, during the Middle Ages, it was used as a form of currency. In 1991, Serge Renaud, M.D., the Director of the French National Institute of Health and Medical Research, coined the term "French paradox." It's widely known that the French generally consume more fat, smoke more, and exercise less than Americans yet are less prone to vascular disease. Renaud theorized that part of the advantage enjoyed by the French was due to their famous national passion for red wine.

Antioxidant compounds in wine seem to lower blood pressure, reduce cholesterol, and make your blood vessels more flexible, thereby inhibiting atherosclerosis. For example, men who consume moderate amounts of red wine enjoy a 30 percent reduction in their risk of dying from any cause, including cardiovascular disease, coronary artery disease, and all types of cancer. What's a moderate amount? Maybe one to two glasses per day of red wine. Hey, let's not allow ourselves to get carried away with this news!

It's been found that the beneficial effects of red wine are due primarily to its high concentration of phenolic compounds. These compounds are actually flavonoids and have powerful antioxidant properties. The antioxidant protection of phenolic compounds may even be stronger than those found in both vitamins E and C combined because they help protect the LDL (bad) cholesterol from oxidation. These phytonutrients are commonly found in the skins and seeds of red grapes.

But that's not all. Recently, red wine got credit for providing another line of defense, known as resveratrol—yet another flavonoid that covers the skins of grapes and resists disease. It's actually a natural fungicide that helps protect grapes from bacteria. Resveratrol, which is found in both red grapes and red wine, helps to prevent clot formation in the coronary arteries. It's also been shown to help increase the levels of HDL (good) cholesterol, and resveratrol has recently been shown to inhibit the growth of cancer cells in the laboratory. More research is still needed to determine how it may affect the growth of cancer cells in humans.

Red wine can apparently also help us preserve our vision—provided that we don't drink too much and start seeing double. Compared to those who drink beer, liquor, or no alcohol at all, people who consume moderate amounts of red wine are at lower risk for developing age-related macular degeneration—the leading cause of blindness in the elderly population.

The Broccoli Connection

Would former President George Bush have been re-elected had he only listened to his mother when she told him to eat his broccoli, rather than proclaiming his dislike for broccoli and his right not to have to eat it as chief executive? Those remarks undoubtedly cost him the vote of the nation's broccoli growers, not to mention the votes of a lot of mothers who had been trying to persuade their kids to eat broccoli. Beyond that, however, he mocked a valuable nutritional ally whose role in the fight against cancer should be emphasized—a major gaffe for a guy who wanted to go down in history as the "education president."

Despite the ex-president's sentiments, however, it turns out his mother was right—and you'd be well-advised to listen to her by incorporating 2 or 3 cups of fresh broccoli into your diet each week. Broccoli, which is a member of the crucifer family, contains high quantities of an anticancer phytochemical known as sulforaphane. Broccoli contains even more of this anticancer agent than cabbage, cauliflower, kale, or Brussels sprouts.

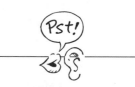

Healthy Hints

The sales of organic wines have been growing, both throughout the United States and around the world. These wines are not only grown with all-natural fertillizers and without chemical pesticides, but they contain fewer sulfites, a common food additive, and are friendlier to the environment. This may be especially important for those who suffer side effects when consuming high amounts of sulfites, which are generally used to preserve and prevent browning of the wine. Such side effects can include difficulty breathing, dizziness, headaches, and abdominal pain.

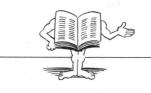

Body Language

Sulfurophane actually belongs to a group of compounds known as *isothiocyanate*, which are also found in mustard, wasabe, and horseradish. These foods also have anticancer effects.

Sulforaphane seems to stimulate the enzymes that block the formation of cancerous growth. And the latest scoop? Fresh broccoli sprouts actually have the highest activity of cancer-inhibiting enzymes of any of the cruciferous vegetables. Try mixing these into your salad or using them in a vegetarian sandwich.

Berry, Berry Best

Blueberries are commonly associated with wholesomeness and childhood memories. But they can also be a boon to us as we get older. That's because they contain a compound known as anthocyanosides, which can help slow vision loss and protect against macular degeneration. The deep blue pigment in blueberries is also found in bilberry extract, an herb that is currently used in Europe for all sorts of eye disorders, including cataracts, diabetic retinopathy, night blindness, and retinitis pigmentosa.

Blueberries can also protect you against chronic urinary tract and bladder infections by blocking bacteria's ability to cling to the cells of the urinary tract.

Try adding some blueberries to your breakfast cereal or simply eating them for dessert in a fruit salad. Cranberries, too, can help ward off urinary infections. About 1 to 2 cups per day should be enough to do the trick.

The Roots of Relief

Ginger has been used in China, India, and other Asian countries for more than 25 centuries to help with digestion, nausea, and motion sickness. Most people use it very gingerly, at best, or perhaps not at all. But obstetricians are increasingly turning to ginger to help fight morning sickness—you know, that terrible nausea and vomiting that occurs early during pregnancy. In a recent study, 70 percent of the pregnant women who took ginger found it to be effective. They used 250 mg of ginger root extract four times per day to help relieve their attacks of vomiting.

And for motion sickness? Take 1,000 mg of ginger in capsule form about a half hour before boarding your plane, train, auto, or boat. You might need to repeat the dosage if symptoms recur. Ginger may also function as an antiinflammatory and help reduce symptoms of rheumatoid arthritis because it seems to block the formation of inflammatory substances known as leukotrienes. In addition, it's a strong antioxidant.

One of the beauties of this spice is that you can incorporate either fresh or powdered ginger into your cooking. You may find that using ginger works better than some of the nonsteroidal, anti-inflammatory drugs that your rheumatologist may have recommended for you. Better yet, unlike such drugs, ginger doesn't seem to produce negative side effects.

Suffering from migraines? Again, try ginger, which may be effective at both preventing and relieving migraine headaches without the side effects of stronger prescription medications.

Note from Your Doctor

An active ingredient in ginger, gingerol, is chemically similar to aspirin. Researchers at Cornell University Medical College found that ginger could help reduce the stickiness of your platelets and cut down on your chances of forming a blood clot. Also, like aspirin, ginger fights headaches. For migraine headaches, try 500 to 600 mg (about one-third of a teaspoon) of powdered ginger mixed with plain water. You can repeat the dose up to four times per day before reaching for the aspirin bottle.

Cloves, ginger, cumin, and turmeric all prevent blood platelets from clumping abnormally. All these spices are thought to reduce the production of thromboxane, a strong promoter of platelet aggregation, which is what happens when platelets start sticking together.

Potent Remedies

It is often said that garlic and onions help ward off diseases, and this may be true in a very fundamental sense. Eat enough of either, and people—coworkers, family, friends, and fellow subway riders—are sure to keep their distance. Encouraging all these folks to maintain a healthy space between you and them—without having to be so rude as to ask them to—is one sure-fire way to keep from being exposed to the latest strains of flu or whatever other infections they may be carrying.

Apart from such considerations, garlic and onions have a long history of helping people stay healthy, not only by fighting infections and viruses, but by lowering blood pressure and cholesterol and preventing your platelets from becoming too sticky. And, of course, they can make your food taste a lot more flavorful in the process.

Garlic may also act as a preventative against certain kinds of cancers. Specifically, it's been shown to help slow the growth of prostate cancer cells. While this result occurred only in a test tube, the possibilities look promising for obtaining similar results in "real men."

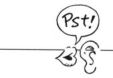

Healthy Hints

Garlic contains several sulfur-containing compounds that have strong antibacterial effects. These compounds allow garlic to destroy germs and fight infections; they may help against fungal bacteria and even viral infections.

Researchers are still at odds as to the exact compound in garlic that provide its beneficial effects—most feel that it's allicin, the sulfur compound produced when garlic is crushed or sliced. That's why it's probably best to include the "real thing" in your diet if you can—at least three cloves per day. If your spouse or "significant other" finds that too objectionable, however, consider supplementing your diet with three to six aged, deodorized garlic capsules per day.

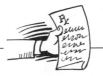

Note from Your Doctor

The history of garlic goes back hundreds of years. Bulbs were placed in the tomb of King Tutankhaman because garlic was thought to ensure eternal life. It was used as a remedy in Europe during the Great Plague and was put in the pillows during childbirth to ensure a successful delivery. It was also believed a deterrent to supernatural creatures, such as vampires. Today, it's still thought of as an agent against infections, heart disease, and cancer.

Green Tea for Two

The British seem to have an instinctive understanding of the protective power of tea. Whenever depicted in a precarious situation—be it on a sinking ship in shark-infested waters or hopelessly surrounded by hostile Zulu warriors—what do they invariably do? Why, take time out for a spot of tea, by Jove!

But whereas "tea" used to mean the standard black variety, it's now widely available in its less mature "green" stage as well (not to mention a whole range of exotic herbal flavors). It's this green tea that's now becoming especially popular among savvy Directors of Prevention everywhere.

Just as you've heard that an apple a day may keep the doctor away, a cup of green tea may keep cancer away. Of course, green tea does tend to be an "acquired taste," meaning it takes a while to get used to its more subtle flavor and color. If you're not feeling bold enough to try it, you'll be happy to know that black tea may have similar effects—although to a somewhat lesser degree. Both green and black tea contain polyphenols, naturally occurring compounds with strong anticancer effects. These may protect against breast, skin, lung, stomach, prostate, and colon cancer.

Polyphenols work by inhibiting cancer-causing genes and by neutralizing cancer-causing chemicals. They may also help prevent strokes; a recent study showed that men who had the highest intake of polyphenols were 73 percent less likely to suffer a stroke compared to men who had little polyphenol intake. Green or black tea may also protect you against heart disease and make you less likely to experience or die from a heart attack.

Four primary polyphenols are found in green tea: epicatechin (EC), epicatechin gallate (ECG), epigallocatechin (EGC), and epigallocatechin gallate (EGCG). In a recent study, green tea extract was found to have 20 times the antioxidant punch of vitamin C. The main antioxidant activity is thought to come primarily from its high content of EGCG.

Women who drink green tea have been shown to be at decreased risk for cancers of the upper digestive tract, the colon, and the rectum. It appears that drinking two or more cups of tea per day can reduce your risk of cancer by 10 percent.

If you are sensitive to caffeine and need to avoid it even in small quantities, you may have to lay off green tea as well as black tea. Although green tea contains only about a third of the caffeine found in black tea—and much less than is found in coffee—it still may be too much for some caffeine-sensitive individuals.

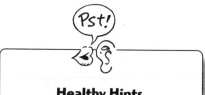

Healthy Hints

If drinking tea is not your cup of tea, green tea extracts are now available in supplement form. Look for one with at least an 80 percent polyphenol content.

Tomatoes: The Lycopene Link

Pizza lovers, rejoice. I have the news you've been waiting for.

The next time you feel the urge to chow down on pizza, only to be given a disapproving look by your spouse, child, or parent, tell them it may be better for you than they think. A recent study published in the *Journal of the National Cancer Institute* found that men who ate at least 10 servings of tomato-based foods per week were up to 45 percent less likely to develop prostate cancer. Those eating four to seven servings per week enjoyed a 20 percent reduction.

That's because tomatoes are rich in another antioxidant phytonutrient, known as lycopene. In addition to protecting against colon and cervical cancer and reducing your risk of cardiovascular disease, lycopene can help to keep bad LDL cholesterol from becoming oxidized and promoting atherosclerosis.

Nor is cooking tomatoes such a bad idea—in fact, it seems to make them even more protective than raw tomatoes or tomato juice. It could be that when tomatoes are heated during cooking, the cells burst and release more lycopene. Lycopene's effects are also enhanced when tomatoes are processed in oil.

I'm not suggesting that you go hog wild in placing orders with your neighborhood pizza parlor. I'd prefer you think in terms of including more fresh tomatoes, tomato juice, tomato sauce, and tomato paste in your diet. You don't like tomatoes? In that case, you might want to opt for red grapefruit and watermelon. They're also sources of lycopene, only in smaller quantities.

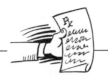

Note from Your Doctor

Eating tomato products not only can help men avoid prostate cancer, but it also can help protect women against cervical cancer. Women who have the highest blood level of lycopene have been shown to be five times less likely to develop precancerous changes in the cervix than those with the lowest blood levels of lycopene.

Lycopene is actually a carotenoid, just like beta carotene. It appears, however, that lycopene is much more protective against vascular disease. To help prevent oxidation by your LDL cholesterol—one of your basic responsibilities as Director of Prevention—consider eating lycopene-containing foods in combination with vitamins C and E. Lycopene can also prevent the formation of cholesterol in the first place.

Beans, Beans, They're Good for Your Heart

I've already told you about some of the wonderful properties of soybeans in helping protect you against the ravages of aging. But what about other beans? They, too, are loaded with phytochemicals and can help prevent disease. For example, navy, kidney, adzuki, lentils, chickpeas, pinto, black, and lima beans are all rich in phytochemicals. Let's look at a few of the phytochemicals contained within beans and the diseases they may protect you against:

➤ Phytosterols: prevent colon cancer

➤ Phytoestrogens (for example, Genistein and Daidzein): prevent breast cancer and reduce symptoms of menopause

➤ Saponins: prevent cancer cells from multiplying, lower blood cholesterol

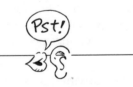

Healthy Hints

Most people can lower their blood cholesterol by eating two-thirds of a cup of oat bran cereal or a cup of beans each day. Such simple dietary changes should be tried before you resort to taking cholesterol-lowering drugs, which tend to have side effects.

Eating a cup of cooked dried beans daily may help lower your cholesterol by as much as 20 percent, increase your good HDL cholesterol by 9 percent, and improve the HDL-to-LDL ratio by up to 17 percent. Because beans can have such a strong impact in reducing your risk of vascular disease, you should try incorporating dried beans into your daily diet on a regular basis.

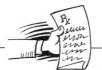

Note from Your Doctor

The protection beans offer from breast cancer is due to their high-fiber content as well as phytoestrogen, which helps block the activity of cancer-causing estrogen.

On the average, Hispanic women eat three-quarters of a cup of beans six days per week, compared to twice per week for white American women. This may account for why women who live in the Caribbean or Mexico are known to have less breast cancer than women living in the United States. Beans contain several anticancer compounds, known as protease inhibitors and phytates, that can reduce the risk of breast cancer.

The Least You Need to Know

➤ Soy products contain phytoestrogen to protect against heart disease, cancer, and osteoporosis.

➤ Flavonoids in fruit and vegetables can lower cholesterol and prevent heart disease and cancer.

➤ Phytochemicals are naturally occurring substances in fruits and vegetables that have strong antioxidant activity to protect against free radicals.

➤ Red wine can be beneficial for lowering cholesterol; cooked, dried beans may lower cholesterol level and prevent cancer.

➤ Using seasonings such as ginger and garlic in your diet can improve your health and digestion.

➤ Tomatoes contain lycopene, which can protect against heart disease and prostate and cervical cancer.

Part 2
Supplements Made Simple

There is a lot of talk about vitamins, minerals, and supplements in the news every day. It is often overwhelming and contradictory. Let's make it simple. To ensure optimum health and longevity, take your vitamins everyday, just like your mother always nagged you to do. It would be great if we could get all of the nutrients we need for survival from our diet. But that is not realistic—taking supplements, however, is.

Plain and simple, let's make sense of the world of supplements available to us. In the following five chapters, you will get the information you need to pick and choose the bouquet of supplements that is right for you.

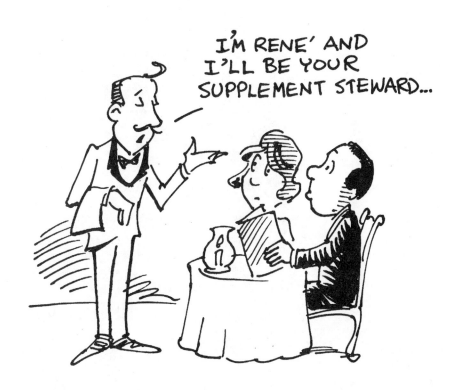

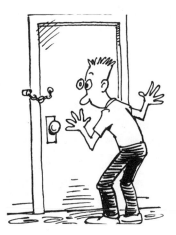

Chapter 6

Nutrients Knocking at Your Door

In This Chapter

➤ Who needs nutritional supplements and why

➤ Different kinds of supplements

➤ The difference between pharmaceuticals and nutrients

➤ How to determine your own nutrient needs

Knock, knock. Who's there? Nutrient. Nutrient who? Nutrient good for you. As nutrients are gaining more popularity than ever, a greater percentage of the population is now taking supplements on a regular basis. Are supplements for you? Probably so. Let's explore some of the reasons why they're knocking at your door.

Who Needs Supplements?

Almost every one of you reading this book could improve your health with the use of nutritional supplements. A substantial amount of medical information today indicates that to obtain optimum health and prevent disease, our bodies need optimum doses, not minimum intakes, of vitamins and minerals. Nutritional supplements have been associated with protection against such diseases as osteoporosis, heart disease, birth defects, macular degeneration, cataracts, infectious disease, and cancer.

Note from Your Doctor

In a recent survey of 8,000 adults, only 1 percent consumed diets that met the minimum requirements of the USDA's food guide pyramid. It's quite obvious that the American diet fails to meet the current dietary guidelines or the nutrient recommendations for vitamins and minerals. This also puts more emphasis on the importance of supplementation.

Which groups of people are most likely to need nutritional supplements?

➤ People who are doing strenuous exercise or burning excessive amounts of calories.

➤ People ingesting large quantities of alcohol.

➤ Those taking prescriptions or over-the-counter medications.

➤ Those who are exposed to environmental pollution, toxins, heavy metals, or pesticides.

➤ People who smoke cigarettes or are exposed to secondhand smoke.

➤ People with certain medical conditions that put a greater demand on their metabolism due to their disease process. This can include some of the diseases of the gastrointestinal tract, such as celiac disease, ulcerative colitis, or Crohn's disease.

➤ Those with infections that can deplete the stores of their vitamins and minerals.

➤ People who are recuperating after significant stress, trauma, burn, or surgery. These processes also deplete the body of its nutrient stores.

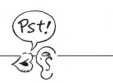

Healthy Hints

The "normal American diet" might not be so normal. In one recent report, only 12 percent of the people tested were found to have normal levels of vitamins in their blood stream.

Add to this list the special nutritional needs of children and teenagers, pregnant and lactating women, and those undergoing chemotherapy, and you can see why I believe that almost all of us can benefit from nutritional supplementation. Even if you're eating what you think is an ideal diet, your food is so devitalized and depleted of the beneficial vitamins, minerals, and fiber that it is difficult for you to get everything you need from your food supply alone. Our food today is processed, milled, refined, and transported, which all take away some of the key components that are so vital for our health. That's probably why more than 40 percent of our population now takes nutritional supplements on a regular basis. As one of my colleagues, internationally renowned immunologist R.K. Chandra, M.D., says, "The era of nutritional supplements to promote health and reduce illness is here to stay."

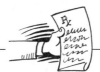

Note from Your Doctor

Have you ever thought of how you would define the word "health"? You might think that health is freedom from disease. But does the mere absence of disease equate with being in good health? Obviously not. The World Health Organization recently defined health as a state of complete physical, mental, and social well-being, not merely the absence of disease or infirmity.

Who's taking nutritional supplements, besides you and me? According to the recent surveys, at least 40 to 50 percent take supplements on a regular basis. And it's not just the general population—even health care practitioners are now jumping on the bandwagon. According to a recent survey of 600 dietitians, nearly 60 percent were found to use nutritional supplements. At a 1994 American College of Cardiology meeting, nearly two out of three of the 700 physicians in attendance reported taking supplements, though many are still reluctant to recommend them to their patients. Forty-four percent of the cardiologists, 38 percent of all nurses, and 47 percent of pharmacy students take nutritional supplements.

Numerous common medical diseases could probably be prevented with supplementation. Let's touch on a few:

➤ Calcium and vitamin D and osteoporosis: Substantial support now indicates that increasing your intake of calcium and vitamin D could help protect you against bone loss and osteoporosis. Unfortunately, most of you probably fall short in obtaining adequate levels of calcium from your diet. Anyone over the age of 50 should try to consume at least 1,200 mg of calcium per day and 400 IU of vitamin D. If you're older than 70 years old, 600 IU of vitamin D would be even better.

➤ Folic acid and birth defects: In my opinion, all women of childbearing age should take folic acid, not only during pregnancy but preferably two or three months prior to conception. This all-important B vitamin has been shown to markedly lower the risk of babies being born with neural tube defects such as spina bifida, cleft palate, or anencephaly. It's also advisable to take a multivitamin in addition to at least 400 mcg of folic acid per day.

➤ Folic acid and heart disease: Taking a multivitamin containing folic acid can also have a beneficial effect on your risk of heart disease and stroke. A recent study concluded that approximately 56,000 deaths from heart disease could be prevented each year if all Americans took folic acid.

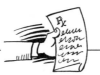

Note from Your Doctor

Only about 35 percent of the elderly population have an immune system similar to their younger peers. Supplementing with a multivitamin containing minerals has been shown to reduce the number of sick days by 50 percent. Deficiencies in nursing homes run rampant, and supplementation should be strongly considered. Vitamin E supplementation has been shown to greatly benefit the immune system in people over the age of 65. If you have low levels of vitamin C, your risk is 11 times greater than people at the highest levels. Beta carotene is not far behind: Those with low levels are at seven times the risk.

➤ Vitamin E and heart disease: Support for vitamin E increases exponentially every month. In fact, of the 44 percent of the cardiologists who take an antioxidant, 90 percent also take vitamin E. Doses as low as 100 IU per day have been associated with a 40 percent reduction in heart disease. And even if you already have heart disease, don't leave out E. Taking just 400 to 800 IU per day might reduce your risk of a new heart attack by 77 percent. Vitamin E can also help protect the bad LDL cholesterol from becoming oxidized, thereby preventing more damage to your arteries.

➤ Cataracts and antioxidants: Simply taking an antioxidant supplement containing vitamins E, C, and beta carotene may protect you against cataracts. It may be possible to prevent or postpone the onset of cataracts by 50 to 70 percent simply by supplementing with antioxidants. A high intake of antioxidants—especially those of the carotenoid family—could reduce the risk of age-related macular degeneration, the leading cause of age-related blindness in the United States. Carotenoids lutein and zeaxanthin are particularly protective. Women who take vitamin C supplements for at least 10 years have been shown to reduce their risk of developing cataracts by 77 percent, compared to women who do not use these supplements.

➤ Antioxidants and cancer prevention: The area of antioxidant and cancer prevention is certainly gaining wider recognition and popularity. While nutritional supplements may not cure cancer, mounting evidence suggests that it can protect against cancer. Vitamin E might guard against prostate cancer and improve your outcome, should you be diagnosed with this common problem. Vitamin E has also been associated with the reduced risk of colon cancer in both men and women. Those who took 200 IU or more per day over 10 years have a 57 percent reduction in the risk compared to nonusers of vitamin E. Selenium, along with vitamin E, may reduce your risk of lung, colorectal, or prostate cancer. In one recent study, the risk to the group treated with selenium was so reduced that the blinded phase of the trial was stopped early so that all participants could begin taking it. While vitamin C might be considered somewhat controversial in its association with cancer prevention and treatment, it is widely accepted that vitamin C reduces the risk of stomach cancer.

These are just a few of the examples of well-documented research studies that support the prevention of disease with nutritional supplements. And what about cost? Taking supplements on a regular basis could greatly reduce our degenerative diseases, improve our quality of life, and lower our health care costs. Let's take a look at some of the recent evidence.

➤ According to the Pracon study commissioned by The Council for Responsible Nutrition, Americans could potentially save $8.7 billion on the treatment for five major diseases if we consumed optimal amounts of antioxidants, vitamin C, vitamin E, and beta carotene. This included heart disease, stroke, cancer, and cataracts.

Note from Your Doctor

A prenatal multivitamin/mineral supplement is an absolute must for pregnant women. In a 1998 *American Journal of Epidemiology* report, those women who took vitamins early in pregnancy greatly reduced their odds of delivering premature or low birth weight babies. By reducing these conditions, supplementation can also reduce the rate of later developmental problems and increase health over the entire lifetime.

➤   We could reduce the number of hip fractures by up to 20 percent per year if we supplemented with calcium and vitamin D. This would mean 40,000 to 50,000 fewer hip fractures and an annual savings of $1.5 billion to $2 billion per year. Not bad, is it?

➤   By taking antioxidant supplements, including vitamins E and C, we could save $3.5 billion per year by reducing the number of cataract surgeries.

➤   By taking just 100 IU per day of vitamin E, we could save up to $8.4 billion due to vitamin E's capability of reducing the incidence of heart disease. If we took 400 IU of vitamin E, we could avoid the half-million hospitalizations for nonfatal heart attacks each year, saving us $14 billion.

There's no question that nutritional supplementation may be one of the safest, most effective, and most cost-efficient ways of improving our health care delivery system, improving your quality of life, and keeping you well, vibrant, and at optimum performance.

Deficiency Versus Dependency

If you're not eating properly, if you're under stress, or if you're smoking too many cigarettes or drinking too much alcohol, your gas tank may be empty. You may be on your way to developing a vitamin or mineral deficiency. But before you get to that point, you might have what I call a marginal deficiency. This means that you might start exhibiting signs of low-grade symptoms before you have the obvious symptoms that go along with severe deficiency. For example, before your blood levels are so low that your doctor calls your B_{12} level deficient, you might experience poor memory, lack of concentration, poor balance, and numbness or tingling in the legs, and you might forget what you ate for dinner the previous day. This can happen even before your blood levels are found to be deficient.

Meanwhile, taking a supplement in this example may prove beneficial. Even though you don't yet have a vitamin deficiency, a more subtle or marginal deficiency should indicate that it's time to begin supplementation.

Do you have to be deficient to take a vitamin supplement? I've already mentioned numerous examples of how supplements can be preventive and therapeutic. As it turns out, many of you probably unknowingly have vitamin dependencies. This means that your body may actually use up a particular vitamin or mineral more rapidly than other people do. Basically, your body is dependent on this nutrient. A simple example of this would be someone who is taking diuretic medications to help lower his or her blood pressure. If you are doing so, your body requires more potassium and magnesium, which are washed out through the urine due to the medication. In addition, many children with learning disabilities have a dependency on vitamin B_1 (thiamine). Their brain and their body have a greater demand for this B vitamin than most other children without this condition. Vitamin dependencies, marginal deficiencies, and obvious deficiencies are all good reasons to supplement your diet with extra nutrient supplementation.

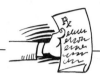

Note from Your Doctor

I've always been intrigued by the notion that most physicians are more than willing to prescribe anti-inflammatories such as Ibuprofen for headache or arthritis, or they might suggest a calcium channel blocker if you have a history of heart disease. Yet they may be reluctant or resistant to recommending or prescribing a vitamin supplement because they feel that you're not deficient. When was the last time your doctor checked you for a deficiency of Ibuprofen or a calcium channel blocker? Or what about the doctors who are quick to recommend and prescribe an antidepressant or antianxiety drug but refuse to recommend B-complex, Kava, St. John's wort, or some other natural remedy because "you're not deficient." I find this lack of logic disturbing.

Are All Supplements Created Equal?

Vitamin supplements come in various forms. At times, I think that's just to confuse us. They may come in tablets, capsules, or liquids. Some people find that one form is more agreeable than another. For example, if you have trouble swallowing pills, then a liquid form may be your first choice. For children, I frequently recommend either a chewable supplement or a liquid to be placed in either juice or water. Try to find supplements that are free of artificial colorings, dyes, or sugar—there's no need to add those extra ingredients in vitamin supplements. If you're allergic to certain foods, you should look for nutrients that are made without wheat, dairy, soy, corn, or yeast products. You can usually find these either in a health food store or through mail-order companies.

When choosing a multiple vitamin, I usually recommend finding one that contains all the B vitamins, along with at least 500 mg of vitamin C and 200 IU of vitamin E. Supplements usually also contain vitamins A and D, along with a variety of trace minerals. The whole area of mineral absorption is quite complex and falls beyond the scope of this book. However, if you have a heart condition, or if you have high levels of iron in the blood, be cautious and try to find a multivitamin that does not contain iron. It is generally easier for you to absorb and assimilate calcium in either the citrate or amino acid chelate form. As for magnesium, I generally recommend either magnesium, aspartate, gluconate, glycinate, or amino acid chelate.

What about the difference between natural and synthetic vitamins? This is a question that my patients frequently ask me. The naturally occurring form of vitamin E (D-alpha) is more absorbable and biologically active than the synthetic form (DL alpha tocopherol). As for vitamin C, there may not be a significant difference between natural and synthetic sources; however, as a rule I suggest that you purchase natural supplements whenever possible, since they generally exclude coal tars, artificial colorings, preservatives, sugars, and other additives.

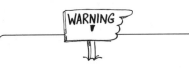

Totally Toxic

I generally do not highly recommend either time-release or sustain-release vitamins, especially for vitamin C. This form of vitamin C does not raise blood levels as rapidly as the non-time-release form. Furthermore, the vitamin might not be released and absorbed as efficiently as it's supposed to be. Each person has a different absorptive capability, so a quick-release, non-time-release supplement is usually best.

When taking supplements, I suggest you follow these guidelines:

➤ Take most of your supplements with food, unless told otherwise. The meal will generally help enhance absorption and assimilation and will reduce your chances of indigestion that can occur when supplements are taken on an empty stomach.

➤ Drink a large glass of water, as opposed to juice, coffee, or other beverage.

➤ Keep your vitamin supplements out of extreme heat. Store them either in a cool, dark cabinet or in the refrigerator.

➤ Keep an eye on the expiration date on the bottle to ensure that they maintain their potency.

Are Your Medicines Making You Mad?

Although prescription medications are absolutely necessary at times, you should be aware of certain factors and precautions when taking pharmaceuticals. First, medications are not benign. They have potential side effects; they may make you feel tired, dizzy, weak, or depressed. Some may even contribute to lack of sex drive (maybe that's why 40,000 prescriptions for Viagra are written each day), gastrointestinal symptoms such as loose bowels, constipation or abdominal cramping, and hives, itching, and headaches.

Unfortunately, overprescription of medications is a great problem and may cause harm. According to a 1998 issue of the *Journal of The American Medical Association*, more than two million Americans become seriously ill each year as a result of the toxic side effects of correctly prescribed medicines that are taken properly. I'm not talking about overdoses or even interactions between one medicine and another; these are people who are taking their medications as prescribed for medically indicated conditions. Of the more than two million people who suffer serious reactions, 106,000 die from those reactions.

It is astounding to note that this high number of drug side effects makes this at least the sixth—and perhaps even the fourth—leading cause of death in the United States. The study went on to say that one out of 15 hospital patients can expect to suffer from a serious reaction to a prescription or over-the-counter medication; about 5 percent will eventually die from it. If these numbers are accurate, then the number of people dying each year from drug side effects may be exceeded only by the number of people dying from heart disease, cancer, and stroke—and may be greater than the number dying from lung disease, pneumonia, or diabetes. I was shocked to see this report and I feel it is imperative that you become aware of these statistics. This lends even more credence to the view that preventive medicine and nutritional intervention should be tried first, before more invasive and potentially toxic pharmaceuticals are used.

A fundamental difference also exists in how pharmaceuticals work (assuming that they really do work) and how nutrients and other more natural therapies may benefit you. First, drugs should work only by inhibiting or by blocking a particular enzyme or metabolic step within your body. For example, calcium channel blockers and beta blockers both work by slowing or stopping normal bodily processes. Ibuprofen and other anti-inflammatories work by inhibiting prostaglandins and other inflammatory substances. But these medications don't just work at one particular site in the body—they have a much greater range, which contributes to their side effects. On the other hand, nutrients work by facilitating or assisting your body in carrying out natural metabolic processes. Natural therapies are generally much more gentle on the body and have a much lower risk of creating side effects.

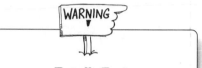

Totally Toxic

More bacteria are becoming resistant to antibiotics as a result of physicians inappropriately prescribing antibiotics. In a recent study published in the *Journal of the AMA*, antibiotics were prescribed for 44 percent of the pediatric patients with a simple cold, 46 percent of those with upper-respiratory tract infections, and 75 percent in those with bronchitis. Unfortunately, these conditions frequently do not benefit from antibiotics and are probably contributing to the rise in antibiotic-resistant bacteria.

Drugs can also interact with vitamin absorption from either supplements or food. For example, many antibiotics can inhibit the absorption of fat-soluble vitamins A, D, E, and K. Cholestyramine, a drug often prescribed to help lower cholesterol levels, can block the absorption of vitamins A, D, and K, as well as essential fatty acids. Birth control pills can increase your requirements for vitamin B_6 and folic acid. Furosemide, a commonly prescribed diuretic, can deplete your body of calcium, magnesium, potassium, and zinc, all key minerals for normal cardiac function. Aspirin can cause iron, potassium, and folic acid shortage. Tetracyclines deplete vitamin C, zinc, iron, and calcium from your body.

Ask your pharmacist for a written printout describing the possible side effects and drug nutrient interactions before taking any medications.

The following chart offers a brief overview of some of the vitamins and minerals that might be depleted from your medications.

Medication	Possible Vitamin or Mineral Deficiency
Acetaminophen	C
Antacids	A, B_1, folic acid, zinc
Antibiotics	B_2, B_3, folic acid, C, D, E, K, calcium, iron, magnesium, potassium, zinc
Anticonvulsants	B_6, B_{12}, folic acid, D, K, calcium, magnesium
Anti-inflammatories	B_6, B_{12}, folic acid, C, D, calcium, iron, phosphorous, potassium, zinc
Anti-psychotics	B_2, B_{12}, D
Birth control pills	B_6, folic acid, C
Digoxin	calcium, magnesium

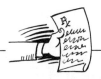

Note from Your Doctor

In 1997, the most prescribed drug in the United States was Premarin (which is used to replace estrogen in post-menopausal women), with a total of 45 million prescriptions. Synthroid, a thyroid replacement drug, was second with 36 million prescriptions. An antibiotic, Trimox, was third, followed by Lanoxin, a heart medicine; Hydrocodone with APAP, a pain killer; Prozac, an antidepressant; and Albuterol, a bronchodilator.

What About Antioxidants?

Antioxidants are a group of vitamins, minerals, or enzymes that help scavenge unwanted free radicals, which can be damaging to your cells. These free radicals are not like protesting college students or demonstrators that you might find on a college campus. Free radicals are generated when you are exposed to toxins and pollutants in the environment, such as auto exhaust, pesticides, or ozone. They can also be formed by eating too much fried or fatty foods, being exposed to excessive sunlight or radiation, or undergoing a particular ongoing health condition such as cancer, heart disease, or diabetes. Antioxidants, however, come to the rescue and deactivate or destroy these free radicals to prevent further damage.

A variety of different antioxidants occur in food and supplements. Many of these were discussed in Chapter 5, and we'll talk about them again in Chapter 7. Some of the most potent antioxidants include vitamin C, vitamin E, betacarotene, selenium, zinc, glutathione, Pycnogenol, grape seed extract, garlic, lipoic acid, and COQ_{10}; most of the phytochemicals also have potent antioxidant activity. Antioxidants have a profound effect in reducing the risk of heart disease, stroke, and cancer. They have also been associated with reducing your susceptibility to cataracts and age-related macular degeneration, as well as slowing the aging process. Before you know it, antioxidants will be a household name, and they should be a part of your daily food intake and a health-enhancing supplement program.

Assessing Your Nutrient Status

Having your doctor assess your nutrient status may be more difficult than breaking into Fort Knox. Unfortunately, most physicians aren't too familiar with the best ways to check your levels of vitamins, antioxidants, and trace minerals.

Several labs are now quite adept at doing nutritional analyses of nutrients with only one or two tubes of blood. Although this type of technology is relatively new and therefore still moderately expensive, it will offer great benefit in the prevention of disease. Most of my patients have deficiencies of at least one nutrient and frequently have marginally low levels of two or more. It is now also possible to evaluate the amount of free radicals your body forms, as well as antioxidant protection against these damaging molecules.

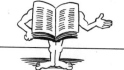

Body Language

Some of you may already be familiar with *hair element analysis*. This is an assessment tool used primarily to screen for toxic and heavy metals such as lead, cadmium, and mercury. Although this technique is controversial, some have found it useful in looking at one's calcium, magnesium, zinc, chromium, and selenium status. To fully interpret it, however, a practitioner must be skilled and educated on the intricacies of hair analysis.

The Least You Need To Know

➤ Nearly everyone has some form of nutrient deficiency or dependency.

➤ Taking nutritional supplements is one of the most effective, safest, and least expensive ways to improve our health and keep us energetic.

➤ Be aware of the differences among various kinds of supplements, and choose the ones best suited for your needs.

➤ Take charge of your health by learning more about the effects and side effects of your prescription medications.

Chapter 7

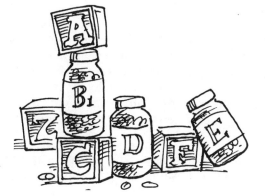

The ABCs of Vitamins

In This Chapter

➤ The impact of vitamin A and beta carotene

➤ The power of the B vitamins, 1–12 and more

➤ The versatility of vitamin C

➤ How vitamin D can strengthen your bones

➤ Vitamin E's antioxidant effect

Vitamins are everywhere these days. They're in supermarkets. They're in department stores. They're in drug stores. They're in health food stores, and they may even be in convenience stores. Which ones do you need? Which ones shouldn't you take? How do you choose how much to take and when, and do you really need them in the first place?

These are some of the questions that I'll address in this chapter as we discuss some of the most important aspects of the water-soluble and fat-soluble vitamins. The water-soluble vitamins include the B-complex family and good ol' vitamin C. Water-soluble vitamins are not stored in the body, and any excess is simply washed out. On the other hand, fat-soluble vitamins, such as vitamins A, E, and K, can be stored in the body and can build up if you take too much.

Both water-soluble and fat-soluble vitamins are important parts of metabolism, and they help the body function more efficiently. They work as enzymes and promote normal growth and development, create energy for your cells, and are an important part of preventing disease and enjoying good health.

Beginning with A and Beta Carotene

Just as the old adage says, an apple a day will keep the doctor away—and a carrot a day may keep infections and cancer away. One medium-sized carrot contains about 10,000 IU of vitamin A. This amount of vitamin A may protect against infections, cardiovascular disease, cancer, and even HIV infections. It also may keep your eyes healthy, reduce your risk of cataracts and macular degeneration, and keep your skin looking vital and healthy. A relative of vitamin A, beta carotene, is converted into vitamin A in your body. It, too, has unique antioxidant activities and protects against some of the same diseases.

Vitamin A is a powerful protector of the immune system and is quite effective against viral infections affecting the mucous membranes. For example, it can be used for sore throats, colds, flu, bronchitis, and sinusitis.

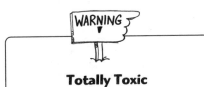

Totally Toxic

Because vitamin A is stored in the liver, it can be toxic in high doses. Early signs of toxicity include bone pain, headaches, nausea, fatigue, blurred vision, and vomiting. This, however, may not occur unless you're taking more than 100,000 IU per day for a few months. Fortunately, these side effects are completely reversible by stopping the vitamin A supplements.

In addition, vitamin A seems to help reduce the severity and frequency of respiratory infections. (I often recommend vitamin C, zinc, and echinacea to accompany vitamin A during times of sinus and respiratory infections.)

Vitamin A may also help nourish the skin. It is frequently used as one of the ingredients in a variety of cosmetic products, and it may help cases of acne. The therapeutic dose for vitamin A in regard to treating acne may be quite high, though, so beta carotene may be a viable alternative—as an added bonus, beta carotene may also help to protect against skin damage from excessive sun.

Vitamin A and beta carotene also help nourish the eyes. Maybe that's why Bugs Bunny ate so many of those healthy carrots. He wanted to make sure Elmer Fudd didn't catch him.

Vitamin A and beta carotene are both important in preventing cataracts and age-related macular degeneration, both leading causes of blindness in the elderly population. Interestingly enough, both vitamins can mop up those free radicals and prevent damage to the lens and retina of your eye.

A variety of good food sources for vitamin A exist besides carrots. Think about eating more fresh fish, such as mackerel, cod, halibut, salmon, and shark. Other good sources include cheese, eggs, and dairy products. On the other hand, beta carotene is found primarily in dark green and yellow-orange fruits and vegetables. Perhaps Popeye was on a good cancer-protection program. Carrots, sweet potatoes, peaches, kale, spinach, apricots, cantaloupe, squash, turnips and dandelion greens are all rich sources.

Note from Your Doctor

If you are a tobacco chewer, the appearance of small whitish growths on the mucous membranes inside your mouth may be a sign of leukoplakia, a premalignant cancer in the mouth. This is frequently a precancerous condition that can be prevented—and possibly even treated—with beta carotene.

As has been mentioned, both beta carotene and vitamin A have antioxidant effects and may play a role in protecting the body against some forms of cancer. Low levels of these nutrients have been associated with a greater risk of cancer, involving those that affect the esophagus, mouth, prostate, cervix, breast, bladder, colon, and stomach. Interestingly, vitamin A may work well in people receiving chemotherapy by making the treatment more selective against a tumor and protecting against possible toxic side effects of the therapy. A recent study suggested that vitamin A and beta carotene may also benefit people with melanoma, a serious form of skin cancer.

In the war against heart disease, beta carotene can also play an important role. It has been shown to alleviate chest pain and may increase levels of the protective HDL cholesterol. In a recent study, patients who took 50 mg (approximately 85,000 IU) of beta carotene per day realized a 50 percent reduction in heart attacks, strokes, and deaths due to heart disease when compared to those who did not take the supplement.

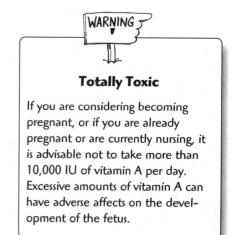

Totally Toxic

If you are considering becoming pregnant, or if you are already pregnant or are currently nursing, it is advisable not to take more than 10,000 IU of vitamin A per day. Excessive amounts of vitamin A can have adverse affects on the development of the fetus.

Beta carotene may also have an important impact on the outcome of AIDS patients. Up to 70 percent in AIDS patients may be either deficient or in the lower percentile of their beta carotene content. When supplemented with 180 mg per day, a significant improvement was noted in the cells of the immune system of HIV-infected patients.

A recent controversial study investigated the effect of beta carotene on lung cancer. A study in Finland found that beta carotene supplements may actually increase the risk of lung cancer in heavy smokers and asbestos workers. This study directly conflicted with numerous previously published findings—and came as a shock to the medical research community. Researchers had expected to see a decrease in those taking the supplements.

However, this 1995 CARET (Beta carotene and Retinol Efficiency Trial) has been criticized on several fronts. First, the amount of beta carotene may have been insufficient to show a favorable response. Second, supplementing occurred only with beta carotene and not with the full spectrum of the other carotenoids. This may be an example in which antioxidant nutrients are more effective when taken together rather than in isolation.

The majority of the evidence still points to beta carotene as a strong anticancer nutrient, and people with high beta carotene levels are generally afforded protection. Perhaps this study tells us only that cigarette smokers should not take beta carotene.

The Benefits of the B's

There are a large group of B vitamins, many better known for their numbers. For example, vitamin B_1 (thiamin), vitamin B_2 (riboflavin), vitamin B_3 (niacin and niacinamide), vitamin B_5 (pantothenic acid), vitamin B_6 (pyridoxine), and vitamin B_{12}, (cobalamin). Then we have more B vitamins that are not associated with numbers. These include folic acid, choline, inositol, and biotin. All the B vitamins work together as a well-balanced team. They seem to improve energy, reduce stress, help with relaxation, and maintain good brain functioning. In addition, each of the individual B vitamins also has its own capabilities and qualities. Let's take a look at some of these.

Vitamin B1 (Thiamin)

Let's talk about some of the benefits of B_1. B_1 can help improve your heart function and may be protective against *congestive heart failure* and *cardiomyopathy*. All doctors recognize that alcohol can deplete vitamin B_1 from your body, so this problem is particularly troublesome if you are a heavy alcohol user. Supplements of B_1 have also helped many kids with low learning capacities and behavioral problems, and it has been used successfully in psychiatric hospitals to treat certain kinds of depression, to elevate mood, and to improve memory.

I have also used thiamin in conjunction with the other B vitamins to help reduce the pain associated with shingles and migraine headaches. Thiamin helps burn carbs as well so that you can utilize them more efficiently for energy.

Junk food junkies are often low in thiamin because processed foods have most of their vitamin B_1 removed. Even when the label says "fortified," the product still may not contain as much thiamin as was originally present.

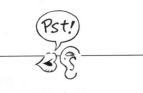

Healthy Hints

If you're breastfeeding, nursing, taking birth control pills, or eating too many sugary foods, refined carbohydrates or alcohol, you have a greater need for vitamin B_1.

Vitamin B₂ (Riboflavin)

Just like thiamin, riboflavin is also important for energy production, and it's particularly important in the maintenance and nourishment of the eyes, because a deficiency of vitamin B_2 can cause you to be sensitive to light. This nutrient may also protect against the formation of cataracts. If you're low in B_2, you may notice blurred vision or eye tearing, burning, or irritation. If you have cracking at the corners of your mouth, (a condition known as *cheilosis*), think about extra B_2.

I have also used B_2 to help with chronic migraines. When combined with vitamin B_6, it might provide relief from the pain of carpal tunnel syndrome.

Plentiful quantities of B_2 can be found in whole grains and cereals, assuming they are not refined. Other good foods to consider include dark green leafy vegetables, nuts, poultry, fish, eggs, lean meat, spinach, broccoli, asparagus, Brussels sprouts, and avocados.

Vitamin B₃ (Niacin and Niacinamide)

To further confuse the picture, there are actually two forms of vitamin B_3: niacin and niacinamide. Both have similar functions, yet some of the benefits are quite different.

Note from Your Doctor

If you're red in the face after taking niacin, you're not alone. Most niacin supplements can cause facial flushing, warmth, and itching, which can last for 30 to 60 minutes. It will, however, eventually wear off. To best avoid this, consider taking inositol hexaniacinate in which the niacin is bound to inositol. You can also take aspirin or a fish oil capsule 30 minutes prior to niacin to lessen or prevent the flushing reaction. Niacinamide, on the other hand, will not cause facial flushing, but probably won't improve your cholesterol metabolism, either.

Niacin should be considered when you're chowing down those French fries, ice cream sundaes, and fried chicken, or if you're a Sunday afternoon couch potato and smoking like a chimney. Why? Because niacin might be one of the best ways of controlling your blood cholesterol level. It's been shown to do the following:

➤ Lower your bad LDL cholesterol by up to 20 percent

➤ Raise that good old HDL cholesterol by up to 30 percent

➤ Reduce your triglyceride levels anywhere from 20 to 50

Quite powerful, isn't it? Niacin can be used either by itself or in conjunction with other cholesterol-lowering drugs. It has also been shown to help prevent the occurrence or recurrence of heart attacks. Niacin also seems to help people live longer following a heart attack.

For niacin to be effective in lowering your cholesterol and improving your other blood fats, it's important to discuss this first with your doctor. The dosages that are necessary are fairly high—generally in a range greater than 1,000 mg per day—and it's important that your build up your intake very slowly.

It may, in fact, actually help people with diabetes, especially the insulin-dependent diabetes mellitus. Niacinamide might protect the pancreas and help in the manufacture of insulin.

Insulin-dependent diabetes mellitus (also known as Type I diabetes), usually affects children and young adults under the age of 35. These people simply do not produce enough insulin from the pancreas and usually require insulin injections most of their lives.

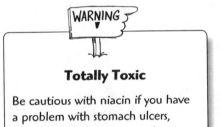

Totally Toxic

Be cautious with niacin if you have a problem with stomach ulcers, gout, or diabetes; it can make any of these conditions worse.

I have also been impressed with the ability of niacinamide to help with osteoarthritis. This type of arthritis frequently comes on as you get older and may be called "wear-and-tear arthritis." It generally takes about three months to notice the beneficial effects at dosages up to 2,000 to 3,000 mg per day. People with osteoarthritis frequently develop little nodules in the joints at the end of the fingers, known as Heberden's nodes; the bumps may favorably respond to niacinamide supplementation. In my experience, even though the nodules do not disappear, niacinamide seems to slow the progression of osteoarthritis and reduces the symptoms.

Foods containing vitamin B_3 include eggs, poultry, meat, nuts, whole grains, legumes, seeds, and seafood.

Vitamin B₆ (Pyridoxine)

Vitamin B_6 is perhaps one of the most important B vitamins. It plays a role in metabolizing amino acids; helps your liver to get rid of excessive toxins, medications, and alcohol; keeps your immune system strong; and lately has been proven to be a big factor in protecting against heart disease. And that's not all. B_6 can help with premenstrual tension. Others have found it to help against carpal tunnel syndrome, arthritis, and recurrent kidney stones. That's not too shabby for one B vitamin!

Even though the RDA for vitamin B_6 is only 2 mg per day, most of the scientific evidence points toward greater quantities to protect you from a variety of diseases. Even so, the average American is still frequently deficient in vitamin B_6, especially people in the following groups:

➤ Women using birth control pills

➤ Alcoholics

➤ Residents of nursing homes

➤ Pregnant and breastfeeding women

➤ Asthmatics using Theophylline medications

Vitamin B_6 is important in helping to form healthy red blood cells, and it can be a cause of anemia that is often not considered by many physicians. Furthermore, B_6 has been shown to help prevent hardening of the arteries and lower your risk of heart attack or stroke. It does this by lowering the level of a blood amino acid known as homocysteine, which, when elevated, can cause premature plaque and damage to your arteries.

Although it may be considered somewhat controversial, B_6 has also been helpful in treating some cases of psychiatric and emotional disorders, including depression and schizophrenia. How does it help? B_6 is necessary for the production of serotonin and other important neurotransmitters in the brain that are helpful in reducing depression. Many antidepressant drugs on the market also work by elevating your serotonin levels.

B_6 may also help your immune system by protecting it against those ugly germs, including viruses and bacteria. If you're over the age of 60, you may consider taking B_6 to help maintain good immune system functioning. People with AIDS are also frequently deficient in B_6.

If you get headaches, feel tired or weak, and have muscle cramps after leaving a Chinese restaurant, consider taking some extra B_6. This nutrient helps to metabolize monosodium glutamate (MSG) so that symptoms can be greatly reduced.

B_6 may also help guard against rheumatoid arthritis and carpal tunnel syndrome. In this condition, you may experience pain in the hand due to compression on the nerve that runs through the wrist. Vitamin B_6 can be helpful if you're prone to a type

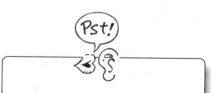

Healthy Hints

Vitamin B_6, folic acid, and B_{12} all play a vital role in cutting your risk of heart disease, stroke, and heart attack by reducing your homocysteine level.

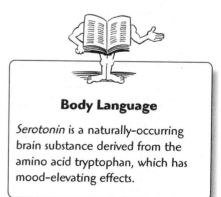

Body Language

Serotonin is a naturally-occurring brain substance derived from the amino acid tryptophan, which has mood-elevating effects.

of kidney stone known as calcium oxalate. This is the most frequent type of kidney stone and, when combined with magnesium, B_6 often cuts down on the number of stone attacks.

As you can see, vitamin B_6 is very important. The following list will help you find good sources of pyridoxine in your diet:

➤ Eggs

➤ Beans

➤ Soy products

➤ Avocado

➤ Bananas

➤ Poultry

➤ Fish

➤ Cantaloupe

➤ Cabbage

Note from Your Doctor

In addition to birth control pills, a lot of frequently prescribed medications may also deplete B_6 from your body. Most of the anti-inflammatories—including aspirin, prednisone, and colchicine—have this effect. Other medications include antiseizure drugs, such as Dilantin, the estrogen replacement Premarin, and the tuberculosis drug Isoniazid. And cigarette smoking? That, too, depletes vitamin B_6.

Vitamin B_{12} (Cobalamin)

Vitamin B_{12} is perhaps best known not for its ability to improve your energy (although it has been found to ward off fatigue), but for its ability to produce red blood cells and to prevent anemia. It also plays an important role in protecting against Alzheimer's disease, mental confusion, moodiness, and depression.

B_{12} can also be helpful if you are diabetic and troubled with peripheral neuropathy: It may help restore normal nerve transmission and get rid of those pins and needles or numbness that diabetics too often experience. I have also used B_{12} injections along with vitamin B_1 to help treat the pain associated with shingles. And as I mentioned in relation to B_6, B_{12} is an important part of lowering your homocysteine level, that amino acid that could accelerate plaque formation and heart disease.

B_{12} offers another impressive ability to help treat asthma, especially in children and younger adults. Multiple Sclerosis and Lou Gehrig's Disease (amyotrophic lateral sclerosis) are two other neurological conditions that may respond to B_{12} therapy. Many of these conditions respond better when B_{12} is given by injection rather than taken orally.

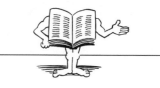

Body Language

Peripheral neuropathy is the term associated with the complications of long-standing diabetes; it's often caused by free radicals damaging the nerves. Not only might B_{12} be helpful, but combining it with B complex and folic acid should be considered.

Folic Acid

Folic acid has gained a lot of notoriety of late because it can help protect fetuses against birth defects and neural tube defects, including spina bifida, cleft palate, cleft lip, and anencephaly. These defects occur during the first trimester of pregnancy, when the spinal cord or brain never completely closes properly. Unfortunately, it took about 20 years for pediatricians and The Center for Disease Control to recognize how important folic acid was and to urge all pregnant women to take this invaluable B vitamin.

In fact, I would suggest that *all* women of childbearing age who are even considering becoming pregnant begin supplementing with folic acid, especially because the brain and spinal cord begin to develop and form during those first weeks after conception, and you may not realize that you're pregnant for four to eight weeks.

Among one of the newer developments, folic acid has been found to protect against heart disease by lowering your level of homocysteine. And if you're trying to prevent a stroke, peripheral vascular disease, or carotid artery disease, folic acid should probably be a part of your treatment plan. It's simple and inexpensive enough to take, and nontoxic. Most importantly, it wards off all three of these tragic medical conditions.

Troubled with an abnormal Pap smear? Has your doctor told you that you have cervical dysplasia? Well, folic acid to the rescue once again. Folic acid has been found to help stop or reverse cervical dysplasia, a precancerous condition probably due in part to insufficient folic acid in the cells of the cervix, which somehow makes them more susceptible to cancer.

Folic acid is primarily found in dark green, leafy vegetables such as spinach, kale, asparagus, and broccoli. It is also found in high quantities in liver, Brewer's yeast, and whole wheat products.

Note from Your Doctor

Experts estimate that just 1 mg per day of folic acid could probably cut the number of heart attacks by 50,000 per year, and that high homocysteine levels may be associated with up to 25 percent of the cases of heart disease. You should keep your homocysteine level below 10 micromoles per liter, and all women of childbearing age should consider taking at least 800 mcg of folic acid per day. This is the same dose I recommend for vascular disease prevention.

So What's Left?

A few other B vitamins are probably worth mentioning. Pantothenic acid, vitamin B_5, is also helpful against emotional and physical stress and helps support the all-important adrenal glands so that you can cope with stressful situations more easily. I have also found it to be an excellent antiallergy nutrient that helps many of my patients with rheumatoid arthritis, osteoarthritis, or plain old stiffness and muscle aches and pains. It comes in handy as well if you're a body builder or if you're doing heavy exercise or long-distance running; B_5 may help improve your performance, to some degree.

Biotin, one of the few B vitamins without a number, is good for infants who have cradle cap or inflammation of the skin. For adults, biotin can help keep skin and hair healthy and may also be used in cases of peripheral neuropathy in diabetics. Two other closely related B vitamins, choline and inositol, can help improve your brain function, may help with relaxation, and has been reported to help in some cases of Alzheimer's disease, though research on this is relatively sketchy.

By now, I hope you get the point. Meet the B family and make them your friends. They're all important parts of feeling good and staying in good health. If you're considering taking an individual B vitamin, consider talking to your doctor first. I usually recommend backing up any of the specific B vitamins with a general B-complex as well, to keep them in balance.

Note from Your Doctor

In my practice, I have been using inositol as an alternative means of treating anxiety, depression, and even obsessive-compulsive behaviors. The amounts you need to take, however, are generally much larger than what's in your typical tablet or capsule in the health food store. The minimum dosage to be effective seems to be at least 6,000 mg per day, while some may require as much as 12,000 mg before you see a good response.

C is for Citrus

Of all the nutrients that you're probably most familiar with and have heard so much about, C wins the prize. It's versatile, helps many parts of your body, is safe and inexpensive and causes no significant side effects. I think virtually everyone should consider taking this all-important nutrient.

Vitamin C or ascorbic acid is one of the mainstays in improving the immune system's response. It helps mobilize forces when you're under attack by unwanted germs and helps gobble up and kill foreign bacteria, viruses, and other harmful invaders. Just 300 mg per day was found to cut the death rate from heart disease and other causes by up to 40 percent, compared to people taking 50 mg per day. Vitamin C also has a mild antihistamine effect and should be a part of your antiallergy approach. If you're getting colds, sore throat, and flu, it may help reduce the duration of the cold and cut down on the severity as well.

A lot of debate has focused on the use of vitamin C for cancer. At this point, it's quite clear that vitamin C probably has a strong antioxidant affect and can guard you from a variety of cancer-causing substances. For example, if you're a cold-cut craver and eat roast beef, corned beef, or pastrami every day for lunch, you're increasing your risk for getting gastric cancer due to nitrosamine formation, which occurs when nitrates are converted to nitrites. Fortunately, vitamin C (along with vitamin E) can help prevent this biochemical reaction. Low levels of vitamin C have been associated with cancer of the lung, pancreas, colon, cervix, mouth, esophagus, and stomach.

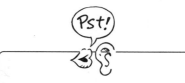

Healthy Hints

Even though the RDA of vitamin C is only 60 mg per day, its antiallergy affect is generally seen at dosages greater than 1,000 mg per day. This level is generally well-tolerated and nontoxic.

Vitamin C probably isn't a *cure* for cancer, but it seems to help cancer patients maintain better health and tolerate their chemotherapy or radiation more effectively. But first and foremost, you should be eating plenty of foods rich in vitamin C to protect you against cancer in the first place. What foods are best? Consider citrus fruits such as lemons, oranges, and grapefruits, as well as melons, berries, tomatoes, and green vegetables.

In the presence of vitamin E, vitamin C may help protect the bad LDL cholesterol from becoming oxidized. If LDL does become oxidized, it promotes more buildup of cholesterol inside your arteries.

Just taking vitamin C may keep you out of the cardiologist's office. A study indicated that taking 500 mg of vitamin C per day could help prevent the reblockage of arteries after undergoing an angioplasty. Because approximately one out of three patients must have this procedure repeated within one year, vitamin C should be a part of every cardiac patient's preventive maintenance plan. Just 1,000 mg per day of vitamin C may also be effective to lower your blood pressure. If your blood level is low, you may be prone to hypertension.

If you're stressed out to the max, you also might have a greater need for vitamin C. Vitamin C helps support one of your major stress organs, the adrenal glands. And if you're under constant attack by chemicals in the environment, C can help you metabolize those toxins a little quicker. C can also help your gums heal after a dental extraction and may protect you against periodontal disease. If you've been troubled with bleeding gums—especially after flossing or brushing your teeth—think C. If you're having surgery and trying to get your wound to heal a little quicker, once again, think C. I have also found it useful in protecting the lungs against air pollution and can cut down on a number of wheezing episodes and asthma attacks.

Note from Your Doctor

When taking vitamin C, it's probably best to divide it up throughout the day because vitamin C is water-soluble and is rapidly excreted from the body. At the onset of cold or flu symptoms, you may want to consider taking 500 to 1,000 mg every hour for the first several hours. It's probably best to taper off slowly once you have improved.

More evidence of late tells us that vitamin C (when combined with vitamin E) can prevent cataract formation or can slow the progression if the cataracts have already formed. Just 500 mg per day may be able to cut your risk of cataract formation by an astounding 77 percent. Because it's a strong antioxidant, vitamin C can gobble up those free radicals in the lens of the eye before damage occurs.

Don't Forget D

Avoiding the sun? Concerned about wrinkles and sun-damaged skin? I am too. But remember that a little bit of sunlight isn't so bad. In fact, it's necessary for you to form vitamin D so that your calcium can be absorbed more efficiently.

Unfortunately, as you age, your body doesn't form vitamin D as efficiently; in addition, your intestinal tract becomes less able to absorb vitamin D. Vitamin D and calcium work as a team and may help to reduce your risk of hip fractures—according to one study, by 40 percent.

It's also useful in osteoarthritis, the wear-and-tear type of arthritis that frequently affects your knees or fingers. And dermatologists are now becoming more interested in the ability of vitamin D to help control psoriasis, a chronic skin condition that causes skin flaking.

Are you deficient in vitamin D? Quite possibly. According to a recent report from Harvard Medical School, as much as 40 percent of the general population in the U.S. may be deficient in vitamin D. In fact, in patients being admitted to the hospital, the numbers were even larger. Fifty-seven percent of all patients were vitamin D deficient and 22 percent were severely deficient. And nearly one-half of these people took vitamins on a regular basis.

Unfortunately our food supply is generally low in vitamin D. You can find it in fish liver oil or in herring, tuna, salmon, sardines, mackerel, sea bass, and swordfish. Is milk a good source of vitamin D? Believe it or not, natural milk has almost no D in it at all. But before it comes to our supermarkets, milk is typically fortified with vitamin D—that is, the manufacturer adds it.

What about vitamin D and its impact on cancer? It appears that people who are deficient in vitamin D are at greater risk for cancer of the colon, breast, or prostate. Supplementing your diet with 200 to 400 IU of vitamin D may give you some protection.

Totally Toxic

Not only may the elderly be deficient in vitamin D, but vegetarians, people who drink excessive amounts of soda, dark-complected people, and hermits who stay indoors all the time are also at risk for vitamin D–related problems.

E Is for Everyone—Almost

There is probably not a nutrient on the market that has gotten as much recognition and publicity in the last several years as vitamin E. Most of the uproar about vitamin E has been related to its strong antioxidant effect—especially in relation to preventing heart disease and cancer, the two leading causes of death in the United States. It's been estimated that if everyone took adequate quantities of vitamin E, we could probably cut our health care costs by up to $8 billion per year. That's not bad for a substance that may cost less than 20 cents per day.

Vitamin E for your heart? You betcha. According to two recent reports from Harvard, just 100 IU per day of vitamin E over two years reduced the incidence of heart disease by 41 percent, compared to nonusers of vitamin E. When the researchers looked at nearly 40,000 male physicians, they saw that vitamin E was able to cut the risk of heart disease by 37 percent. If that's not good enough, a British researcher found that 400 to 800 IU of vitamin E could dramatically reduce the death rate from heart disease by 47 percent and the occurrence of a heart attack by 77 percent. E has been helpful in cases of angina pectoris and can cut the episodes of chest pain. It can keep your blood from becoming too thick and can assist the platelets from becoming sticky and clumping. This also reduces the risk of a blood clot.

Body Language

Angina pectoris is a common condition associated with lack of oxygen being carried by the blood to the vessels of the heart. This can cause chest pain, chest heaviness, or tightness in the chest.

Due to its strong antioxidant affect, vitamin E has a favorable impact on your cholesterol level. Along with vitamin C, it may help reduce your level of bad cholesterol and increase the good HDL. It can also protect the LDL cholesterol from becoming oxidized and can protect you against damaging plaque build-up.

Vitamin E may also offer cancer protection. Generally, the higher your blood level of vitamin E, the less risk you face of getting cancer. Vitamin E may be protective against the following forms of cancer:

➤ Lung

➤ Esophageal

➤ Colon

➤ Breast

➤ Cervical

Vitamin E has also been used in a variety of conditions with success. These can include the following:

➤ Menopausal symptoms: Vitamin E may help reduce those hot flashes and night sweats and helps serve as a natural estrogen-replacement therapy.

➤ Parkinson's disease: When vitamin C was combined with 3,200 IU of vitamin E, patients with Parkinson's disease saw a reduction in symptoms.

➤ Alzheimer's disease: Vitamin E may protect against deterioration of Alzheimer's disease in dosages of 2,000 IU per day.

➤ Immune strengthening: Vitamin E supplements can help improve your immune response, especially in the elderly population.

➤ Improved vision: When combined with vitamin C, vitamin E may reduce your risk of developing cataracts and macular degeneration, two of the leading causes of blindness.

➤ Fibrocystic breast disease: Many women have noted that vitamin E supplements can help soften the hard nodules of fibrocystic breast disease. (It's also important to reduce the intake of caffeine and chocolate.)

Totally Toxic

Eating cured meats such as bacon and fried foods? Smoking cigarettes and living in a polluted area? Consider protecting yourself against those damaging free radicals with vitamin E.

I usually start patients out with 400 IU of vitamin E and may increase to 1,600 units, if I feel it's necessary. Vitamin E is remarkably safe; if you're a cigarette smoker, or if you're engaging in heavy aerobic exercise and jogging near a polluted highway, your need for vitamin E may be on the higher side. It's difficult to get all the vitamin E you need through your diet alone, and that's why vitamin E supplements may be necessary. The best sources of vitamin E are vegetable oils (such as sunflower or safflower oil), wheat germ oil, and nuts.

Note from Your Doctor

A variety of forms of vitamin E are known as tocopherols. The natural form is known as D–Alpha Tocopherol, while the synthetic form is called DL Tocopheryl Acetate. You might want to look for the natural mixed tocopherols, which contain not only the alpha but also the beta, gamma, and delta forms of tocopherol.

And Tag-Along K

Vitamin K is useful if you've cut your finger or scraped your knee. It plays a role in the production of certain blood clotting factors in your body. But don't think that the only valuable effect of vitamin K is that it helps blood clotting. That's true, but it has some very important functions that you should know.

One of the most important and new discoveries is the relationship between vitamin K and osteoporosis. Recently, it has been discovered that low blood levels of vitamin K can accelerate bone loss and contribute to osteoporosis, but all is not lost. Boning up on vitamin K can strengthen your bones and reduce your risk of bone fractures.

If you're looking to stay with K, try spinach, cabbage, tomatoes, broccoli, or turnip greens.

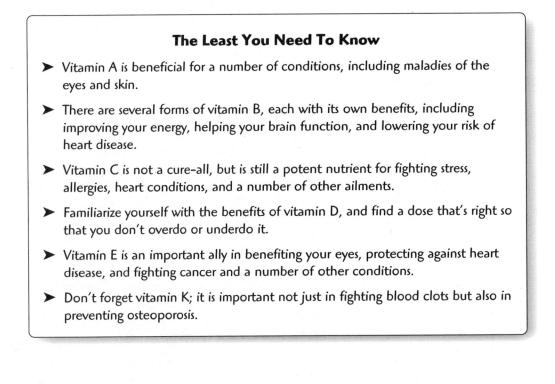

The Least You Need To Know

➤ Vitamin A is beneficial for a number of conditions, including maladies of the eyes and skin.

➤ There are several forms of vitamin B, each with its own benefits, including improving your energy, helping your brain function, and lowering your risk of heart disease.

➤ Vitamin C is not a cure-all, but is still a potent nutrient for fighting stress, allergies, heart conditions, and a number of other ailments.

➤ Familiarize yourself with the benefits of vitamin D, and find a dose that's right so that you don't overdo or underdo it.

➤ Vitamin E is an important ally in benefiting your eyes, protecting against heart disease, and fighting cancer and a number of other conditions.

➤ Don't forget vitamin K; it is important not just in fighting blood clots but also in preventing osteoporosis.

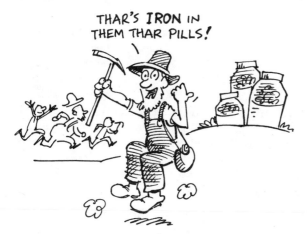

THAR'S IRON IN
THEM THAR PILLS!

Chapter 8

Minding Your Minerals

In This Chapter

➤ Do you need more minerals in your diet?

➤ Boron, the overlooked mineral

➤ Other key minerals and their benefits

➤ Learn how to "think zinc"

Numerous minerals in our food supply are necessary for good health. They help enable normal metabolism and work with vitamins and enzymes in your body to help prevent disease. Minerals, like vitamins, come from our food supply and are stored in the body in places such as the bone, muscle, and heart. If your diet is short in minerals, your body begins to age more quickly than normal. In some cases, taking minerals in supplement form can also be highly beneficial. Let's talk about some of the key minerals you need.

Assessing Your Mineral Status

Checking your cholesterol level is pretty simple, and checking your blood count is fairly easy, too. But checking the level of the different minerals in your body is not as easy. We are still learning the best ways to evaluate whether you have enough minerals in your body. A regular blood test might look at the serum levels of calcium, magnesium, or potassium, but it generally won't measure some of the other important minerals, such as zinc, selenium, boron, or chromium. Without these other minerals, you won't feel up to snuff.

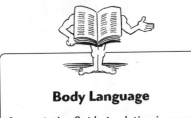

Body Language

Serum is the fluid circulating in your blood vessels outside your blood cells.

I'm a strong believer that mineral assessment is important, perhaps as important as measuring your red and white blood cell count, or your cholesterol level. But getting a doctor to check your levels can be a real chore. Some labs do a great job of testing all the different trace minerals with one tube of blood—and, better yet, some labs measure your minerals within the red blood cells themselves, not just in the *serum*. Because most minerals do their job inside the cells, it makes a whole lot more sense to measure them where they do their work, that is, in the red cells or white cells themselves. Just checking your mineral levels in the serum is often not enough to give you a complete picture.

As discussed in Chapter 2, your body might show signs of low minerals. For example, little white spots on your fingernails or problems with your sense of taste or smell can be a sign of a zinc shortage.

Does Your Diet Do You Right?

Hopefully by now you've thought about cutting your intake of those soft drinks, donuts, chocolate bars, and candy. Hopefully you've started to eat more fresh vegetables, fruit, lean meats, chicken, fish, whole grains, and a variety of beans. These foods are certainly a lot higher in all the trace minerals and will help protect you from mineral deficiencies. (Mineral deficiencies probably occur more frequently than you or possibly even your physician would think. I have noted at least one mineral deficiency in more than 15 percent of my patients, and about 20 percent of my patients have mineral levels that I consider suboptimal.)

Eating too much white bread or other forms of white flour, such as white rice or crackers, can also contribute to mineral shortages. Let me give you an example. When whole wheat is refined and processed and made into white flour, the following losses can occur:

➤ Chromium: 87 percent

➤ Manganese: 90 percent

➤ Copper: 66 percent

➤ Zinc: 82 percent

➤ Iron: 81 percent

➤ Magnesium: 83 percent

As you can see, not much is left in white bread—and not only are the minerals removed, but vital vitamins and fiber are also removed. If you ask me for change of $1.00 and I kept 83 cents and gave you back 17 cents, as in the example of magnesium, you probably wouldn't be too happy. So when choosing the type of bread that you eat or the pancakes that you make, choose whole grains so you're not short-changed.

Bone Up on Boron

Boron is probably one of the more important of the lesser-known minerals. Like calcium, boron helps keep your bones strong and can be useful in preventing osteoporosis. It helps you absorb your calcium more efficiently, and it can help a post-menopausal woman naturally raise her estrogen level. If you have been considering taking hormone-replacement therapy but are concerned about the possible risks and side effects, boron should be considered.

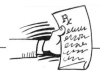

Note from Your Doctor

Who needs boron? Probably those with symptoms of arthritis, osteoporosis, and menopausal hot flashes. Boron may be helpful either in place of or in addition to hormone-replacement therapy.

Most of the time, I recommend 3 mg per day. At this level, boron can help you use vitamin D more efficiently, which also helps strengthen your bones. And 3 mg per day can help you retain calcium so you don't lose as much through your urine. It may also be helpful in reducing the symptoms of arthritis. To boost your boron intake, think about eating more raisins, dates, grapes, apples, peaches, cheese, and dark green veggies.

Calcium: More Than Just Milk

"Drink your milk to strengthen your bones." That's what I was told, and I'm sure you were, too. But building strong bone requires more than just calcium. It also involves getting enough magnesium, zinc, boron, copper, manganese, silica, folic acid, vitamin D, and perhaps other nutrients as well. Calcium is the most abundant of our trace elements. Most of your calcium, approximately 99 percent, is stored in your bone, teeth, and nails.

Calcium plays an important role in preventing bone loss and osteoporosis. Whether you realize it or not, bone is living tissue and is continually being broken down and reformed. As you get older—perhaps over the age of 30 or 40—you are constantly breaking down and forming new bone. The key is to form new bone more quickly than it's being broken down. Calcium can help slow the breakdown of bone and prevent osteoporosis. And calcium works along with other vitamins and minerals to strengthen your bones.

Those of you who don't like milk or dairy products can consider a lot of nondairy sources of calcium. The following list of foods are good nondairy sources of calcium:

➤ Dark-green leafy vegetables

➤ Nuts and seeds

➤ Salmon

➤ Sardines

➤ Tofu

➤ Soy products

➤ Broccoli

➤ Kale

➤ Turnips

➤ Collard greens

➤ Mustard greens

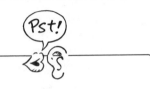

Healthy Hints

Unfortunately, close to 50 percent of the population ingests less than 500 mg of calcium per day, far below the recommended 1,200 mg per day. Make it a priority to get enough calcium through your diet or through supplements.

Besides strengthening your bones, calcium can help improve other parts of your body as well. It may help lower high blood pressure, usually in the 1,000 to 1,500 mg per day range. Calcium may be used in conjunction with your blood pressure medications and at times could be a factor in getting you off antihypertensive medicines. Interestingly enough, calcium supplements may also guard against cancers of the colon, pancreas, and uterus. In addition, calcium seems to help people relax and may be useful to induce sleep. Not only do post-menopausal women have a greater need for calcium, but also those who are pregnant or are nursing require at least 1,500 mg per day.

Chromium in Control

The use of chromium has been impressive in helping control blood sugar, especially in Type II, non–insulin-dependent diabetes. Chromium seems to help diabetics utilize their insulin more efficiently so that their blood sugars can be better controlled.

Type II diabetics who take upward of 1,000 micrograms per day of chromium picolinate will be able to stabilize their blood sugar level within two to three months. Chromium may also help you raise your good HDL cholesterol and reduce bad LDL and triglycerides. Some people find that this may decrease body fat; it certainly may speed your metabolism, especially if you're doing regular exercise.

If you're getting those sugar blues and feel down in the dumps, are weak or tired, or experience palpitations or shakiness if you haven't eaten for a few hours, you might be experiencing hypoglycemia. Chromium often helps level out your blood sugar and alleviates symptoms if you have hypoglycemia. Unfortunately, hypoglycemia frequently develops into diabetes later in life, which is even more reason to get a handle on it now so that you can prevent blood sugar problems later in life.

As I mentioned earlier, the milling and refining of grains removes 87 percent of the chromium that was originally present.

Unfortunately, chromium is not replaced when foods are enriched. Good sources of chromium include Brewer's yeast, whole grains, mushrooms, beans, meat, and peas.

Pumping Iron

Iron is a double-edged sword. Too much of it can lead to heart disease, joint pain, abnormal behavior, and a toxic liver. On the other hand, too little iron has been associated with a low blood count and anemia. This could translate into feeling tired and sluggish, looking pale, and running out of breath. Low iron is certainly a more common problem than excessive amounts.

If you have heavy menstrual periods, or if you're vegetarian and avoid all animal meats, you are at greater risk for developing iron deficiency. If you're pregnant or nursing, you may also have greater needs for iron. Perhaps the best test to see whether you need iron is a serum ferritin level, which helps measure how much iron is stored in your body. Before taking any iron supplements, you should discuss this first with your doctor. Iron supplements may be better absorbed when you take them in combination with vitamin C, but be aware that iron can also cause constipation or intestinal upset. Different forms of iron supplements are on the

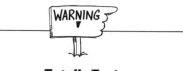

Totally Toxic

Most of our soil is low in chromium, which leads to chromium-depleted food and, in turn, has led to a chromium deficiency in 90 percent of our population. And chromium deficiency has been associated with sugar cravings, which deplete your stores of chromium even further.

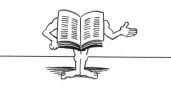

Body Language

Hypoglycemia means low blood sugar. You can feel tired, weak, or depressed when your sugar drops too low. Eating small, regular meals and avoiding sweets can be helpful.

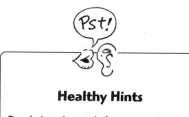

Healthy Hints

Don't be alarmed if your stools look dark or turn black after taking iron supplements. This is a frequent and natural phenomenon.

market. I prefer either ferrous fumerate or ferrous gluconate—generally speaking, they are easier to absorb and better tolerated than ferrous sulfate.

If you take too much iron, it can trigger a rusting-like reaction in your body. We call this free radical damage, because too much iron can oxidize and damage your tissues. Some research indicates that excessive iron can cause damage to the bad LDL cholesterol, which can initiate more damage to your arteries. Therefore, be cautious when considering taking iron, and discuss this with your doctor first.

Magnesium the Magnificent

Who would believe that the most important mineral for your heart is magnesium? I would. Magnesium has many beneficial effects on your body, most important its beneficial impact on vascular disease. Unfortunately, close to 80 percent of Americans don't get enough magnesium in their diet. No wonder we see so much heart disease.

Let's look at a few beneficial properties attributed to magnesium:

➤ Magnesium supplements can lower blood pressure.

➤ Magnesium has been shown to help with angina and chest pain.

➤ Magnesium can help reduce spasms of the heart vessels.

➤ Magnesium supplements can help in cases of congestive heart failure.

➤ Magnesium can keep your platelets from clumping together and triggering a blood clot.

➤ Magnesium supplements may increase your HDL cholesterol and lower LDL cholesterol.

➤ Magnesium can help regulate an irregular heart rhythm.

These are only a few of the benefits attributed to magnesium. It's also essential in people who have diabetes or problems with insulin resistance. If you are magnesium-deficient, which occurs all too often, not only are you prone to diabetes, but you will also be prone to the complications of diabetes. Taking nutritional supplements may help regulate your blood sugar more efficiently, and it may help reduce your requirements for diabetes medications.

If you have high blood pressure, you may want to have your doctor check for magnesium shortage. A large percentage of hypertensive people have low levels of magnesium in the red blood cells. Magnesium can also work as a natural calcium channel blocker and may substitute for some of the commonly prescribed antihypertensive medications.

Note from Your Doctor

Magnesium has been found to help in cases of migraine headaches, asthma, fibromyalgia, and chronic fatigue syndrome. In my own practice, I have found it useful in helping with premenstrual tension, insomnia, leg cramps, recurrent kidney stones, hypertension during pregnancy, muscle spasms, and osteoporosis. Now you can see why it's my favorite mineral!

You can get magnesium from a lot of different foods, such as bananas, peas, dried beans, green vegetables, seafood, nuts, wheat germ, rice, and oatmeal. Unfortunately, a large percentage of our population is at risk for magnesium deficiency. If you're taking diuretics, birth control pills, or antibiotics, you are particularly at risk.

Many different forms of magnesium supplements exist on the market. Make sure you don't take too much, as it can cause loose bowels or diarrhea. My preferred forms include magnesium citrate, gluconate, aspartate, or glycinate, which seem to be absorbed better than some of the other forms that you may have seen (such as magnesium oxide or carbonate). If you're confused about how much magnesium to take in relation to calcium, you're not alone.

Most of the time I suggest a calcium-to-magnesium ratio of 2:1. At times, however, equal amounts of calcium and magnesium may be beneficial. This is where a detailed history, physical exam, and laboratory studies help give us the answer.

Don't Sell Selenium Short

If you're looking to cut your risk of cancer, you might want to consider taking selenium supplements. Recently, a long-term study indicated that 200 mcg of selenium could reduce the occurrence of cancer by 40 percent—and better yet, decrease the risk of dying from cancer by 50 percent. This was a major breakthrough in cancer research. A significant reduction in cancer of the prostate, lung, and colon occurred in people who took selenium supplements for 10 years. If you are at high risk for cancer, you should certainly consider supplementing with this inexpensive trace mineral.

Selenium also works as a natural antioxidant, and it's an important part of another enzyme, called glutathione peroxidase, which helps protect us against free radicals and the ravages of aging. Note that selenium and vitamin E work together and have a synergistic and additive effect.

Totally Toxic

Be careful if you supplement with selenium; it can be toxic in high doses. I usually do not recommend taking more than 600 mcg per day, while the more ideal dose is probably 100 to 400 mcg on a regular basis.

Interestingly enough, in different populations around the world where soil selenium levels are low, cancer rates are generally much higher. To top it off, cancer patients generally have lower selenium levels in their bloodstream than healthy people. As you can see, selenium is one of the most important minerals to protect against cancer.

Selenium may also help in a few other conditions: It may help improve skin conditions such as seborrhea dermatitis and acne. If you are bothered by the odors of different chemicals, selenium may help you tolerate that smelly perfume or those new carpets. In addition, selenium may protect you against heart disease. And if you're on certain chemotherapy, such as Adriamycin, selenium may protect your heart against the toxic side effects, just as magnesium may also have some anti-inflammatory effects and help relieve some of your arthritic symptoms. This does not happen overnight, however, and you may have to take it for at least six months before you feel the benefits.

You can get selenium from broccoli, garlic, meat, mushrooms, seafood, chicken, wheat germ, and whole grains. As with chromium, however, our soil is frequently low in selenium and supplements may be useful, especially if you had cancer or have a family history of cancer.

Think Zinc

Zinc is perhaps my second favorite mineral, behind magnesium, because it is an important component of enhancing and boosting your immune system's response to infection. Zinc helps you produce antibodies and get rid of those little critters such as viruses and bacteria. You may find it useful if you get frequent colds or sore throats. Zinc throat lozenges are particularly effective in cutting down the number of days of the common cold in adults.

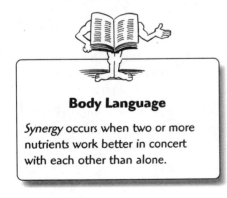

Body Language

Synergy occurs when two or more nutrients work better in concert with each other than alone.

If you've lost your sense of taste or sense, think zinc. If you've lost your desire for food, or if the food has lost its taste, think zinc. Zinc may also be useful in people who are suffering from eating disorders such as anorexia or bulimia.

For men who are troubled with prostate enlargement, zinc has been helpful in reducing the frequent urge to urinate. When you combine zinc with essential fatty acids and the helpful herbs saw palmetto and Pygeum africanum, you give your prostate a good chance to avoid medications or surgery.

Note from Your Doctor

Zinc is quite helpful if you'll be undergoing any kind of surgical procedure. It can help you recover more quickly and may help heal your incision sooner. I have also used it on the skin of people with leg ulcers or who have other kinds of wounds or infections. It may help in treating some skin disorders, such as acne, especially if you're deficient to begin with. I've also found it to be helpful in some cases of eczema and psoriasis.

You should be aware of a few other conditions that may also respond favorably to zinc supplementation. Because zinc works as an antioxidant, it can be useful to help treat and prevent macular degeneration. Zinc is found in fairly high concentrations in the iris and retina of the eye, so it may be useful in cataract prevention, the reduction of inflammation of the optic nerve, and treatment of night vision. Zinc also can protect you against problems associated with toxic metals, such as lead and cadmium, to which you may be exposed through drinking water, auto exhaust, or cigarette smoke.

As mentioned earlier, a sign of zinc deficiency can include small white spots in the fingernails. Children are particularly prone to this problem, and increasing their intake of eggs, soy products (such as tofu and tempeh), sunflower seeds, whole grains (such as rice, oats, and whole wheat), lean meats, poultry, seafood, cheese, almonds, and dried beans are all part of my Think Zinc program.

The Least You Need to Know

➤ Determining your mineral level is a critically important step toward good health, but it is often overlooked.

➤ Boron and calcium are important minerals for bone formation.

➤ Your iron intake should be watched carefully. Too much is not healthy, but the right doses bring a multitude of health benefits.

➤ Selenium is a strong antioxidant and protects against cancer.

➤ Magnesium is magnificent: Familiarize yourself with the advantages of having a good intake in your diet.

Chapter 9

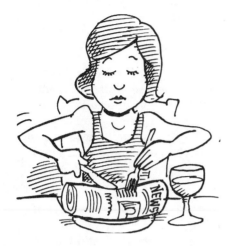

Nutrients in the News

In This Chapter

➤ Recent developments in nutrient information

➤ The benefits of CoQ$_{10}$ and glutathione

➤ Essential fatty acids and quercetin

➤ Alpha-lipoic acid and 5-HTP

This chapter discusses what you need to know about "Nutrients in the News." These nutrients have been reported to help with everything from arthritis to heart failure, to insomnia, to memory, to fatigue. They're actually not vitamins, minerals, or herbs, so I'm simply calling them Nutrients in the News. They are very powerful and can certainly boost your energy and immune system, and quite simply make you feel a whole lot better.

Alpha-Lipoic Acid

Alpha-lipoic acid: Sounds pretty serious doesn't it? Some simply call it lipoic acid. But don't be alarmed, it won't burn your skin, your eyes, or your stomach. Let me tell you what it will do.

Alpha-lipoic acid is a strong antioxidant that can help defend you against some of the complications of diabetes. It has been used for more than 30 years in Europe for Type I

Totally Toxic

Lipoic acid is very safe and has virtually no side effects. However, if you are diabetic and taking insulin or other sugar-lowering medication, lipoic acid can reduce your blood glucose level, thereby lowering your need for medications. This can be of great value to you, but talk to your doctor before taking this nutrient.

and Type II diabetes, and a dose of about 600 mg per day might help improve symptoms of diabetic neuropathy. Alpha-lipoic acid may reduce the leg pain seen in diabetics and improve your ability to utilize sugar.

Lipoic acid is also a wonderful protector for the liver, and I have used it in numerous cases of hepatitis and alcoholic liver disease. It works very efficiently with other antioxidants, such as glutathione, vitamin E, vitamin C, and CoQ_{10}. I feel it's an important nutrient for anyone who has heart disease because it may be a more potent antioxidant for your arteries than even vitamins C or E.

Alpha-lipoic acid should also be considered as part of the natural therapy for anyone who is HIV-positive. It may have the ability to inhibit HIV replication and can protect the liver if you are on any conventional AIDS medications.

CoQ Who?

To put it quite simply, CoQ_{10} is perhaps the most important nutrient to help protect your heart. It's actually a fat-soluble compound that functions as an antioxidant. CoQ_{10} is also known as ubiquinone and is nontoxic. Your body's production of CoQ_{10} peaks around age 20, and it's all downhill thereafter.

There are a host of benefits for cardiac function. Here are just a few.

➤ CoQ_{10} can help strengthen the heart muscle and treat *cardiomyopathy*, a life-threatening condition that often requires a heart transplant.

➤ CoQ_{10} can help strengthen the heart muscle in cases of congestive heart failure. It can improve the pumping action of the heart and reduce symptoms a lot more quickly.

➤ CoQ_{10} may help reduce your blood pressure and decrease your requirements for prescription medications.

➤ CoQ_{10} has been valuable in cases of irregular heart rhythms and mitral valve prolapse.

As if that's not enough, CoQ_{10} has been helpful in cancer treatment. It has shown promise in improving the outcome in patients with breast cancer and lung cancer. It may not cure their disease, but they are much healthier for a whole lot longer. I have also used CoQ_{10} to help lower high blood sugar in diabetic patients. Let's take a look at what dosages may be required for different diseases.

➤ Congestive heart failure: 60–200 mg per day

➤ Cardiomyopathies: 100–300 mg per day

➤ Angina pectoris: 60–300 mg per day

➤ Cancer: 100–400 mg per day

➤ Diabetes: 60–100 mg per day

➤ Hypertension: 60–100 mg per day

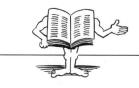

Body Language

Cardiomyopathy is a serious condition characterized by weakening of the muscles of the heart so that the heart no longer pumps blood as efficiently. It is often caused by either a virus or too much late-night drinking—alcohol, of course.

Although small amounts of CoQ_{10} exist in organ meat, such as heart and kidney, along with red meats and nuts, the amount of CoQ_{10} to be effective and therapeutic cannot be obtained solely from foods. That's why supplementation is important.

CoQ_{10} can also improve energy and reduce fatigue. It's been particularly helpful in marathon runners or those who want to improve their exercise performance. It stimulates the mitochondria of your cells so that you can derive oxygen more efficiently.

Essential Fatty Acids Are Essential

Essential fatty acids are just what they sound like: They're essential, they're fats, and they're acids. Essential fatty acids are actually the good fats that your body needs. There are two major categories, known as Omega-3 and Omega-6 oils. We have to get both of these from our diet because our body doesn't manufacture them. Unfortunately, many of you are probably not getting enough through food intake and may be showing signs of EFA deficiency.

Omega-6 Fatty Acids

Omega-6 fatty acids are found in polyunsaturated oils (such as corn, safflower, sunflower, and soy bean oil) and in the seeds of black currant, borage, and the evening primrose plant. I frequently have turned to primrose oil capsules or borage oil capsules to help treat patients complaining of PMS (premenstrual syndrome). These nutrients seem to relieve mood swings, irritability, and breast tenderness and swelling. They can also help improve the appearance of your nails, skin, and hair, especially if you're already troubled with dry, flaky skin and hair. Primrose oil may also help the liver metabolize alcohol and other toxins, and it has been useful in some cases of eczema and in children who have attention deficit disorder.

107

Omega 3 Fatty Acids

On the other hand, the Omega-3 oils are primarily found in cold water, fatty fish (such as salmon, tuna, cod, halibut, mackerel, and sea bass). These oils seem to help with lowering blood pressure and triglycerides and have been used successfully to treat rheumatoid arthritis, Crohn's disease, and ulcerative colitis.

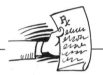

Note from Your Doctor

Fish oil concentrates usually contain a mixture of eicosapentaenoic acid (EPA) and ocosahexaenoic acid (DHA). DHA is valuable in nourishing the retina and brain and has been very helpful in improving learning capacity in children. It naturally occurs in breast milk, so breast-fed babies may develop better visual acuity at an earlier age than formula-fed infants.

Healthy Hints

NAC has been used in the treatment of HIV and has been shown to increase the low T helper cell count so often seen in this condition. When vitamin C and NAC are combined, a more powerful effect occurs to interfere with replication of the virus. NAC is also associated with slowing the aging process, and can protect the eye, heart, and nervous system from progressive deterioration.

Glutathione Goes After Free Radicals

By now, you're probably pretty familiar with vitamin C, vitamin E, CoQ$_{10}$, and other antioxidants. But one that you may not be familiar enough with is glutathione. This very strong antioxidant can mop up those damaging free radicals and protect you from cancer, heart disease, and the ravages of aging. Glutathione is actually made up of three amino acids: cysteine, glutamic acid, and glycine.

Glutathione can help protect you against toxins in the environment and help the liver get rid of medication residues. It helps your immune system by activating your white blood cells to help fight infections.

Even though some foods contain small quantities of glutathione (including fresh fruits, vegetables, and meats), it is not particularly absorbable. In addition, supplements of glutathione are also hard to assimilate. Therefore, I usually suggest either reduced glutathione or its close relative, N-acetyl cysteine (NAC). NAC is much easier to absorb and is an effective way to boost your glutathione level.

The Arthritic Answer: Glucosamine Sulfate

Of all the substances I've used to treat arthritis over the years, glucosamine sulfate is probably the most effective. This substance helps nourish your cartilage and may even help repair it. This is particularly useful if you're troubled with osteoarthritis, which often comes with advancing age.

Glucosamine sulfate is particularly safe and has almost no side effects. I haven't found it to be 100 percent effective, but it sure helps in most cases. I usually suggest 500 mg three times per day, though it might take two to three months before you notice the benefits.

You might notice several different forms of glucosamine in the health food store. Glucosamine sulfate seems to be the most effective form, although some people have benefited from glucosamine hydrochloride or N-Acetyl Glucosamine.

Relaxing with 5-HTP

It's baaack! Well, sort of. As you may recall, several years ago, the amino acid tryptophan was recalled by the FDA after a contaminated batch was manufactured in Japan and eventually ended up on the shelves in our health food stores. Unfortunately, several people died and numerous others were injured.

Tryptophan has been used as a natural sedative and tranquilizer. It was very helpful for inducing sleep and reducing depression and anxiety. Quite logically, the FDA recalled tryptophan; but quite illogically, tryptophan has never made it back to our shelves. But guess who's coming to dinner? His cousin, 5-HTP (that's 5 hydroxytryptophan). 5-HTP is now available. I have been using 5-HTP as a substitute for some of the overly prescribed antidepressants on the market.

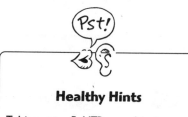

Healthy Hints

Taking extra 5-HTP can elevate your level of serotonin, a naturally occurring mood enhancer. Taking 100 to 200 mg before bedtime can do the trick.

Medicinal Mushrooms

Mushrooms can add great flavor to your foods; some, such as portobella mushrooms, can give you that meaty texture and flavor that you desire. In some Asian countries, mushrooms are quickly becoming an important part of their fight against cancer.

I've been particularly impressed with the extracts of three different forms of mushrooms that have medicinal properties: shiitake, reishi, and maitake. All have shown some promise in treating cancer, bolstering the immune system, providing relief for allergies, and improving the outcome and stamina in people with cancer.

One of the specific mushroom extracts that I have become particularly fond of in helping to improve the health of my cancer patients is polysaccharide K (PSK). This substance has been shown to increase the survival rate in people with lung cancer, colon cancer, and stomach cancer. PSK contains a naturally occurring extract of a fungus called coroiulus versicolor, which somehow may interrupt tumor growth.

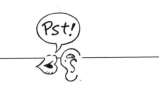

Healthy Hints

It's virtually impossible to obtain 10 mg of NADH from your diet alone—you'd probably have to eat four or five pounds of steak on a daily basis. And then you'd end up in my Totally Toxic sidebar!

NADH

Tired of feeling those afternoon blues? Trying to find ways to boost your energy? Nicotinamide adenine dinucleotide (NADH) may be the answer.

NADH fuels the Krebs cycle, one of the major biochemical cycles in our body where you burn fat and sugar to be converted to energy. If you're healthy, your body probably makes enough NADH on its own. However, with disease or advancing age, NADH begins to decline on its own. Recently, people with chronic fatigue have benefited greatly after taking NADH supplements. I usually recommend about 10 mg per day; for diseases of aging, such as Parkinson's disease or Alzheimer's disease, taking 10 mg before breakfast for three months may elicit striking improvements.

Quercetin: The Allergic Response

If you're tired of that runny nose, constant sneezing, or itchy and watery eyes, you might consider taking the star of the flavonoids: quercetin. Quercetin might be used as a substitute and an alternative for some of the common decongestants or antiallergy medicines you might be taking.

In plants, there are actually more than 500 different flavonoids, which enhance all antioxidant functions. Quercetin is one that's been well-studied and found to have numerous benefits as an anti-inflammatory, antiheart-disease, and perhaps even an anticancer nutrient. A recent report found that people who ate foods rich in quercetin—such as apples, onions, tomatoes, green peppers, broccoli, and tea—were less prone to heart disease. It's believed that quercetin can protect your bad LDL cholesterol from damage by free radicals, thereby protecting your cholesterol from oxidation.

Consuming onions in your diet may reduce your risk of stomach cancer by up to 74 percent.

Note from Your Doctor

For quercetin to help protect you against allergies and heart disease, you'd probably have to take it in supplement form. The amount in food is inadequate to do the trick. I usually recommended 500 mg two or three times per day, frequently combined with vitamin C, vitamin E, and other antioxidants.

Pycnogenol and Grape Seed Extract

Pycnogenol contains substances known as proanthocyanidins and other flavonoids from the bark of the French Maritime pine tree. Its bioflavonoid concentration is 85 percent, while grape seed extract may be a little more highly concentrated, at 92 to 95 percent. Not only is grape seed perhaps more concentrated, but it also is generally less expensive.

Pycnogenol and grape seed extract also help some allergic patients. Both function as antioxidants and anti-inflammatories, especially because they're high in proanthocyanidins (PCOs). The PCOs help neutralize free radicals and should be a part of a strong antioxidant program.

PCOs seem to help strengthen the capillaries and improve circulation. They have been particularly useful in helping with varicose veins, improving blood flow to the brain, healing bleeding gums, protecting against bruises, and reducing heavy menstrual bleeding.

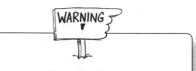

Totally Toxic

Several years ago a report suggested that quercetin may be cancer-provoking. This report has subsequently been deemed unfounded and, overall, quercetin is believed to have a strong protective effect against cancer, heart disease, and allergies.

P.S. Don't Forget the PhosphatidylSerine

Can't remember anything? You're already reaching the A and L in Alzheimer's disease and trying to prevent making it to Z? PhosphatidylSerine (P.S.) may be the most effective brain nutrient to improve nerve transmission and your memory. In fact, it may actually improve mental capacity and performance in people with Alzheimer's disease and Parkinson's disease.

This brain enhancer is an important component of nerve tissue, composed of about 60 percent fat. As you get older, you may have more needs for this all-important nutrient. I usually suggest 300 to 500 mg per day—and make sure you take it for at least six months. Don't stop too early; I find that some of my patients become discouraged after two or three weeks and discontinue it prematurely.

What's on the Horizon?

As if all these nutrients aren't enough, probably another dozen are also making their way onto the scene. That's not to say that they're not important, but the jury is still out on most of these. I'll mention some of the more important nutrients and the possible roles they play:

➤ Creatine has been reported to enhance athletic performance and increase lean muscle mass.

➤ Pyruvate may increase energy and be helpful for chronic fatigue syndrome.

➤ Dimethylglycine (DMG) is thought to be an energy enhancer. Others feel it enhances the immune system and may help improve the attention span in autistic kids.

➤ Octacosanol may help increase endurance during heavy exercise and benefit certain degenerative neurological diseases, such as Parkinson's disease, Lou Gehrig's disease (ALS), and multiple sclerosis (MS).

➤ Gamma-oryzanol is extracted from rice bran oil and has been reported to promote healing of a gastric ulcer, to improve cholesterol metabolism, and to reduce hot flashes and night sweats associated with menopause.

➤ Cetyl myristoleate (CMO) has been reported to improve symptoms in people with both osteoarthritis and rheumatoid arthritis.

➤ MethylSulfonyl methane (MSM) has been found to be an antiallergy and antiarthritis substance. Some say they also feel more energetic upon taking it.

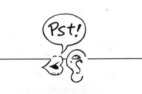

Healthy Hints

When working to improve your brain function and memory, consider not only P.S., but also other nutrients such as B_{12}, C, E, ginkgo, and antioxidants. But if you have a problem with memory, you must remember to take the supplements in the first place.

Even though data supports these nutrients on the horizon, research is still limited. As we begin to learn more about these products, they may offer us more promise. In the meantime, keep your eyes and ears open, maintain an open mind, and let's see where we end up.

> ### The Least You Need to Know
>
> ➤ We learn more everyday about the benefits of "new" nutrients.
>
> ➤ Getting essential fatty acids in our food or dietary supplements is important because our bodies cannot produce them on their own.
>
> ➤ Glutathione is an important antioxidant.
>
> ➤ NADH can help boost your energy level.
>
> ➤ By staying informed, you can keep an eye on new developments that might help you improve your nutrition.

Chapter 10

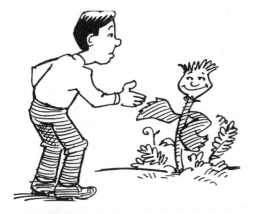

An Introduction to Botanicals

In This Chapter

➤ The healing power of herbs

➤ The benefits of bilberry, echinacea, and ginseng

➤ Ginkgo biloba and peppermint oil

➤ Kava and hawthorn

The hot news about healing herbs is spreading like weeds. I guess that makes sense, since many medicinal herbs are like weeds anyhow. More of you have probably been hearing about the healing power of herbs, and in this chapter we'll touch on some of the most important ones.

Herbs are becoming more popular with every passing day. If you lived in Germany, there is a 40 percent chance that your doctor would recommend herbs before turning to prescription medications. Better yet, many of these herbs are covered by The National Health Care Insurance Program.

The Healing Power of Herbs

Why do people look at you so strangely if you tell them you're treating your cold with echinacea? Or that you're using St. John's wort for depression or maybe even helping your memory with ginkgo? Even though you may be more familiar with treating these conditions with a variety of medications, the reality is that 80 percent of the world's population depends on herbs to treat many of these and other common ailments.

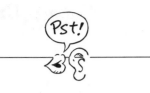

Healthy Hints

Although herbs can be very effective in helping to treat a variety of health conditions, they work best when used in combination with a comprehensive treatment plan, including proper nutrition, diet, and healthful lifestyle practices.

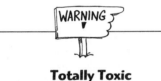

Totally Toxic

Before self-diagnosing a medical problem and taking herbs on your own, find a skilled health care practitioner who is experienced at prescribing herbs. Do not discontinue any of your medications without first discussing it with your doctor.

➤ Nearly one-third of our prescription medications are actually derived from plants. These include digitalis, pain killers such as codeine and morphine, colchicine, antispasmodics, and some forms of chemotherapy.

➤ The sales of herbs in Germany are in excess of $5 billion per year. (I suspect that as we become more educated, America will not be too far behind.)

➤ The annual sales of ginkgo biloba in Germany and France exceed $600 million. Ginkgo is one of the most commonly prescribed drugs in these countries for the treatment of vascular disease.

➤ The sales of saw palmetto berry to help treat an enlarged prostate gland exceed $3 million per year in France.

As comedian Yakov Smirnoff used to say, "Only in America—what a country." What are we doing wrong? And what are they doing right? Let's talk amongst ourselves.

Hardly a day goes by when you don't hear something about the latest benefits of garlic or ginger or perhaps ginseng. You walk down your supermarket aisle or near the check-out counter, and you see it splashed all over the tabloids. Can you believe everything you read? Of course not, but the evidence in favor of the healing power for a variety of botanicals and medicinal herbs continues to mount.

Herbs have been reported to help a variety of everyday health conditions that affect many of us, including:

➤ Improving eye sight

➤ Preventing infections

➤ Mitigating migraine headaches

➤ Boosting memory

➤ Improving energy

➤ Helping the heart

➤ Relieving stress and anxiety

➤ Detoxifying the liver

➤ Helping the bowels

➤ Shrinking the prostate

➤ Alleviating sneezing attacks and allergies

➤ Minimizing depression

➤ Reducing menopausal hot flashes

They can't do it all, but they sure seem like they could do a lot.

Selecting and Shopping for Herbs

It's confusing. You walk into your local health food store, pharmacy, or even some department stores and see herbs everywhere. They come in tablets, capsules, teas, tinctures, and maybe even stuff that looks like twigs and dirt from your neighbor's yard.

To confuse the picture even more, they come in different potencies and strengths.

When purchasing herbs, make sure the label states *standardized extract*. You can rely more on the potency of an herb found in its standardized form. You can feel more comfortable that the active constituents within the herb are really there. For example, when purchasing St. John's wort, keep you eyes open for the label to indicate that it is standardized to .3 percent Hypericin, the active compound with the antidepressant properties. (The term *standardized extract* means that your herb contains a standardized level of the active ingredients.)

Although many liquid extracts and tinctures are dissolved in alcohol, some new products on the market are prepared alcohol-free. Instead, water is used as a substitute. These generally taste a whole lot better and may appeal more to your taste buds. I frequently also recommend freeze-dried extracts in powdered forms, which can be purchased in capsules and taken at meal time.

We're still struggling to make sure that the herb contained in the bottle is the same as what is stated on the label. Quality control is still not standardized in this country, but most of the more reputable herbal manufacturers and suppliers are doing a fairly good job of policing themselves. Many will provide you with documentation to the authenticity of their products, should you inquire.

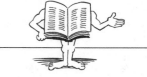

Body Language

Tinctures are made when an herb is soaked in a solvent (typically alcohol) for several hours—or even days. The remaining solution is then pressed out, yielding a tincture. *Extracts* are usually made by distilling the alcohol from the tincture, thereby making an extract more concentrated.

Bilberry: The Eyes Have It

Remember I told you earlier to make sure you include a variety of berries, such as blueberries, raspberries, or cranberries, in your diet? These fruits might be able to improve your eyesight and protect you against visual problems because they all contain bilberry. The deep purple pigment in bilberry contains a flavonoid compound known as anthocyanosides. These are strong antioxidants that can help protect your eyes from free radical damage. Bilberry extracts may help treat many eye disorders, including these:

➤ Cataracts and macular degeneration

➤ Diabetic retinopathy

➤ Night-time visual disturbances

➤ Poor visual acuity

In one remarkable study on 50 patients, bilberry (combined with vitamin E) stopped the progression of cataract formation in 97 percent of the people in the study. Bilberry may also help you with nearsightedness and may improve your overall vision.

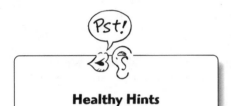

Healthy Hints

When eyeing the bilberry label, look for a standard extract of 25 percent anthocyanosides. The effective dose for most eye disorders is 250 to 500 mg per day.

In my opinion, anyone trying to prevent the progression of cataracts should consider bilberry. With more than 4 million Americans developing cataracts, cataract surgery has become the No. 1 surgical procedure in people over the age of 65—that's 600,000 surgeries per year! We could probably save a big chunk of the $4 billion dollars spent each year on cataract surgery.

Eye disorders are not the only conditions helped with bilberry extract. This nutrient has also been useful in helping lower elevated blood sugar levels in diabetics and can reduce high levels of cholesterol and triglycerides. It may even strengthen the small fragile capillaries in your legs and help get rid of those ugly varicose veins.

Echinacea: Nature's Antibiotic

Are you amoxicillined and penicillined out? Or perhaps Ciproed and Biaxined to the max? Are you sick and tired of taking antibiotics around the clock? If so, you might want to consider turning to echinacea.

The herb is perhaps best known as an infection fighter. It can help prevent viral and bacterial invaders and treat recurrent colds, ear infections, respiratory infections, flu-like symptoms, and chronic vaginal yeast infections. Better yet, it doesn't have the side effects or cost of some of those prescription antibiotics. Quite simply, echinacea stimulates the immune system and activates your defenses to spark your white blood cells to gobble up and conquer those foreign invaders.

Not only can echinacea help you fight a cold, but it is also effective at decreasing the frequency of cold symptoms. If you start taking two or three capsules two or three times per day for 10 to 14 days, chances are that you'll get rid of that little bugger a lot quicker. If you're hoping to boost your overall immunity and cut down on recurrent infections, you can take echinacea for six to eight consecutive weeks, followed by a one- to two-week rest period. If you're still symptomatic, you can repeat this cycle.

Feverfew: Migraine Medicine

Feverfew has a very impressive ability to help treat and prevent migraine headaches. If you're looking for an alternative to aspirin, Feverfew may be the answer; you may also reduce the frequency and severity of migraines. I usually recommend 100 to 200 mg per day, which should have a guaranteed concentration of at least .2 percent parthenolides, Feverfew's active compound. Be patient with it, since it might take four to six months to really notice the benefits.

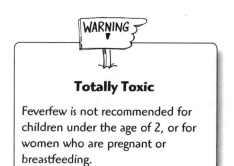

Totally Toxic

Feverfew is not recommended for children under the age of 2, or for women who are pregnant or breastfeeding.

Ginkgo Biloba: Memory Booster

What is the oldest leaf-bearing tree in North America, lives as long as 1,000 years, and grows as tall as 122 feet? The answer is...ginkgo biloba. This very popular herb accounts for more than 1 percent of all of the pharmaceutical purchases in Europe. And why not? Here's what it can do:

➤ Improve memory loss that frequently comes on as you age

➤ Improve circulation to your extremities and to the carotid arteries leading to your brain

➤ Reduce ringing in your ear (known as tinnitus)

➤ Delay the progression and help with symptoms of Alzheimer's disease

➤ Protect your brain tissue from free radical damage after suffering from a stroke (and therefore help you recover more quickly)

➤ May help with male impotency by improving blood flow to the erectile tissue

➤ Can have an anti-inflammatory effect and be useful in the treatment of allergies and asthma

Some other benefits are less well researched, but ginkgo might also help against premenstrual tension, depression, and dizziness because it's such a powerful antioxidant and an enhancer for blood circulation. I have been using dosages anywhere from

120 mg to 360 mg per day, usually in capsule form. Make sure you purchase a standardized extract containing 24 percent concentration of flavone glycosides.

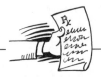

Note from Your Doctor

Of all the research performed on herbal therapies, ginkgo biloba is perhaps the most well documented in scientific literature. There are at least 280 clinical reports and eight separate textbooks published on ginkgo alone illustrating its therapeutic effects. This research suggests that ginkgo biloba is highly safe and nontoxic, and it seems to be devoid of any serious side effects. As far as we know, it does not interact adversely with any prescription medications, except possibly Coumadin.

Ginseng: For the Weary and Stressed

Ginseng is a wonderful antistress and antifatigue herb. It has been widely used in Asian countries for many centuries, possibly dating back more than 4,000 years. The two most common forms include panax ginseng, also known as Korean or Chinese ginseng, and Siberian ginseng. Both have similar properties.

Ginseng is effective at strengthening your immune system and perhaps stabilizing your blood sugar. It seems to help with mental and physical stress and also helps with endurance. People who take ginseng feel that they recover from colds and flu-like symptoms a little more quickly.

Overall, ginseng is remarkably safe and well-tolerated, and rarely does it cause any side effects. Some have found, however, that in very high doses it contributes to insomnia, irritability, or anxiety. And some women find that high doses of ginseng causes some mild breast tenderness. If this happens to you, simply reduce the dosage or stop the treatment altogether, and the symptoms will usually subside fairly quickly.

Hawthorn: Helping Healthy Hearts

Hawthorn is perhaps the most important herb for a healthy heart. It has so many great benefits that it should be a part of almost any household, especially when you consider that coronary artery disease and related problems (such as hypertension, heart failure and angina pectoris) are the number-one cause of death in America.

Hawthorn exhibits great results for a variety of ailments involving the cardiovascular system. These include the following:

➤ Increases blood flow to the coronary arteries of the heart

➤ Helps lower blood pressure in hypertensive patients

➤ Improves the pumping capability of the heart, which can be helpful if you have congestive heart failure and are looking for additional therapies to Digoxin

➤ Improves circulation to the legs, especially if you've been told that you have a condition known as peripheral vascular disease

➤ Helps treat angina pectoris and chest pain

Due to its high content of flavonoids, hawthorn is a potent antioxidant. It can be used with virtually no side effects or long-term risks. It may take one to two months to see the full benefits, however. My usual doses are from 160 to 480 mg per day.

Hawthorn appears to be safe if you are pregnant or nursing. If you're already taking digitalis, however, you should discuss hawthorn with your physician since it may have an additive affect with the medicine.

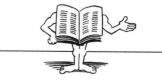

Body Language

Peripheral vascular disease is generally caused by a lack of oxygen due to insufficient circulation of blood to the legs and feet. If you have this condition, you may feel pain or cramping in the legs when walking or exercising; stopping your activity can reduce the discomfort.

Kava: Controlling Anxiety and Stress

Looking for that answer to your daily stress? After seeing patients all day and then writing this book all evening, I've been reaching for the bottle of Kava. This nutrient does a great job in helping with anxiety and stress. It seems to lift your spirits and improve your ability to think clearly—and it simply puts you in a good mood. Some have called it the natural tranquilizer or the natural alternative to Xanax.

Kava can also be helpful against depression and insomnia, and may even help with muscle relaxation. Make sure you find a standardized concentration of the active ingredients, known as kavalactones. You may want to think about taking about 100 to 200 mg of kavalactones per day as a natural anxiety reliever. If you're having trouble sleeping, take it about one hour before bedtime. Even if you take kava during the day, it shouldn't make you fall asleep. In fact, it may make you feel calmer and happier. Try to find an extract of kava standardized at 70 percent kavalactones.

Do not take kava for more than three months without seeking medical advice. If it's not helping with stress or anxiety by that time, other options or other underlying problems should be considered. Also, avoid it if you're pregnant or nursing.

Note from Your Doctor

Kava has been used in the Pacific islands as a key component in a beverage used in religious and social rituals. The beverage is prepared by grating the stem of a kava plant, mixing it with water, and then straining it. The beverage creates a relaxed feeling in those who drink it.

Milk Thistle: Liver Cleanser

Milk thistle is undoubtedly the most important liver-detoxifying herb that I am aware of. I have used it for many clinical conditions including these:

➤ Cirrhosis of the liver

➤ Elevated liver enzymes

➤ Hepatitis

➤ Side effects from drugs or drug intoxication

➤ Sensitivities to pollution and chemicals

➤ Liver disease induced by excessive alcohol intake

I have found milk thistle in dosages from 100 to 600 mg per day to be an important part of helping the liver function better and clearing wastes from the body. As more of our population continues to be diagnosed with hepatitis C, milk thistle should be thought of as one of the most important aids for maintaining healthy liver cells.

When buying milk thistle, make sure you purchase the standardized extract of 70 percent silymarin; it is extremely well tolerated and produces almost no side effects at all. It can even be used in pregnant and lactating women. In some people, however, it may have a mild laxative effect.

Peppermint Oil: Irritable Bowel Be Gone

Have you ever used those after-dinner mints upon leaving the restaurant to help calm your stomach? Or were you aware that antacids are frequently flavored with peppermint? It's not just for good looks or taste. Peppermint oil capsules can help soothe irritable bowel syndrome and reduce abdominal pain and distention, painful or frequent bowel movements, symptoms of indigestion (such as gas or nausea), and mucous in stools.

Peppermint oil may also be useful in treating the common cold. You may note that it's frequently added to throat lozenges and topical nasal decongestants. Some find that it helps to improve their nasal or upper chest congestion. You can also prepare peppermint tea by using 1 to 2 teaspoons of the dried leaves per 8 ounces of warm water.

Saw Palmetto: Prostate Protection

Saw palmetto has to be the king of the prostate protection. More than 20 well-documented studies show that the extract of saw palmetto berries is a useful therapy in treating benign prostatic hyperplasia (BPH), a condition resulting from the enlargement of the prostate gland, which can cause pressure and obstruct urinary flow. In fact, saw palmetto may even be superior to Proscar, currently the most popular pharmaceutical agent for treating this condition. While Proscar may help about 40 percent of the men who take it, saw palmetto may be effective in nearly 90 percent.

Not only might it shrink a swollen prostate gland, but saw palmetto may also reduce painful urination and prevent you from running to the bathroom all night long. Most men have found that it also improves their urinary flow rate. It seems to work by blocking an important enzyme that would otherwise increase prostate size.

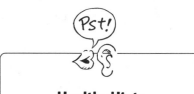

Healthy Hints

An enteric-coated capsule is the preferred form when taking peppermint oil. This helps prevent the oil from being released in the stomach and will deliver the peppermint to the small and large intestine.

Healthy Hints

It may take one to two months of 160 mg twice per day before you notice benefits from saw palmetto. When combined with stinging nettle and Pygeum africanum, the effect on the prostate gland may be even better.

St. John's Wort: Diminishing Depression

Are you ready to throw out your Prozac, Zoloft, Wellbutrin, or Paxil? Don't do it just yet, but St. John's wort may be the most perfect natural antidepressant that you can find. In fact, it works so well that it's the most prescribed treatment for depression in all of Germany, outnumbering any prescription drugs commonly used worldwide.

What can it do for you? St. John's wort is an excellent mood enhancer. It seems to pick up your spirits, especially if you're suffering from mild to moderate depression. The usual dosage falls in the range of 300 to 900 mg per day. And now there's some research indicating that 800 mg three times per day may even help with more severe depression. What about side effects? Well, they're anywhere from two to three times

123

less than those caused by most of the standard antidepressant prescription medications. St. John's wort works by enhancing the same naturally occurring brain substances (such as serotonin, epinephrine, and dopamine) that a drug such as Prozac might affect. Why not try something natural and safer first before starting on conventional antidepressant therapy?

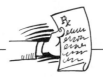

Note from Your Doctor

Do scientific papers support the use of St. John's wort for depression? You betcha. In fact, the *British Medical Journal* published a report examining 23 scientific studies on more than 1,700 patients. They found that extracts of hypericum were more effective than a dummy pill in treating depression, were as effective as standard prescription antidepressants, and had fewer side effects compared to standard medications.

St. John's wort may also have a mild antiviral effect and could be helpful in ridding your body of the common cold or flu symptoms a little more quickly. It is available in capsules, tinctures, and tablets. Try to purchase the standardized extract of .3 percent hypericin, the active ingredient found in St. John's wort.

Stinging Nettle: Nothing to Sneeze at

Tired of all that sneezing, itchy eyes, itchy nose, or other hay fever symptoms? Tired of taking those decongestants and antihistamines that sometimes don't help anyhow? You might want to consider trying stinging nettle during the allergy season to help prevent and treat your allergy symptoms. Nettle has an anti-inflammatory effect by cutting down on your production of prostaglandins. During allergy season, consider taking 200 mg of nettle leaf capsules two to three times per day, or 2 to 3 ml of a tincture three times per day.

When combined with saw palmetto and pygium africanum, stinging nettle may also be helpful if you're troubled with BPH. A 240 mg capsule of the root extract on a daily basis might help do the trick.

The Case of Doris and Her UTI

Doris had come to my office because she was experiencing urinary pain, burning, and having to empty her bladder every few minutes. Her lower abdomen was tender, and I recommended that she have a urinalysis performed. Lo and behold, her study indicated that she had a urinary tract infection caused by the most frequent urinary bacteria known as E. Coli.

No problem, right? Simply write out a prescription for an antibiotic, and tell her to take two pills each day and see me in a week. But that wasn't the case with Doris. She refused to take any antibiotic because she had a long history of allergic reactions to almost all medications. Herbal remedies to the rescue. I recommended that Doris take echinacea, goldenseal, and garlic for their strong antibacterial-like effect, along with an herb known as uva ursi, which has a wonderful antiseptic and anesthetic-like effect on the urinary tract. Just for good measure, I asked Doris to take some extra vitamin C and drink a glass or two a day of fresh cranberry juice.

Within three days, all her symptoms had cleared. She was pain-free and was no longer running to the bathroom every few minutes. Perhaps more remarkable was the fact that when I rechecked her urinalysis 10 days later, the bacteria was completely gone. This case illustrates an example of how natural medicines can help you with a very common medical condition. Please talk to your doctor before trying this treatment, however.

As you can see, the benefits of all these botanicals are numerous and cover a wide variety of health conditions. If you've only been keeping up on the benefits of vitamins and minerals, you should probably read and reread the information in this chapter to give you a wider arsenal of weapons against illness and stress.

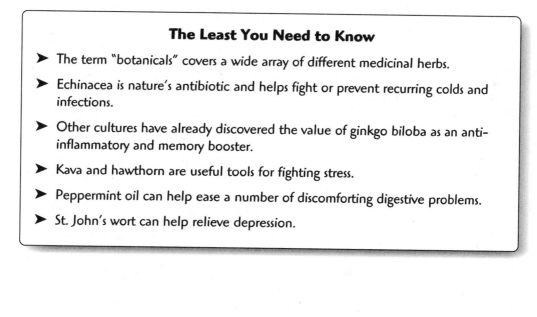

The Least You Need to Know

➤ The term "botanicals" covers a wide array of different medicinal herbs.

➤ Echinacea is nature's antibiotic and helps fight or prevent recurring colds and infections.

➤ Other cultures have already discovered the value of ginkgo biloba as an anti-inflammatory and memory booster.

➤ Kava and hawthorn are useful tools for fighting stress.

➤ Peppermint oil can help ease a number of discomforting digestive problems.

➤ St. John's wort can help relieve depression.

Part 3
Combating the Diseases of Aging

Chronic and debilitating diseases are certainly no fun. And they certainly defeat the purpose for living longer and healthier. There is a whole world of options out there to help you in conquering these individual ailments. It all begins with strengthening your immune system to ensure optimum health.

Let's take a closer look at some of the leading incapacitating diseases associated with aging and address treatment options. While I can't take the place of your own physician, I can try to provide you with an opportunity to explore adjunctive treatments to help in prevention and treatment.

Chapter 11

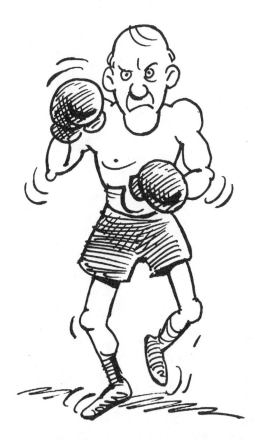

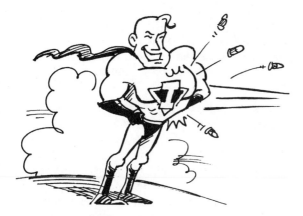

Strengthening Your Immune System

> **In This Chapter**
>
> ➤ The causes of a weakened immune system
>
> ➤ The signs of a weakened system
>
> ➤ Behaviors you should avoid
>
> ➤ Nutrients that can strengthen your system

Are you troubled by recurrent ear infections, sore throats, colds, and flus, or are you constantly on antibiotics, decongestants, or antihistamines? If so, you are probably bothered by a weak immune system—and there is something that you can do about it. No, it won't require surgery or more medications, at least not most of the time. The immune system is unique; it is unlike other organs that you may be able to touch, feel, or listen to.

For example, a stethoscope is effective at listening to your heart or lungs. An otoscope is used to look into your ears. A reflex hammer makes sure your reflexes are intact. But the immune system is much more complex and less well understood than many other parts of your body. Still, it helps ward off infections, like little Pacmen, so that you're not constantly sick.

How the Immune System Works

The skin and mucous membranes of your body function like linemen on a football team, preventing your body from the invading bacteria and viruses. The immune system is also responsible for gobbling up and repairing insults before they become cancerous. We are all constantly exposed to bugs, viruses, and bacteria, but we don't all get sick. Why? Some of us have stronger immune systems than others. That's why some of us never miss a day of school or work and others of us are always out sick. You see, it's not just what critter your body is exposed to, but also the condition of your body at the time of the exposure. You are the Director of Prevention. Put it on your resume. Provide a healthy environment to enable your immune system to do its job properly.

Causes of Immune Dysfunction

Let's talk about what you can do to prevent your body from fumbling and turn it into an all-star team. The next time your Aunt Frances lights up a cigarette, insist that she put it out. Or if Uncle Bob wants to take you to the local bar to get you drunk, tell him "no thanks." Both heavy exposure to cigarette smoke and intoxication can weaken your immune system. Your immune system is made up of numerous antibodies, whose job is to act like Pacmen and attack foreign invaders. Numerous white blood cells known as neutrophils team up with the antibodies to kill their opponent. Several environmental and nutritional factors may interfere with the cells of the immune system, leading to immune dysfunction.

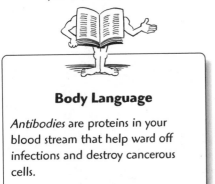

Body Language

Antibodies are proteins in your blood stream that help ward off infections and destroy cancerous cells.

What do Sugar Smacks, Apple Jacks, and Captain Crunch have in common? Yes, they are all breakfast cereals, but that's not what I had in mind. They are all loaded with sugar, which can also gum up the immune system. For example, eating just 3 ounces of sugar may result in a 50 percent reduction in the ability of the white blood cells to gobble up and kill viruses and bacteria for up to five hours.

And if you're looking for antibiotics every time you go to your doctor, you're also asking for trouble. The frequent use of antibiotics makes bacteria stronger and more resistant to other antibiotics—making you more susceptible to those beasties.

Your food intake also plays an important role in immune function. Deficiencies of B vitamins such as folic acid, B_6, B_{12}, and pantothenic acid, or shortages of vitamins A or C, may also set you up for recurrent infections. If you have trouble with your sense of taste or smell or poor wound healing (both signs of a zinc deficiency), your diet may also be contributing to your "Pacman deficiency state."

The Sugar Connection

Unfortunately, all forms of sugar have been associated with weakening the immune system. This applies to not only plain table sugar but also to honey and fruit juice.

Be careful and read labels, as sugar seems to creep into so many different foods. This includes not only breakfast cereals but also sodas, pies, cakes, ice cream, donuts, and chocolate, all the things you're probably saying yum to!

Food Allergy Facts

Whenever I see someone complaining of chronic ear infections, a runny nose, excessive mucous, nasal congestion, or simple colds, I always consider the possibility of food allergies. Food allergies seem to contribute to so many different symptoms, most notably unexplained recurrent infections. It has been estimated that up to 60 percent of the chronic undiagnosed illnesses may be associated with food allergies.

Totally Toxic

The average American probably ingests 4 to 5 ounces of sugar per day, so it's no wonder that you may be chronically sick. And that's assuming that you're *average*. I see many patients who are chocoholics, alcoholics, and sugarholics—who end up turning into antibiotic-holics.

The interesting thing is that food allergies don't necessarily have to cause hives or swollen lips or diarrhea—they can affect virtually any part of the body. If you continually eat those foods to which you may be sensitive, you are overwhelming your immune system and depleting your Pacmen.

Hundreds of patients are found to be allergic to common foods:

➤ Chocolate

➤ Corn

➤ Eggs

➤ Milk

➤ Oranges

➤ Peanuts

➤ Shrimp

➤ Soy

➤ Strawberries

➤ Sugar

➤ Tomatoes

➤ Wheat

➤ Yeast

Simply removing them from the diet can reduce the frequency of ear infections and nasal congestion. I would recommend a thorough evaluation by a nutritionally oriented physician skilled at diagnosing food allergies if you are troubled by recurrent infections.

Toxins in the Environment

Did you ever wonder what you are really breathing in every day or wonder what that cloud of smog really consists of? Do you notice a brown-colored ring in the bottom of your toilet, sink, or bathtub?

Yuck. You're constantly exposed to environmental toxins that have an adverse effect on the immune system. Although chemical agents are frequently tested for potential effects to cause cancer, they are rarely tested to see whether they are contributing to your headaches, nasal congestion, sinus infections, earaches, or perhaps chronic fatigue. And one of the areas that is greatly neglected is the possible role that environmental toxins may have on your immune system. For example, if you can't wait to call in the exterminator to get rid of those little pests crawling around in your house, you may be depressing your lymphocytes, thereby making your immune system susceptible to viruses and bacteria. The frequent spraying of insecticides and pesticides in schools, homes, and the workplace is now becoming a real matter of concern. Unfortunately, those little beasties are becoming more resistant to chemicals as the years go on, necessitating the use of more potent pesticides every few years.

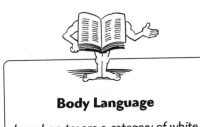

Body Language

Lymphocytes are a category of white blood cells that develop into T cells, B cells, and natural killer cells to help fight infections. They comprise 20 to 40 percent of the total white cells.

Pesticides, unfortunately, get stored in your fat tissue and can weaken your immune system. Unless you are eating organically grown foods, you are probable exposed to pesticides on a fairly regular basis, even though you may not think about it. This also lends more support to the ingestion of organically grown foods whenever possible.

What do you think about heavy metal? I am not talking about the music here, but rather heavy metals in the environment. For example, some of you may be exposed to lead if you live in an old home or work in an old office building. Old paint and the solder found in copper water pipes are potential sources of lead. Cigarette smoke contains another heavy metal, called cadmium, while dental fillings and contaminated fish contain trace amounts of mercury. All three heavy metals are potentially toxic and can inhibit the formation of antibodies and weaken the ability of your white blood cells to gobble up and kill bacteria.

Even substances such as paint thinners or carpet cleaners can depress your immune system by decreasing the number of natural killer cells. And medications such as aspirin, acetaminophen, ibuprofen, or even steroids can depress your ability to form antibodies. Steroids such as cortisone can reduce the number of lymphocytes and make your neutrophils more sluggish so that they don't travel to a site of infection as rapidly. Obviously, there is a time and place for these medications, but that's exactly my point. These should be used only when necessary, and other options and alternatives should be considered first.

To avoid exposure to lead, avoid situations where people are smoking, and don't hesitate to ask smokers to put out their cigarettes. This will help you avoid cadmium exposure. Attempt to eat fish from cold waters, such as salmon, cod, tuna, mackerel, or halibut in place of warm-water fish such as flounder, shrimp, crab, lobster, or scallops. Warm-water fish are generally higher in mercury content than cold-water fish.

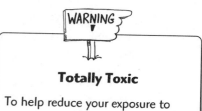

Totally Toxic

To help reduce your exposure to lead, let the faucet run for at least 30 seconds before using the water.

Is Your Immune System Weak?

How do you know if you have a weakened immune system? It's quite simple. You may be experiencing frequent infections, such as colds, flu, sinus infections, or ear infections. You commonly see this at the beginning of the school year, when kids may catch everything coming down the pike. If you have unexplained fatigue, or if your cuts, bruises, or wounds are slow to heal, this may be a result of a weak immune system, too. And if you've been off and on antibiotics for weeks or months at a time, it sounds to me like you're going to need some immune support.

How to Enhance Your Immune Response

If your grandmother told you to eat your breakfast so you'd grow to be big and strong, she was right. If your eating habits are lousy, you may be more prone to nutritional deficiencies, which can translate into a weakened immune system. Unfortunately, deficiencies of some key vitamins and minerals are not as uncommon as you might think. If your diet is low in specific nutrients, or if you're cooking your foods at too-high temperatures or storing your foods so long that they are no longer fresh, you may be susceptible to further nutrient depletion.

Nutrients Necessary for Immune Support

Foods such as broccoli, peppers, oranges, grapefruit, spinach, papaya, and strawberries are all high in vitamin C. Low levels of vitamin C can cause poor wound healing, bleeding gums, or easy bruising. If you're getting recurrent infections, think about your vitamin C intake. If you're not eating enough fresh fruits and vegetables, your immune system will suffer, making you more susceptible to infections. Vitamin C protects against free radical damage and can help guard against environmental pollution and toxins.

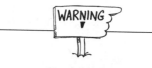

Totally Toxic

Your body loses approximately 25 milligrams of vitamin C for each cigarette that you smoke. Give your body a break by quitting smoking; if you do continue to smoke, be sure to include enough vitamin C in your diet to compensate for this depletion.

I frequently recommend more than the RDA of 60 mg per day of vitamin C for my patients who are experiencing frequent colds, flus, or infections. Optimal doses are probably more in the range of at least 500 mg per day, and I frequently recommend doses from 1,000 to 3,000 mg per day. Vitamin C is water-soluble and very well tolerated. Vitamin C is so safe and inexpensive that it can provide an excellent insurance policy for good health. It can not only prevent the frequency of colds, but also decrease the duration of the common cold. Interestingly enough, the blood levels of vitamin C actually fall when you are troubled with a cold. Vitamin C helps virtually all aspects of the immune system and has a direct effect on killing both viruses and bacteria.

Vitamin A, which is found in carrots, turnip greens, liver, parsley, and spinach, also plays a vital role in maintaining a healthy immune system. It protects against infections by nourishing the lining of your nose, mouth, throat, and gastrointestinal tract. Vitamin A may help stimulate the production of white blood cells so that you have more Pacmen to fight off infections.

Vitamin E has some very interesting qualities. Not only is it good for protecting against heart disease, but it also plays an important role in protecting you against infections. Vitamin E is a strong antioxidant and can protect you against that yucky smog and air pollution. It is particularly important as you get a little older, because it has been shown to stimulate the immune response as you age, thereby protecting you against infections. Vitamin E can help guard the cells of the immune system from being raided by free radicals, and it helps your body respond more appropriately.

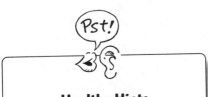

Healthy Hints

If you are an adult, consider taking zinc lozenges when you start to notice cold symptoms. They help you rid your body of these symptoms a little more quickly than if you didn't take them.

A shortage of zinc can also contribute to a weakened immune response. This trace mineral can help protect against respiratory and middle ear infections.

A shortage of zinc can weaken the ability of your white blood cells to double up and kill viruses or bacteria. Consider adding sunflower seeds, pumpkin seeds, green leafy vegetables, greens, almonds, or oysters to your diet to increase your zinc intake. Doses of zinc that may enhance your immune system range from 15 to 30 mg per day. Be careful not to take too much zinc, however, as dosages greater than 100 mg per day may actually suppress your immune system and increase your susceptibility to infection.

If you are deficient in any of the B vitamins, such as vitamin B_1, B_2, B_6, B_{12}, folic acid, or pantothenic acid, you may also be setting yourself up for more frequent colds, infections, and flu-like symptoms. The B vitamin family of nutrients plays an important role in pumping up your immune system and making you less prone to immune dysfunction.

Simply taking a quality multivitamin with minerals can also help protect the elderly against disease by enhancing their defenses against illness. As an insurance policy, I usually recommend that most patients take at least a multivitamin on a regular basis to protect from disease.

Helpful Herbs

The next time you plant your garden, you may want to consider learning more about the use of medicinal herbs. Several different herbs can have a potent effect on improving your immune system function. Perhaps the most well-known herb that has a profound immune-stimulating effect is echinacea. Echinacea can help stimulate those Pacmen, making them more efficient at gobbling up viruses and bacteria. If you have a raging infection, you may want to consider taking echinacea in higher than normal doses for a short period of time. On the other hand, if you're simply trying to prevent disease and strengthen your overall immune system, you can take lower amounts of echinacea for a longer period of time. Echinacea can increase the activity of the white blood cells, especially the activity of the macrophages. This enables the Pacmen to go to work, gobble up those viruses, and get rid of your infection a lot quicker. Echinacea can help you get rid of your colds more quickly—and they're generally less severe if they do occur.

I generally don't recommend that a healthy individual take echinacea for a long period of time, but if you're susceptible to frequent infections and are concerned about your immune system, you may benefit by taking echinacea for up to six to eight weeks, followed by a one- to two-week period when you discontinue it.

Note from Your Doctor

Echinacea appears to be nontoxic and is safe during pregnancy and breast-feeding. It should not be used, however, by people with autoimmune illnesses such as lupus or illnesses such as multiple sclerosis or tuberculosis.

Another important herb that you want to consider if you're sick and tired of taking all those antibiotics is goldenseal. No, that's not a mutant animal that you may find at the South Pole, but rather an important herb that has antibiotic-like activity. Goldenseal may activate the macrophages, thereby stimulating those little Pacmen cells to destroy bacteria and viruses. This herb may be truly valuable in the treatment of strep throat because it seems to inhibit streptococci, the bacteria that causes this all-too-common problem.

That smelly garlic that probably causes you to run away from your neighbor may not be so bad after all. Garlic has antibiotic-like effects and is effective at inhibiting the growth of several different bacteria. Try to eat a half a clove two to three times per day or take four to six capsules as an alternative to antibiotics.

Behaviors Affecting Immunity

It's amazing to me that we're not sicker than we are, considering the all-you-can-eat buffet dinners and the volumes of saturated fat, excess calories, and excess sugar that somehow seems to creep into our diet. Overconsumption and gorging on fats, sugar, and calories actually impairs our immune response. On top of that, most Americans do not consume the minimal requirements of five servings of fruits and vegetables per day, and rarely eat whole grains and beans. So you may not be getting enough of the protected nutrients to support your immune system in the first place.

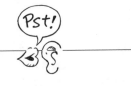

Healthy Hints

A positive attitude can go a long way to support the immune system. In his book *Anatomy of an Illness*, Norman Cousins attributes much of his recovery from illness to laughter, humor, and happiness.

And all of you stress junkies and Type A maniacs are also stressing your immune system. Stress from lack of sleep or from studying for tests can actually weaken your immune response and make you more susceptible to infections. So stress-reduction and other relaxation techniques should be a part of every immune-building program. Try to get at least seven hours of sleep per night because sleep deprivation can suppress immune function.

Obesity is also associated with a lousy immune system and increased risk of overriding different diseases. The arsenal of Pacmen does not work as efficiently in people who are overweight. Because one out of four Americans is obese, getting down to your ideal body weight should not be taken lightly.

Your immune system is responsible for warding off infections and protecting against cancer. Through healthy lifestyle changes, avoiding chemicals, ingesting high quality food, and taking the appropriate supplements of vitamins, minerals, and herbs, you have an excellent chance of restoring the health of your immune system and keeping it strong.

The Least You Need to Know

➤ Sugar, alcohol, and cigarette smoke can all hurt your body's immune system.

➤ Be aware of the possibility of food allergies, especially from foods such as wheat and milk.

➤ Behaviors such as overeating can put a strain on your immune system.

➤ A variety of vitamins and botanicals—including A, B, C, E, echinacea, and goldenseal—can help strengthen your immune system.

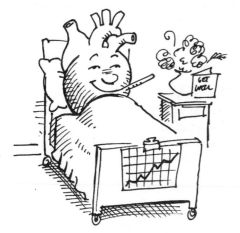

Chapter 12

Healing Your Heart

> **In This Chapter**
>
> ➤ Risk factors for heart disease
>
> ➤ The dangers of high cholesterol and high blood pressure
>
> ➤ Nutritional supplements to heal your heart
>
> ➤ The importance of chelation therapy

Lub-dub, lub-dub, lub-dub. That's the sound of your heart beating approximately 70 times per minute, 24 hours per day, 7 days per week, 52 weeks per year during your entire lifetime. The heart is actually a muscle, hardly any different from the muscles in your upper arms or lower legs. It has to pump blood throughout your body the entire day. Just as you want to keep your bones and muscles strong, let's talk about ways of keeping your heart strong as well. We wouldn't want your heart to fail and for you to suffer from a broken heart.

Let's Get to the Heart of the Matter

If you're like me and most humans, your heart is located in the center of your chest behind your breast bone. (I know some of you may have those emotional times when you "think with your heart," when it may feel like your heart is in your head.) The heart is actually made up of four different chambers; the upper two are called the left and right atria, and the bottom two are the left and right ventricles. We rely on our hearts for more than just love. We count on our hearts to beat consistently throughout the day. It pumps blood, which carries oxygen throughout our body and to all the tissues and cells. The beating of the heart is an involuntary response based on nerve impulses and muscle contractions. If the nerves become diseased or the heart muscle begins to deteriorate, the heart might beat irregularly or chaotically. This can cause you to feel lightheaded or dizzy, or have chest discomfort. It can also give you the sensation of palpitations, in which case you might feel a skipping, jumping, racing, or thumping sensation.

The heart muscle itself derives its nourishment from blood vessels called coronary arteries. These arteries are responsible for providing oxygen and nutrients to the heart muscle itself. However, if they become diseased, you may suffer from a heart attack, angina pectoris, or an arrhythmia. A variety of other diseases also can affect the heart, including congestive heart failure and cardiomyopathies.

Is Heart Disease Inevitable?

Unfortunately, even in light of all our miracle medicines and invasive cardiac treatments, heart disease still remains the number-one cause of death in the United States. To demonstrate how enormous this problem really is, take a look at some staggering statistics. According to the American Heart Association:

➤ One person every 33 minutes dies from heart disease.

➤ More than 60 million Americans have some form of heart disease; that's 25 percent of our entire population.

➤ Fifty million people have high blood pressure.

➤ Nearly 100 million Americans have cholesterol levels higher than 200 mg/dL, putting them at high risk for heart disease.

➤ Having diabetes or hypertension can double your risk of heart disease. If you have both hypertension and diabetes, your risks for heart disease can increase fourfold—and, worse yet, if you're a cigarette smoker and have either diabetes or hypertension, your risk for heart disease increases eight times.

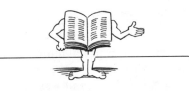

Body Language

Angina pectoris is caused by a lack of blood supply going to the heart, usually resulting from a buildup of plaque. With angina, you may feel chest tightness, pain, heaviness, or squeezing that is relieved by rest or medication.

Heart disease is actually a general term to describe a variety of different problems that can arise within the heart. For example, if the vessels supplying the heart, the coronary arteries, become clogged with plaque (which can block the flow of oxygen and blood), atherosclerosis, or hardening of the arteries, results. If this becomes severe, you can suffer from angina pectoris—in the worst of circumstances, it can progress to a heart attack. In this condition, the muscles of the heart are damaged, resulting in death to the heart muscle.

That's all the bad news. But there is some good news here as well. You can take certain measures to help reduce your risk of suffering from heart disease. First and foremost, perhaps, is the quality of your foods and dietary intervention. Several major risk factors increase your risk of heart disease:

➤ High cholesterol

➤ Cigarette smoking

➤ Hypertension

➤ Sedentary lifestyle and lack of exercise

➤ Obesity

➤ Excessive stress

➤ Diabetes mellitus

➤ Family history of heart disease

➤ Being a male

Cardio Treatment

How is cardiovascular disease treated? Most commonly, in conventional medicine, it is treated with medications. Most of the medications are geared toward reducing the load or pressure against which the heart must pump. The main classes of drugs to treat most cardiac conditions include diuretics, beta blockers, calcium antagonists, ACE inhibitors, and nitrates. Each of these categories of medications has its benefits and risks, so try a non-pharmacological approach first. This should include alcohol and sodium restriction, weight control, regular exercise, smoking cessation, and a low-fat, low-cholesterol, high fiber, whole foods diet.

One of the most common procedures performed today is the cardiac catheterization, or cath. This procedure involves the insertion of a tube and wire into the arteries of the heart, followed by an injection of dye. This is usually performed by a cardiologist in a hospital setting, where he or she can visualize the anatomy of your coronary vessels and valves and see the pumping action of the heart. The goal is to help identify plaque buildup or blockage in your arteries. These procedures can also identify diseased valves or diseased heart muscle. More than one million caths are performed each year in the United States.

Unfortunately, however, it has been estimated that half the catheterizations may actually be unnecessary—or could at least have been postponed. In other words, many of these patients could have been treated with medications or other means. On top of that, catheterizations frequently lead to the next procedure, either a bypass or a balloon angioplasty. More than 400,000 bypass surgeries and angioplasties are performed each year.

The coronary artery bypass surgery is a surgical procedure in which a blood vessel is removed from either the leg or inside the chest and is used to bypass the diseased

141

artery supplying blood to the heart. On the other hand, the balloon angioplasty involves the insertion of a balloon into the heart vessels. The balloon is then inflated to compress and reduce the blockage of the plaque buildup. The problem is that both these procedures carry potential risks, such as stroke, heart attack, irregular heart rhythm, bleeding, or rupture of a blood vessel. In addition, many times these procedures simply fail, and a second or even a third or fourth angioplasty or bypass may be necessary. That's why you, as the Director of Prevention, should do your best to prevent disease in the first place rather than subjecting yourself to surgery or other invasive procedures in the future.

Heart Healthy Hints

Fortunately, you can modify several risk factors by changes in your diet, exercise, and other lifestyle changes. For example, following a low-fat, high-complex carbohydrate diet, as discussed in Chapter 4, can help reduce your cholesterol and blood pressure. Actually, heart-healthy hints are not that different from tips I would give you to prevent cancer, osteoporosis, or most other chronic degenerative diseases. From a dietary standpoint, you should do your best to follow these recommendations:

➤ Minimize your intake of saturated fat, typically found in animal products such as milk, cheese, beef, eggs, chicken, lamb, and pork.

➤ Eat a diet that consists primarily of plant-based foods, including whole grains, beans, legumes, fresh fruit, vegetables, pastas, cereals, and rice.

➤ Be cautious not to consume large quantities of sugar or salt.

➤ Try to avoid processed foods, such as white flour and white rice.

➤ Use butter and oil sparingly because these contain primarily fat. Even though margarine is partly polyunsaturated, it, too, should be minimized.

Zero in on Exercise

Being physically active is a vital part of maintaining healthy heart function. Regular stretching and some form of aerobic activity (including walking, jogging, bicycling, tennis, volleyball, basketball, swimming, or rowing) can all help strengthen your heart muscle and reduce your blood pressure. Taking a brisk walk every day is a good habit to start. If your time is limited, try to walk during your break at work or during lunch. You will feel better at work, and your work performance will probably improve. Don't hesitate to do some mild weight-lifting to help strengthen the muscles throughout your body and improve your sense of vitality. In Chapter 22, we'll discuss exercise in greater detail.

Note from Your Doctor

If you're over the age of 35 and are considering starting an exercise program, it's probably best to first talk to your doctor about an exercise prescription. If you have a history of high blood pressure or cardiovascular disease, a stress test might be a good idea before initiating an exercise program. This is the treadmill test that you've probably heard of, where the doctor can monitor your blood pressure and heart rhythm during exercise.

Relaxing from Stress

If you're feeling stressed out every day and are under a lot of pressure, try to get involved in a relaxation program. Relaxation can also help reduce blood pressure and relax the walls of the arteries. This helps improve blood circulation from the heart to the rest of your body. It may also help you sleep better, reduce headaches, reduce muscle spasms, and feel more at ease with yourself. We will be discussing more about the different types of stress-reduction techniques that you should make a part of your everyday life in Chapter 21.

Controlling Cholesterol

As mentioned earlier, cholesterol is a fatty, waxy type of substance that can build up in your coronary arteries and other blood vessels in your body to obstruct blood flow. After the cholesterol hardens, it can restrict the amount of oxygen being supplied throughout your body. Hardening of the arteries is also known as atherosclerosis, which is a factor that contributes to coronary artery disease. Keeping your total cholesterol level below 200 mg/dL is certainly advisable.

As your cholesterol level increases beyond 200 mg/dL—and especially above 240 mg/dL—your risk of developing heart disease increases. In most individuals, the cholesterol level begins to rise if one's diet is too high in total fat or saturated fats, or if one eats foods that are high in cholesterol. It is possible to reduce cholesterol levels by doing the following:

➤ Eat at least 20 to 30 grams of total fiber, with a variety of both soluble and insoluble types of fiber included. Try to incorporate oatmeal, oat bran, rice bran, barley, brown rice, figs, prunes, raisins, apricots, broccoli, cauliflower, potatoes, chickpeas, soy beans, and lima beans into your diet.

➤ Lean more toward a vegetarian diet, including the diet emphasized in the Pritikin or Ornish program, as discussed in Chapter 4. This has been found to be helpful in reducing your total cholesterol and raising the HDL "good cholesterol."

➤ When choosing dairy products, try to select low-fat or fat-free products, including milk and cheese. You can also substitute dairy products with soy milk, rice milk, tofu, or soy cheese.

➤ Exercise regularly.

➤ If you are overweight, lose a few pounds to help improve your cholesterol metabolism.

➤ If you are a cigarette smoker, minimize your smoking—and eventually eradicate this habit. Cigarette smoking can produce high amounts of free radicals, which have been associated with heart disease, hypertension, and high cholesterol levels.

➤ Some nutritional supplements also may be of benefit. These include vitamin C, vitamin E, chromium, magnesium, lecithin, niacin, and garlic.

Medications: The Only Answer?

Numerous prescription medications on the market can help lower your cholesterol level as well. These include lovastatin (Mevacor), simvastatin (Zocor), pravastatin (Pravachol), gemfibrozil (Lopid), atorvastatin (Lipitor), fluvastatin (Lescol), colestipol (Cholestid) and cerivastatin (Baycol). Before you start with cholesterol-lowering drugs, however, try diet, lifestyle changes, exercise, and nutritional supplementation. You may experience side effects to cholesterol-lowering drugs, such as liver inflammation, constipation, gastrointestinal upset, insomnia, reduced sex drive, and headaches.

Efforts to lower blood cholesterol levels have become big business. Too many times a doctor may recommend that you take a prescription drug to help reduce your cholesterol level without stressing the importance of lifestyle changes and dietary modifications. More than nine million Americans are currently taking cholesterol-lowering drugs, and most of these people have never been instructed to try more natural therapies first. By reducing your intake of saturated fats and cholesterol—together with weight reduction, exercise, and perhaps a small amount of red wine intake—it may be quite possible to reduce both your LDL and total cholesterol.

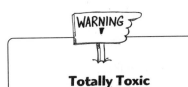

Totally Toxic

Niacin has historically been a very efficient B vitamin to help reduce total cholesterol and LDL levels. However, it can cause itching, flushing, and redness of the skin if you're not careful with it. Start with very low doses, in the 100 mg per day range, and slowly build up. Always take niacin with meals. If the reaction is unbearable, you might want to try a form of niacin known as inositol hexaniacinate. This form of niacin is less likely to cause side effects and may be easier for you to tolerate.

Foods and Nutrients That Work

One of the most neglected treatments to help bring down your cholesterol level is the use of soy protein powder. Mixing a scoop or two of this powder into some skim milk or soy or rice milk on a daily basis may greatly lower your total cholesterol and LDL cholesterol. In fact, the higher your cholesterol is from the start, the greater the impact soy may have. Soy protein is much safer and much less expensive than most of the medications typically prescribed for lowering cholesterol. As mentioned in Chapter 5, soy contains phytonutrients known as isoflavones. Two in particular—genistein and daidzein—are thought to provide the cholesterol-lowering and tumor-inhibiting effects that are afforded by soy.

Several other foods also may have a beneficial effect on your cholesterol metabolism, as discussed in Chapter 5. Keep in mind that foods containing flavonoids and phytochemicals play a beneficial role in reducing your risk of heart disease and blocking the LDL cholesterol from becoming oxidized. When cholesterol becomes oxidized, it can promote more damage to the arteries, and plaque begins to form. Some foods that you should try to incorporate into your meals include tomatoes, blueberries, watermelon, strawberries, broccoli, ginger, garlic, and dried beans.

Keep in mind that even though cholesterol is a very important factor in your risk of developing vascular disease, it is not the only factor. Even if your cholesterol level is between 150 mg/dL and 170 mg/dL, that does not necessarily mean that you are immune to developing heart disease or suffering a heart attack. One of the major goals should be to prevent the cholesterol that is circulating in your blood from becoming oxidized. This can be accomplished by taking extra supplements of vitamins C and E and by eating foods that contain lycopene and flavonoids.

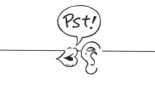

Healthy Hints

Try to incorporate at least 25 grams of soy protein into your daily diet to help bring down your cholesterol level. You can do this by purchasing soy protein powder and making yourself a breakfast shake with 8 ounces of orange juice and a banana; put the ingredients in a blender, and get your day started off with a bang. To get more information about the benefits of soy, contact The American Soybean Association at 1-800-TALK-SOY.

High Blood Pressure: The Silent Killer

At virtually every physical exam, your blood pressure will be checked by your doctor or nurse. Two numbers make up your blood pressure: The top number is your systolic blood pressure, and the bottom number is your diastolic blood pressure. A normal blood pressure should be approximately 120/80. If your blood pressure is found to be

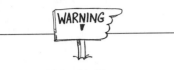

Totally Toxic

If your blood pressure remains elevated for a long period of time, you are at higher risk for kidney disease, heart attack, blindness, and stroke. If your blood pressure is high, your risk for a stroke may be eight times that of people with normal blood pressure, while your risk for heart attack is three times greater. This is why it is so important to control your blood pressure.

greater than 140/90 on more than one occasion, then you have high blood pressure. More than 60 million Americans have been diagnosed with high blood pressure, also known as hypertension. Having high blood pressure is one of the most important risk factors that contributes to heart disease.

Most of the time hypertension is treated with prescription medications. Several classes of drugs are commonly prescribed, including diuretics, beta blockers, calcium channel blockers, vasodilators, and ACE inhibitors. All these medications have their merit, but they also have their side effects. Before going on blood pressure medications, try a more natural approach to see whether your pressure can be brought down this way. To start, there are some dietary guidelines that you should take into account when trying to lower your blood pressure naturally:

➤ Try to maintain your weight in an ideal range, and prevent obesity. If you are overweight, you are at much greater risk for developing high blood pressure and other forms of heart disease.

➤ A diet that is low in sodium and high in potassium can help reduce your blood pressure. Minimize your use of common table salt (sodium chloride). If you insist on using the salt shaker, try using potassium chloride. Furthermore, include several different types of fruits and vegetables in your diet because they generally have a high ratio of naturally occurring potassium to sodium.

➤ Minimize your intake of saturated fats, and try to replace them with polyunsaturated fats or monounsaturated oils. This would incorporate more nuts, seeds, canola oil, olive oil, salmon, and tuna into your dietary plan.

➤ Just as I mentioned in the prior section on controlling cholesterol, always try a natural, nontoxic approach to controlling your blood pressure before beginning medications. Although medications are frequently effective in lowering blood pressure, they have also been known to cause several side effects. The diuretics, for example, may cause depletion of both potassium and magnesium, the same two minerals that help protect you from hypertension and heart disease. Beta blockers such as Inderal, Tenormin, Lopressor, Normodyne, and Corgard, another commonly prescribed group of medications to help lower your blood pressure, may contribute to the nearly 1 million cases of congestive heart failure per year. These medications relax the blood vessels and weaken the pumping action of the heart.

As you get older, perhaps over the age of 65, it is more typical to see the blood pressure begin to rise. It may be acceptable for your systolic blood pressure to rise up to 150, but your diastolic pressure (the bottom number) should still stay below 90. Keep in mind that the intake of caffeine (commonly found in coffee, tea, or chocolate) can raise your blood pressure. Excessive stress, lack of exercise, and cigarette smoking may also raise your BP.

Agonizing over Angina

Angina is caused by a lack of circulation getting to the heart. The full name is actually angina pectoris, which may manifest itself through chest pain, chest discomfort, or chest tightness. This is a common condition that can develop after a buildup of plaque and hardening of the arteries. It's usually caused by a lack of blood supply and oxygen to the cells of your heart muscle. The symptoms may occur after physical activity, eating, exposure to cold, or emotional upset and can be relieved by rest, relaxation, or the drug nitroglycerin.

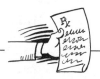

Note from Your Doctor

If you are active in exercise and experience chest pain or angina during your activity, do not try to push through the pain. It is advisable to slow down or completely stop your activity until your discomfort has subsided. The angina that you feel is the heart's way of crying for more oxygen and blood supply, so why stress it any more?

If you still insist on puffing on those cigarettes, it's a real no-no when you have angina pectoris. Keeping slim and fit and maintaining a normal blood pressure and cholesterol are also a part of reducing angina symptoms. Regular exercise can be helpful in improving the function of the heart, but if you are troubled with increasing chest pain or tightness when you exercise, curtail your activity and discuss it with your physician.

Commonly, medications are prescribed to help relieve your symptoms. These can include aspirin, nitroglycerin, nitrates, beta blockers, or calcium channel blockers. The same dietary guidelines provided in the section on controlling cholesterol also apply in helping to reduce the severity and frequency of angina symptoms. This generally includes a low-fat, low-cholesterol, high-complex carbohydrate, high-fiber type of diet.

Although calcium channel blockers are commonly prescribed for angina, I generally lean towards the mineral magnesium, which has a similar effect. Magnesium is nature's calcium channel blocker. This means that it prevents calcium rushing into the cells of the heart, which can cause spasms. Magnesium, on the other hand, can help your blood vessels relax and can reduce stress on the heart muscle. Magnesium provides a much simpler, less expensive, and safer alternative to calcium channel blockers.

As discussed in Chapter 9, I've also had very good success in using CoQ_{10} in my patients with angina pectoris. CoQ_{10} helps improve the body's ability to utilize oxygen and has been very effective in reducing angina symptoms. In fact, it's been so effective that in Japan it is one of the most commonly prescribed substances for the treatment of angina, congestive heart failure, and cardiomyopathies.

Homocysteine and B Vitamins

Have you ever wondered why some people who have a normal cholesterol level and normal blood pressure, and who don't have the typical risk factors for heart disease, may still be troubled with hardening of the arteries or have possibly suffered a heart attack? The answer may lie in the accumulation of a little-known amino acid known as homocysteine. If high levels of this substance build up in your blood stream, you are more likely to develop clogged arteries, high blood pressure, or stroke. All of these factors also increase your risk of a heart attack. Interestingly, three specific B vitamins—B_6, B_{12}, and folic acid—can all play a role in lowering your homocysteine level. Believe it or not, some estimate that up to 40 percent of the cases of coronary heart disease may be associated with elevated homocysteine levels. This amino acid can easily be brought down by taking these B vitamins. In fact, both B_6 and folic acid have been shown to reduce your risk of heart disease and heart attack by nearly 50 percent.

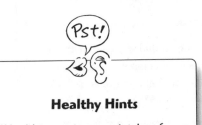

Healthy Hints

Would increasing your intake of whole grains and beans be sufficient to bring down your homocysteine level? Probably not. The latest evidence indicates that you would probably have to supplement with folic acid, B_6, and B_{12} to get your homocysteine below 10, the range that has been associated with a significant reduction in heart disease.

Where have all the B's gone? Because we generally obtain most of the B vitamins by eating more whole grains and beans, we should incorporate more of these foods into our diet. However, nearly 80 percent of these B vitamins are lost when food is processed and refined. For example, when whole wheat is processed and turned into white flour, 82 percent of the B_6, 67 percent of the folic acid, and a significant amount of the B_{12} is lost. So beefing up on the B vitamins is an essential part of bringing down your homocysteine level and reducing your risk of heart disease.

Super Supplements for Super Hearts

A wide range of supplements probably can help to protect the heart and blood vessels and to treat heart disease, should it arise in the first place. Because it is the leading cause of death in the United States, prevention certainly takes a front seat and should be a priority for those who want to live longer. Antioxidants—especially those discussed in Chapter 5, Chapter 6, and Chapter 7—protect our bodies from rusting and aging, so why not protect the heart and blood vessels as well?

Some of the most impressive work in regard to antioxidants has demonstrated the strong benefits of vitamin E in reducing the incidence of heart disease. Taking just 400 IU per day may help reduce your risk by up to 40 percent. That's not bad for such a safe and inexpensive nutrient. Vitamin E has also been useful in reducing the chest pain associated with angina, and it may help increase the good HDL cholesterol.

Vitamin C, too, plays a role in working along with vitamin E, and it may elevate the HDL and bring down the total cholesterol. Both of these nutrients team up to protect the LDL cholesterol from becoming oxidized. In a study of 10,000 people who took supplements of vitamin C, men were able to reduce their risk of dying from coronary artery disease by 42 percent and women by 25 percent. And if you've already had bypass surgery, these two teammates may reduce plaque buildup and prevent progression of your disease. This really comes in handy because so many cardiac patients require a second or even third bypass or angioplasty at times.

As previously mentioned, coenzyme Q_{10} should be thought of for any kind of weak heart or related condition. It's quite safe but unfortunately still very expensive. CoQ_{10} is a fat-soluble nutrient that is vitally important if you are suffering from symptoms of insufficient blood flow to the heart or blood vessels. I also frequently recommend L-carnitine, a nutrient that helps you burn fats more efficiently. This can help alleviate the chest discomfort associated with angina and may help strengthen the weakened heart muscle commonly seen in cases of congestive heart failure or cardiomyopathies. If you use this nutrient, make sure you use L-carnitine and not DL-carnitine. The L-carnitine is the more natural form, whereas the DL-carnitine may interfere with the absorption of the natural form.

Always consider magnesium for almost any cardiac problem. Nearly 50 percent of my heart patients are deficient in magnesium, which is the most important mineral for improving cardiac function. Can you get it all from your foods? Probably not. About 400 to 1,000 mg of magnesium per day is necessary to relieve angina and reduce blood pressure. This amount is almost impossible to obtain from food alone.

The herb hawthorn, which we discussed in Chapter 10, can also be an integral part of healing your heart. Hawthorn can help relax the blood vessels, thereby reducing your blood pressure. It has been shown to improve blood flow and increase oxygen going to the heart. It seems to work as a tonic for the heart and may help the heart pump more efficiently. Some consider it nature's answer to the drug digoxin, which is commonly prescribed for a weakened heart muscle. I have also incorporated an Indian herb, known as guggul, into my cardiac program. This herb may help improve your HDL and lower your LDL and triglycerides. Derived from the commiphora mukul, guggul has been used as a medicinal herb in India for more than 2,000 years. It may lower your total cholesterol and triglyceride levels in a dose of 200 mg three times per day.

Chelation Therapy: The Controversy Continues

I can't think of a more controversial therapy that has been used for more than 40 years in more than 800,000 people than chelation therapy. This treatment (pronounced *key-LAY-shun*) was initially discovered in Germany as a means of treating lead poisoning more than 50 years ago. Coincidentally, many of the patients who were treated were noted to have a reduction in angina, blood pressure, cholesterol, and other cardiac symptoms. Open-minded physicians then began utilizing this therapy to treat many of their cardiac patients, even if they were not found to be lead-toxic.

Lo and behold, these patients also greatly benefited. As a result, more than 1,000 physicians worldwide are now utilizing this treatment as an alternative or additional therapy for their cardiac patients. The treatment itself involves the infusion of an intravenous solution (I promise, it's not too bad) of vitamins, minerals, and a synthetically derived amino acid known as ethylene diamine tetra acetic acid (EDTA) given on a regular basis.

Note from Your Doctor

Chelation is available in an intravenous and oral form. I am not very impressed with oral chelation; it usually consists of a multivitamins, minerals, and antioxidants, along with oral EDTA. Only about 5 percent of the EDTA is absorbed by mouth, and no studies substantiate that oral chelation can help improve vascular disease. On the other hand, intravenous chelation therapy is remarkably effective in reducing cardiovascular symptoms and improving quality of life.

This therapy, although controversial, has been shown to save millions of dollars in health care costs, to reduce the number of bypass surgeries and angioplasties, and to improve the quality of life in thousands of people. It helps remove toxic metal such as lead, cadmium, and arsenic, and rids the body of free radicals, which damage the lining of the arteries. It also removes excess copper and iron from the body, which, when combined with oxygen, can also provoke more free radical damage. Remember, these free radicals can damage your arteries and contribute to plaque buildup.

I have supervised more than 50,000 chelation treatments during my career and have found it to be one of the most important aspects of helping the cardiovascular patient. I have been particularly impressed with its ability to help those with poor circulation or blockage in the legs due to either diabetes or vascular disease. In fact, several patients have been able to cancel their amputation of a toe or a limb after undergoing chelation therapy. If you're troubled with angina and continually rely on nitroglycerin or other medications, chelation therapy may be a treatment for you to consider. I have been most impressed with the fact that not only do symptoms clear up relatively quickly, but medications can be reduced and frequently completely eliminated.

The Case of Irv

Irv was a 68-year-old male who came to my office quite scared. He was told by a cardiologist that he better have a bypass surgery or else. He was a walking time bomb. After undergoing a *cardiac catheterization*, Irv was told that three of his main blood vessels in his heart showed significant blockage. He was not getting adequate circulation to his heart, and he was at risk for an immediate heart attack. He was scheduled for bypass surgery the following day.

But Irv was a fighter. He was a nonconformist. In fact, he didn't believe in the traditional medical model. He happened to be talking to a friend, who told him about the benefits of chelation therapy. He called my office and made an appointment to be evaluated. Irv began his treatments the next day and never felt better. After three months, he was no longer feeling any angina, chest heaviness, uneasiness, or fear. After nine months, an exercise stress test showed significant improvement from his prior study. His cardiologist could not believe the change. In fact, he told Irv, "I don't know what you're doing, but whatever you're doing, continue it." And he did for approximately two-and-a-half years. In addition, he was treated with a variety of oral vitamins, minerals, and antioxidants as well as a low-fat diet and regular exercise.

It is now six years since Irv was initially told that he was a walking time bomb, heard he needed surgery immediately, and opted for chelation therapy. This is not an isolated incident, as physicians such as myself who are skilled in chelation therapy have seen these examples over and over and over again. This treatment appears to improve the quality of life and the general well-being in more than 85 percent of the patients who elect to try it. Considering that virtually all the patients who opt for chelation therapy have previously been diagnosed with some form of disease, that's not bad odds.

Keep in mind that heart disease is preventable, curable, and perhaps even reversible, simply by making better food choices, taking antioxidants and other nutrients, maintaining your ideal body weight, and making healthful lifestyle modifications.

The Least You Need to Know

➤ Keeping cholesterol in the range of 140 to 180 mg/dL maximizes your chances of avoiding heart trouble.

➤ You can help keep high blood pressure at bay by losing weight and keeping sodium intake low.

➤ Super supplements for healthy hearts include vitamins C and E, magnesium, CoQ_{10}, and hawthorn.

➤ Chelation therapy can be an important component in treating cardiac problems.

Chapter 13

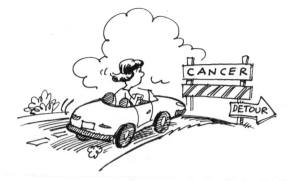

Cancer: The Danger Zone

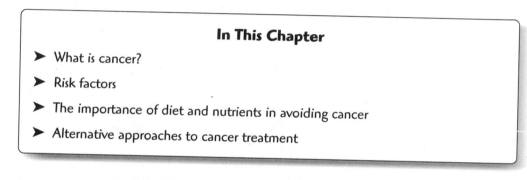

In This Chapter

➤ What *is* cancer?

➤ Risk factors

➤ The importance of diet and nutrients in avoiding cancer

➤ Alternative approaches to cancer treatment

Perhaps the disease that strikes the most fear in our minds is not heart disease or infections or high blood pressure, but rather, the Big C—otherwise known as cancer. Cancer can attack anyone at any age. But as we learn more about health and nutrition, we find that most cancers are preventable. Let's talk about some of the factors that may contribute to cancer—and what you can do to reduce the likelihood of developing it.

Cancer in a Nutshell

Cancer is actually a broad term that we apply to a disease process in which healthy cells lose their capability of functioning properly. Something happens to the cells that causes them to grow out of control, and new *mutated* cancer cells begin to multiply uncontrollably.

When these cells continue to grow uncontrollably this can manifest itself as cancer. The cancer cells copy themselves, the process leads to chaos, and a tumor can form.

Approximately half a million new cases of cancer are diagnosed each year (excluding skin cancer), making this the second-leading cause of death in the United States (second only to heart disease). So, you have every right to be concerned about your risk of developing cancer. Let's take a look at some of the statistics:

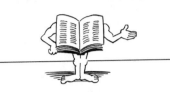

Body Language

When an abnormal change occurs in the genetic material of a cell, the DNA can become altered, leading to an abnormal cell known as a *mutation*.

➤ More than 1,500 people die from cancer every day. This accounts for one in every four deaths.

➤ One American life is lost every 45 seconds as a result of cancer.

➤ The number of new cancer cases and deaths from cancer continues to rise. From 1975 to 1989, new cancer cases rose by 13 percent, and the death rate rose by 7 percent. Although you may have heard that the mortality rates for some less common cancers has declined, the overall cancer rates continue to climb.

➤ Cases of prostate cancer continue to rise; in fact, there has been a 600 percent increase in new cases since 1985. If this trend continues, one out of five males born in the 1990s will likely develop prostate cancer.

➤ The incidence of breast cancer continues to rise, and the disease affects almost one in eight American women now. For comparison, only one in 20 American women was diagnosed with breast cancer in 1960.

Now that you've heard some of the grim statistics, I want to emphasize that up to 70 percent of all cancers are preventable. So once again, you as the Director of Prevention have an important task ahead of you.

Assessing Your Cancer Risk

Probably close to 90 percent of cancers are associated with environmental and nutritional factors. And of these, close to 50 percent are probably directly related to what you eat. You might think that cigarette smoking is the number-one risk factor for the development of cancer—and that's probably true for lung cancer and cancer of the throat and esophagus. No doubt smoking also contributes to cancer of the pancreas, bladder, kidneys, stomach, and cervix.

But perhaps the biggest risk factor for all cancers is diet. We simply aren't getting adequate antioxidant-rich foods, such as beans, fruits, and vegetables. These antioxidants can help protect us against DNA damage and mutations taking place in our cellular makeup. Most of us get only half as much fiber as we should be getting, even though high-fiber diets can help protect against both colon and breast cancer. Fiber helps pull out fat and carcinogens from our intestinal tract and also speeds the movement of food from our mouth to our rectum. This way, intestinal bacteria have less time to produce *carcinogens*.

A high-fat diet may also increase your risk for certain cancers, such as breast, colon, or rectal cancer. Although it's still controversial, most experts would agree that eating a diet high in saturated fats can increase your risk of cancer. But keep in mind that the *type* of fat that you consume is also very important. Saturated fats—those found in animal protein, such as beef, pork, and chicken—generally are believed to be the most troublesome. On the other hand, vegetable oils—such as canola and olive oil or fish oils—may have a beneficial effect and could reduce your risk of developing cancer. Polyunsaturated fats—such as safflower and sunflower oil—oxidize readily, and

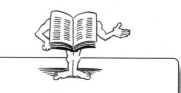

Body Language

A *carcinogen* is a substance capable of changing our cells so that they multiply and divide abnormally. Carcinogens can produce a cancerous growth. They are derived from our food, the environment, or chemicals, or are produced in our body.

increase certain prostaglandins, which in turn can promote breast and prostate cancer. (These different kind of fats are discussed in Chapter 4; you may need to refresh your memory by rereading this chapter.) Eating a diet that is primarily plant-based seems to provide more protective antioxidants and phytonutrients to reduce your risk of developing cancer.

Let's take a look at some of the well-known risk factors for colorectal cancer. This type of cancer claims as the second-highest number of cancer victims, second only to lung cancer. If you're over the age of 50 and have a family history of colorectal cancer or polyps, you face a higher risk for developing colorectal cancer. If you've had a history of benign growths—known as adenomas, ulcerative colitis, or Crohn's disease—you may also be at higher risk.

Breast Cancer

Then there's breast cancer, the leading cause of death among women between the ages of 35 and 54. In fact, after lung cancer, breast cancer is the leading cause of cancer death among women of all ages. With such a dramatic increase in the incidence of this type of cancer, it is imperative to be aware of some of the risk factors:

➤ Women with a family history of breast cancer—especially if it affects her mother, aunt, sister, or grandmother—are at greater risk.

➤ Women who first become pregnant after the age of 35 can be at increased risk.

➤ Women who have never had a baby have greater odds of developing breast cancer. Pregnancy reduces your exposure to estrogen (thought to contribute to breast cancer), so women who have several babies are less likely to develop the disease.

155

➤ Breast-feeding your baby can reduce the risk of developing breast cancer.

➤ If you've had early menstruation or late menopause, both factors can increase your risk of breast cancer. Again, this is thought to be due to prolonged exposure to circulating estrogen.

➤ If you have had previous breast cancer, you can still develop other cancerous growths.

Numerous other risk factors, while not well proven, merit mention:

➤ Women who take hormone-replacement therapy for more than 10 years may be at greater risk for developing breast cancer. This is still an area that's extremely controversial but of great concern. For this reason, many nutritionally oriented physicians recommend a more natural hormone-replacement program than the typically prescribed synthetic forms of estrogen and progesterone. (This is discussed in detail in Chapter 15.)

➤ Some researchers suggest that exposure to pesticides and other environmental toxins (known as organohalogen compounds) can also increase your risk of breast cancer. Higher cancer rates have been found in women who have chemicals such as PCB (polychlorinated biphenyls), DDEs (dichloro-diparacholophenyl-ethylene), DDT, and PBB (polybromenated biphenyls) in their body, compared to women with low amounts or undetectable levels. Commonly these chemical substances are acquired through pesticides sprayed on the food supply or drained into the water supply from farming communities. These substances can promote tumor growth and also suppress your immune system, thereby increasing your susceptibility to disease.

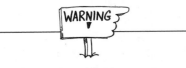

Totally Toxic

If you're trying to prevent breast cancer, I caution you against drinking water on a frequent basis from plastic containers or eating foods from plastic jars. The chemicals found in plastic products have an estrogen–like effect; although it's still controversial, they may increase your susceptibility to breast cancer. Try to use glass containers whenever possible, especially when storing food in your refrigerator.

As with other cancers, a diet that is high in fat, low in fiber, and high in calories may also increase your risk for breast cancer.

Several more controversial factors might trigger the development of breast cancer:

➤ Breast implants, especially the silicone gel implants that were eventually banned in 1992, are a risk factor.

➤ Two types of medications appear to increase breast cancer risk: metronidazole (Flagyl) and nitrofurazone (Furacin and Furoxone). Both drugs have been shown to trigger breast cancer in rodents.

➤ Some of the cholesterol-lowering drugs, such as the fibrates and statins, also have been associated with breast cancer in rodents. More human scientific research to evaluate these medications is probably necessary before prescribing them to women—especially women at high risk for breast cancer. Women taking Pravachol showed a breast cancer rate 12 times higher than women who were not taking it.

➤ Other medications, including hydralazine (Apresaline), a vasodilator used for high blood pressure; spironolactone (Aldactone), a diuretic used to treat high blood pressure and edema; atenolol (Tenormin), a beta blocker to reduce angina and lower blood pressure; antidepressants (such as Elavil and Prozac); tranquilizers (such as Valium); and some chemotherapy medications could contribute to breast cancer. The concern for most of these drugs stems from rodent studies up to this point. These medications still remain controversial, and human studies must be evaluated.

Furthermore, medication to ward off this dreaded disease might not be effective as previously thought. Oncologists are frequently using tamoxifen, a synthetic hormonal drug frequently recommended to reduce the risk of breast cancer, to treat women in conjunction with radiation chemotherapy or surgery. Although a recent study showed that tamoxifen indeed could reduce the risk for women at a very high risk for developing breast cancer, its effect in similar studies has come under fire. Some follow-up studies show that the drug actually afforded no significant preventive effect.

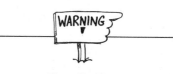

Totally Toxic

Concern remains that tamoxifen can increase your risk of developing blood clots, hepatitis, premature menopausal symptoms, or eye damage. Given these risks, I would advise you to think twice before entering into a tamoxifen treatment trial; instead, use preventive measures (discussed later in this chapter) instead.

Maintaining Lifestyle Modification

For preventing cancer, there's no question that cigarette smoking should be eliminated at all costs. If you are a cigarette smoker, do your best to get into a program that helps ease the cravings for smoking; if you're capable of quitting on your own, so be it. If a spouse, friend, or other acquaintances smokes in your presence, it's best to avoid that as well. Exposure to second-hand cigarette smoke could also increase the risk of developing a variety of cancers.

Also try to minimize your alcohol intake. A recent study showed that drinking just one alcoholic drink per day can increase a woman's risk of breast cancer by 9 percent. One drink equals about 4 ounces of wine, 12 ounces of beer, or a shot of hard liquor. If you drink two to five drinks per day, the risk for developing breast cancer can increase by 41 percent. Drinking that amount of alcohol increases a woman's risk of developing breast cancer as strongly as if she has a family history of breast cancer. Alcohol does this by raising the estrogen levels, and high levels of estrogen have been associated with breast cancer.

Drinking alcohol on an infrequent basis, perhaps one or two times per week, may not put you at great risk. If you already have a family history of breast cancer, however, and if you had your first child after the age of 35 or have never had children, you should consider limiting your alcohol intake even more. Other studies have shown that even drinking only two to three alcoholic beverages per week may increase the risk of cancer of the bladder and esophagus by 20 to 70 percent.

Maintaining a healthy body and preventing obesity should also be a part of a cancer preventive program. For example, if you hold a lot of your extra weight in your belly rather than your hips or thighs, you're at higher risk for developing cancer. (Of course, ideally you don't want to maintain excess body fat in either area.) Along the same lines, exercise is certainly a valuable part of cancer prevention. Physical activity helps reduce your body fat and lowers estrogen levels.

Some very simple tests are now available to help detect various forms of cancer. For example, colorectal cancer—the cancer of either the colon or the rectum—remains the second most common cancer in the United States. In fact, nearly 20 percent—one out of five—of the cancer deaths in the nation are due to colorectal cancer.

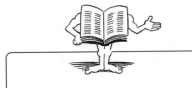

Body Language

A *hemoccult card* generally detects blood in the stool after a small amount of liquid developer is applied to the card. It is advisable not to eat red meat or take aspirin, iron, vitamin C supplements, or non-steroidal, anti-inflammatory agents for at least 24 hours beforehand.

Unfortunately, many of these cancers are diagnosed in a late stage. Early detection is key in all cases to preventing the worst effects of the disease, and a simple test in your doctor's office to check for blood in your stool is a reliable first sign that something may be wrong. If the initial screen turns up abnormal and blood is found, your doctor might suggest a follow-up study to examine your colon with a flexible tube and search for the cause. Your doctor can give you a *hemoccult* card to check for blood in the stool.

In addition to these screening tests, women should have a Pap smear on a yearly basis to rule out cervical cancer. This simple procedure can be performed by your gynecologist or family doctor. Your gynecologist can also discuss the importance of a breast self-exam, which should be done monthly.

As for mammograms, even the experts don't agree on the frequency with which these screenings should be performed. Physicians from The National Institutes of Health recently concluded that not enough evidence existed to recommend screening mammograms for all women in their 40s.

Because mammograms may miss 10 to 15 percent of all breast cancers in women under age 50 (because dense breast tissue may obscure a tumor), researchers at the NIH believed that there was no solid evidence that mammograms at an early age could save lives. However, The National Cancer Institute recommends that women have a mammogram every one to two years, starting in their 40s, and then continue on a yearly basis after the age of 50. Still others, however, advise against mammograms on a regular basis, fearing that radiation delivered directly to the breast tissue may actually increase your risk of developing breast cancer.

As you can see, opinions vary. My advice? Talk to your physician about all the pros and cons of this procedure before making your own decision.

Dietary Decisions

Without a doubt, diet plays an important role in cancer prevention. Try to maintain your ideal body weight, and trim the fat—not only off your body, but also off your plate. Dietary fat, especially saturated fat, seems to be a major factor in the development of several forms of cancer. Dietary fat is associated with higher estrogen levels, traces of pesticides (which can also provoke cancers), and the formation of hazardous free radicals.

On the other hand, dietary fat contains no fiber, which is so beneficial in protecting you against cancer. What's more, saturated fat is deficient in the key nutrients to protect you in the first place. The typical American diet is exceedingly low in fruits, vegetables, whole grains, and beans. Probably close to 60 percent of the cancers in women and 40 percent of the cancers in men are linked to poor nutrition. Consuming a diet rich in fresh fruit and vegetables also offers the benefits associated with vitamins A, C, and betacarotene. These antioxidants have the capability of lowering your risk of breast cancer—and several other forms of cancer as well.

When making your dietary decisions, choose your foods wisely. Try to stay away from the anti-nutrients, such as the processed foods, refined sugar, and soft drinks discussed in Chapter 3. Here's a summary of anticancer dietary tips:

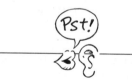

Healthy Hints

One of the most important steps in cancer prevention is to try to maintain your ideal body weight. Curb your calories. Obesity has been associated with cancers of the breast, prostate, colon, uterus, and cervix.

➤ Cut back on the fat. The average American diet consists of approximately 34 percent fat, and that's much too high. Try to reduce your total fat intake to less than 30 percent—and preferably in the 20 percent range. Fat may promote the growth of cancerous cells that can increase your risk of breast, colon, prostate, and rectal cancer. Try to buy more lean meats, take the skin off the chicken, and increase your intake of fresh fish. Limit the amount of cream sauces, gravies, and high-fat desserts. Switch from whole milk to low-fat or skim milk—or better yet, choose soy milk or rice milk. Opt for non-fat yogurt or low-fat cheeses.

➤ Load up on fiber. Try to increase your intake of fiber by eating more cereals, whole grains, beans, vegetables, and fruit. High-fiber diets can substantially reduce your risk of colon and breast cancer. Try to eat at least 25 grams per day, which is twice the amount most Americans are currently consuming. Eat at least five servings of fresh fruit and vegetables per day, along with some beans and grains on a regular basis. Stay away from white bread, white pasta, and refined crackers. Most of the fiber has been stripped out of these foods, so look for the whole-grain varieties.

➤ Color your plate—and I don't mean with crayons. Try to eat a variety of fresh vegetables and fruit of different colors every day. Each of the different fruits and vegetables offers different nutritional value. Try to increase your intake of dark green leafy vegetables, which are good sources of antioxidants, and also yellow-orange vegetables, which are high in carotenoids and flavonoids. The cruciferous vegetables—broccoli, bok choy, cauliflower, and cabbage—have strong anti-cancer properties. Try to incorporate more yellow, orange, green, or red peppers into your diet as well; these are particularly high in vitamin C, fiber, and other antioxidants. (They also make your plate look more interesting.) In addition, try to eat more foods that contain sulfur, such as garlic, onions, and leeks, all part of the allium family. These can help protect you against colon cancer.

The bottom line once again is to eat less fat, more fiber, and a wide variety of fresh fruit, vegetables, and unrefined whole grains.

Macrobiotics in Micro

Several diets have been touted as cancer cures, and though probably no one diet can actually boast that power, strong dietary recommendations can certainly help prevent cancer. One of the diets some have found helpful in easing the process of cancer treatment (and, in some cases, even treating the disease) is the macrobiotic diet.

I certainly don't feel that the macrobiotic diet is a cure-all, nor does much scientific documentation support this diet. However, numerous anecdotal reports point to potential benefits. The macrobiotic diet is based on the fact that we are eating too much protein, too much sugar, and not enough complex carbohydrates. Furthermore, we're eating the wrong kind of food, which is not helping our body to stay in balance. The macrobiotic diet primarily stresses a variety of whole grains, including barley, millet, and brown rice, along with numerous vegetables, beans, soup, soy products, and sea vegetables. Meat and dairy products are greatly restricted and, in some cases, not eaten at all. Seafood is included in small amounts, while sugar and alcohol are completely prohibited. Fruits are permitted if they are in season and grown locally. People who live in a temperate climate are restricted from eating tropical fruits, such as bananas, pineapple, and grapefruit. On the other hand, if you live near the equator, you would be advised to avoid dairy products, as they're not indigenous to your area. Sounds pretty complicated doesn't it?

Because macrobiotics is based on the concept of balance, it goes beyond only dietary recommendations. The underlying idea is that each food—and virtually everything you do in life—has a yin and yang component to it that must be balanced to maintain health.

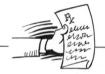

Note from Your Doctor

If you're considering a macrobiotic diet, be sure to meet first with a skilled macrobiotic practitioner who can provide you with the necessary guidelines. It takes a thorough understanding of the philosophy of macrobiotics—and a few quick cooking classes—to learn how to prepare the food to make this a successful diet.

This diet certainly isn't for everyone, and some find that it takes some time to get used to the taste of the food. Still, eliminating sugar, refined carbohydrates, and excess protein is good advice for virtually everyone.

Phytochemicals and Antioxidants

As we discussed in Chapter 5, phytochemicals are rapidly becoming a part of our everyday vocabulary. Even though the specific names of the phytochemicals sound complicated and intimidating, don't let them scare you. These phytocompounds contain a wide variety of cancer-preventing substances primarily found in plant-based foods. Try to incorporate a variety of phytonutrients into your diet to help prevent your development of cancer. Some of the most important phytochemicals that you should be aware of include the following:

➤ **Flavonoids**, present in almost all fruits and vegetables, can help keep potential carcinogens out of the cells so they can't cause damage.

➤ **Indoles** and **isothiocyanates**, which give broccoli, cauliflower, and other cruciferous vegetables their bitter taste, also help keep harmful carcinogens out of your cells.

➤ **Isoflavones**, found primarily in soybeans, tofu, miso, tempeh, and soy milk. They have powerful antioxidant properties and may inhibit tumors from getting started in the first place.

➤ **Monoterpenes**, found in a variety of citrus fruits, can help protect you by interfering with the action of potential carcinogens.

Keep in mind that increasing your soy intake has powerful anticancer affects. Japanese women consume more than 20 times the amount of soy as do Americans, and these high amounts of the isoflavones appear to protect against endometrial cancer, the cancer of the lining of the uterus. Tofu and vegetables may also contribute to significantly lower rates of breast and prostate cancer. Soy is thought to prevent cancer by blocking the harmful effects of estrogen and inhibiting cancer-causing enzymes.

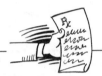

Note from Your Doctor

There are two major forms of tofu; the type you use should depend on your particular recipe. Firm tofu seems to hold its shape better during cooking and is recommended for soups and stews. It can be baked, grilled, or marinated, or simply crumbled into dishes such as salad, brown rice, or lasagna. Soft tofu, on the other hand, is used for cream sauces, soups, puddings, and other dishes when a smooth consistency and texture is more important.

Antioxidants, found primarily in fruits and vegetables, are also important in protecting against cancer. These are the same foods that contain the cancer-inhibiting phytonutrients. Try incorporating fresh spinach salads, strawberries, blueberries, kale, asparagus, Brussels sprouts, watermelon, and cantaloupe into your program. All are high in fiber, contain lots of cancer-inhibiting antioxidants, and are low in fat.

What about supplements? Can they also protect you against cancer? Antioxidant supplements have shown great promise in protecting against cancer formation, and it appears that vitamins E, C, beta carotene, and selenium are particularly protective.

Recently, vitamin C was found to protect against breast cancer and stomach cancer: In evaluating 46 studies, people with low vitamin C intakes face twice the risk for developing cancer of those ingesting greater amounts. Vitamin C is also protective against cancer of the mouth, larynx, esophagus, colon, rectum, stomach, lung, and cervix.

Vitamin C supplements have also been shown to reduce the risk of colon cancer. People who took 200 IU or more of vitamin E per day over 10 years had a 57 percent reduction in their cancer risk, compared to those who did not supplement with vitamin E. Selenium, another antioxidant that works together with vitamin E, can also protect against cancer. In a recent study lasting nearly 11 years, men who took 200 micrograms of selenium per day had a lower incidence of lung, colorectal, and prostate cancer; recently, those who were supplemented with vitamin E were found to have a 32 percent lower risk of developing prostate cancer and a 41 percent reduction in their risk of dying from it.

As you can see, nutritional supplements are here to stay and can provide strong protection against a variety of cancers. That's not to say, however, that you should neglect the importance of eating a healthful diet at the expense of taking supplements. Supplements should be just as their name suggests: They should be used to supplement a healthy diet and not used in place of a cancer-preventive diet.

What Should You Do?

The first step in your fight against cancer is, once again, to step in as Director of Prevention. Remember, cancer is preventable; it is not inevitable. You are certainly at greater risk if you have a strong family history of cancer, and we can't change genetics, but we hopefully can prevent the expression of these genetics through diet, exercise, lifestyle modifications, stress-reduction techniques, and positive thinking. You have the tools to increase your odds of remaining free of cancer. Even so these guidelines will not necessarily make you immune to cancer.

If you're diagnosed with this problem, what should you do? Obviously, you want to seek help from the best oncologist that you can find. Also be sure to seek a second—and possibly even a third—opinion regarding the recommended course of treatment. Explore other avenues and other possibilities. Pick up a book or two on cancer therapies. Read about other possible options available to you. Explore the Internet. Not everything you read might be accurate, but at least you know what might be available to you.

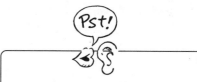

Healthy Hints

When consulting with your physician, don't hesitate to ask questions. Bring a list with you so you don't end up saying later, "Oh, I forgot to ask her . . ."

Tradition, Tradition

One of the common questions that I'm asked is, "Do I need to stop my supplements if I'm undergoing cancer therapy?" This is certainly a controversial area, and probably no definitive answer exists at this point. However, I have suggested to my patients that they continue most of their nutrients, especially if they are under the direction of a knowledgeable and skilled physician.

Many cancer patients—nearly 40 percent—die not from their cancer, but from malnutrition. In addition, chemotherapy and radiation put excessive amounts of stress on your body and can also create an abundance of free radicals.

When you're undergoing these difficult treatments, it is very important to feed and bolster the immune system continually. Contrary to some popular medical beliefs, nutritional supplements do not interfere with either process. In fact, they decrease the side effects and allow the therapy to work more efficiently. My experience has been that people who undergo chemotherapy and radiation and who also use nutritional supplements in addition to their conventional therapy have an improved survival rate and quality of life.

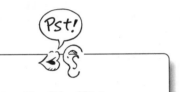

Healthy Hints

If you're experiencing a lot of nausea and vomiting from your chemotherapy, consider taking ginger, either as a tea, capsule, tincture, or root to help curb your symptoms. It's worth a try before taking the antinausea medications.

If you're undergoing radiation and chemotherapy, that doesn't mean you have to throw out all the healthy dietary tips that you've learned. Unfortunately, too many physicians tell their patients something like, "Just drink milkshakes because you need the calories." There are other, more effective and nutritious ways of obtaining calories than drinking milkshakes all day. For example, if you had heart disease, you would eat a heart-healthy diet to help reduce your symptoms and reverse the disease.

By the same token, because most cancers are induced by a poor diet, eating a wholesome foods diet should be part of the treatment plan. Again, go back to basics and remember that you're the Director of Prevention.

Over the Border of Mexico

If you've been diagnosed with cancer and you're not satisfied with your second or third opinion, or if you've already undergone unsuccessful medical treatment, you may consider other options. Even though we have a wonderful medical system in the United States, we certainly don't have all the answers.

Several patients have been successfully treated in other countries. Some may opt to go to Mexico, while others have decided to go to Germany or Switzerland. Each country has its own opinions and viewpoints on preventing and treating active cancers. Going to a spa and receiving therapies, which may not be widely accepted in the United

States, is something to consider if you feel that your options here have been exhausted. Don't hesitate to incorporate acupuncture, massage, yoga, psychotherapy, support groups, homeopathy, and herbal therapies when facing the dilemma of comprehensive cancer therapies.

But remember, one of the first laws of medicine is "first do no harm." Make sure that you're receiving opinions from licensed medical practitioners or other experienced health care professionals. Family support and a positive attitude is absolutely crucial when faced with cancer. Don't hesitate to have your spouse, children, or an acquaintance accompany you to the doctor's office, as these other people may be a very important part of your treatment plan.

Try to play an active role in preventing cancer by following the guidelines outlined in this chapter. Modifying your diet and lifestyle habits can go a long way to keep you cancer-free.

The Least You Need to Know

➤ Cancer is a broad term covering various kinds of cellular dysfunction.

➤ Cancer accounts for one-quarter of all the deaths in the United States.

➤ Diet is the biggest risk factor for developing cancer.

➤ A low-fat, high-fiber diet can help you fight cancer. And don't forget to "color your plate" so that you get the nutrients you need.

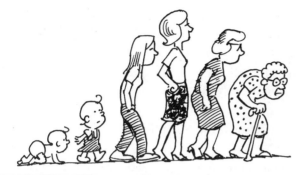

Chapter 14

Osteoporosis

> **In This Chapter**
>
> ➤ What is osteoporosis?
>
> ➤ Who osteoporosis affects
>
> ➤ How diet and exercise can help
>
> ➤ New developments in treatment

Perhaps you've gone to your doctor and proclaimed even before getting measured that you're 5 feet, 4 inches tall. Lo and behold, he measures you and finds that you stand only 5 feet, 1$\frac{1}{2}$ inches. You're in disbelief. You've shrunk 2$\frac{1}{2}$ inches since your early 20s, and now, at age 65, it's the first time you've had your height checked in 45 years. Where did those inches go? Unfortunately, you have become one of the 25 percent of post-menopausal women with osteoporosis. You lost a significant amount of height due to weakening and thinning bones.

In my own practice, I go through this routine with several patients per week. Unfortunately, osteoporosis comes on very slowly—chances are, it may be slowly affecting your spouse as well. For this reason, neither of you realize that each of you are shrinking. Let's find out more about this problem and what you can do about it.

Where Has Your Height Gone?

Osteoporosis involves the loss of bone density, accompanied by a weakening of the bone and loss of height. The bones become more porous and they lose their strength.

This condition is reaching epidemic proportions, and the statistics are absolutely staggering:

➤ More than 28 million Americans either have osteoporosis or are at risk for it. This problem doesn't affect only women, either; although 80 percent of those with osteoporosis are women, one in eight men is affected as well.

➤ Osteoporosis accounts for more than 1.5 million bone fractures per year, with 17 percent of these fractures involving the hips. The spine and the ribs are also frequently affected.

➤ One-third of all women will suffer a fracture from osteoporosis in their lifetime. One out of six men will also suffer a fracture.

➤ Fifty percent of all people who suffer a hip fracture from osteoporosis will never be able to walk independently again. They will require long-term nursing care or other forms of care.

➤ A woman's risk for hip fracture due to osteoporosis is as great as the combined risk of developing cancer of the breast, uterus, and ovaries.

➤ Up to 20 percent of those suffering a hip fracture will not survive their fall and will die of the complications.

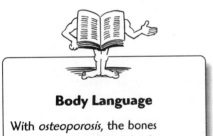

Body Language

With *osteoporosis*, the bones become porous, which leads to weakening of your bones and increases your susceptibility to bone fractures.

As these statistics show, we need to make a sincere effort to prevent and address osteoporosis. The condition affects men and women of all ages, but osteoporosis is much more common in the elderly and in post-menopausal women. Around the age of 35, you continually lose bone mass and your bones become more brittle. This puts you at risk for a fracture that can occur after a fall, or perhaps even simply moving in the wrong direction. Accelerated bone loss begins after the age of 40.

So let's not wait until we're 35 or 40 to prevent osteoporosis. Actually, bone is continually being formed and broken down throughout our lives. As we grow and proceed into our earlier 20s, it is imperative to try to build strong bones during those formative years. Your bones constantly absorb calcium and then release it into the bloodstream. During your younger years, you tend to absorb more calcium than you release into the bloodstream. But after the age of 35 or so, your bones release calcium much faster than they absorb it. When this occurs, you're slowly developing osteoporosis. You tend to lose height and don't stand as straight. You may have seen these little old ladies and men who look bent over and have a hump (called a dowager's hump) at the top of their spine. This, too, is generally due to osteoporosis. Let's look at some of the ways you can prevent yourself from losing stature as you advance in years.

Preventing Osteoporosis in the First Place

Now it's time once again for you to put on your Director of Prevention hat. If we could prevent osteoporosis from occurring in the first place, this chapter would be shorter—or perhaps wouldn't even be necessary. Some of the major risk factors for osteoporosis in women include the following:

➤ Currently experiencing menopause

➤ Having a thin, small-boned frame or small stature

➤ Having a family history of osteoporosis

➤ Early menopause

➤ Eating a calcium-poor diet or a high-protein diet, especially one derived from animal proteins

➤ Having a sedentary lifestyle and inactivity

➤ Taking medications such as steroids, diuretics, antiseizure medicines, or blood-thinners

➤ Smoking cigarettes

➤ Drinking too much alcohol

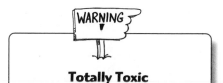

Totally Toxic

As with so many other diseases associated with aging, osteoporosis is more likely to develop in smokers. If you don't smoke, don't start; if you do smoke, find a way to stop.

High intake of red meat can lead to accelerated bone loss because excess animal protein apparently can increase the excretion of calcium in the urine and increase your risk of bone fracture. Try to limit your intake of red meat to no more than 3 ounces per week. In one recent report, those who eat more than five servings of red meat per week significantly increased their risk of arm fractures, compared to those who ate less than one serving per week.

Cigarette smoking also increases your rate of bone loss by decreasing estrogen production in pre-menopausal women, who therefore have difficulties maintaining bone mass. Smokers who smoke one pack per day have 5 to 10 percent less bone density than nonsmokers by the time they reach menopause.

Alcohol intake should be minimized as well, as it interferes with the body's ability to absorb and utilize calcium and vitamin D.

Women seem to be at greater risk for osteoporosis in part because they have 25 percent less bone mass than men. Both men and women lose about 1 percent of their bone mass per year, but this loss accelerates to 2 to 3 percent per year for women during and after menopause.

Note from Your Doctor

Women who have undergone a surgically induced menopause—where their uterus was removed prior to natural menopause—are at greater risk for osteoporosis at an earlier age. To compensate for this, they are usually placed on hormone replacement therapy post-surgically. They should also be particularly conscientious to follow the treatment guidelines discussed in this chapter.

More than Calcium

By now you've probably seen numerous advertisements supporting the use of calcium to prevent osteoporosis. Calcium is, in fact, one of the many important nutrients in the prevention and treatment of bone loss. It's important to start increasing your calcium intake at an early age. As you're growing through adolescence, your rapidly growing bones require more calcium. Unfortunately, the average American ingests just over 500 mg of calcium per day, which falls far short of what your body actually needs.

The latest recommendation by The National Institute of Health is for women between ages 25 and 49 to consume at least 1,200 mg of calcium per day. Post-menopausal women need even more; they should be ingesting at least 1,500 mg daily. Pregnant and lactating women also require 1,200 to 1,500 mg per day. Because it seems difficult for most of use to obtain that much calcium from our diet, calcium supplementation may be necessary. Supplements have been proven effective in reducing bone loss in post-menopausal women.

Calcium Sources

Several different types of calcium are on the market. The most popular appears to be calcium carbonate, which has the largest percentage of calcium. However, this form may not be the most easily absorbed as you become older because people over the age of 60 sometimes do not assimilate calcium carbonate as well as they do calcium citrate. For this reason, I usually recommend the citrate form of calcium for post-menopausal women.

Several different food sources also exist for calcium. Because you also need to be conscientious about the amount of fat in your food, you may want to switch from whole milk to either low-fat or skim milk. Eight ounces of either contains about 300 mg of calcium. One cup of low-fat or nonfat yogurt also contains about 300 mg of calcium.

If you're looking to avoid dairy products, consider a cup of broccoli, collard greens, or turnip greens, all of which provide about 100 mg of calcium. A 3-ounce canned salmon (with bones) contains 180 mg per serving. One ounce of cheddar cheese has 200 mg of calcium, while mozzarella has 150 mg and a cup of low-fat cottage cheese has 138 mg.

If you have difficulty eating dairy foods or if you're a vegetarian, try eating more dark greens, almonds, navy beans, spinach, tofu, chickpeas, or broccoli. These alternatives may not have as much calcium as dairy products, but their calcium content is readily absorbed by the body.

The Vitamin D Dilemma

Simply loading up on calcium isn't the whole answer, though. Bone is living tissue and requires a wide variety of nutrients to maintain its health. Taking a multivitamin with vitamin D should be a part of any bone-building program. Vitamin E also enhances the absorption of calcium, and appears to have its own bone-strengthening properties.

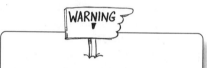

Even though milk is generally fortified with extra vitamin D, it turns out that many people are still quite deficient. Recently, a study at Harvard Medical School found that 40 percent of the American population is deficient in vitamin D. That number was even higher in patients admitted to a Boston hospital, which found that 57 percent of all patients were deficient in vitamin D. Quite surprisingly, 46 percent of those who reported that they took vitamins on a regular basis were still deficient in vitamin D. It wasn't just the elderly who were deficient, either. In those under age 65, 42 percent were deficient in vitamin D; 11 percent were severely deficient.

Totally Toxic

The excessive intake of sugar, refined carbohydrates, and phosphorus frequently found in soda and processed foods can accelerate the loss of calcium from your bones and contribute to osteoporosis. Drinking more than two alcoholic drinks per day may also increase your risk for osteoporosis.

We need vitamin D so that our bones can absorb the calcium. If you're getting insufficient amounts of D, your bones begin to weaken and soften. Too little vitamin D can put the elderly population at risk for a bone fracture. Typically, your body makes vitamin D naturally from exposure to sunlight, and if you get enough sun the sun alone may provide you with enough vitamin D. However, if you live in the northern climates or rarely go outside, or if you apply sunscreen every time you do go outside, you may be at risk for vitamin D deficiency.

Vitamin D is also frequently added to breads and breakfast cereals—but probably not enough to fully absorb your calcium. Think about eating more oily fish (such as salmon, sardines, and tuna), dairy products, and eggs. Most people need at least 400 IU of vitamin D, but the elderly probably require at least 600 to 800 units daily.

In addition to upping your intake of calcium, vitamin D, and a multivitamin, estrogen-replacement therapy is also an effective method for preventing bone loss in menopausal years. Estrogen seems to decrease post-menopausal bone fractures, and discontinuing the estrogen therapy may actually accelerate bone loss. Taking calcium in addition to estrogen may provide even greater benefits. Still, however, some controversy exists regarding the use of estrogen-replacement therapy, as some studies have suggested an increased risk for breast cancer.

Can you improve your bone density solely with natural nutrients? Perhaps. The final answer is not in, but some studies have shown that simply taking good nutritional supplements with adequate calcium, vitamin D, and the herb black cohosh may also enhance bone density and reduce the risk of fractures.

Some additional nutrients are worth mentioning as well. Chapter 12 discussed the fact that high homocysteine levels may contribute to heart disease. High levels of this amino acid can also contribute to osteoporosis, so folic acid, vitamin B_6, and vitamin B_{12} may be helpful.

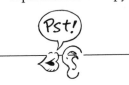

Healthy Hints

Try to minimize your intake of sodium, commonly found in salt. Not only will doing so benefit your blood pressure, but it may also protect your bones. Consuming more than 2,500 mg of sodium per day will increase your calcium excretion in the urine, leading to further bone loss. One study found that cutting sodium intake in half was as beneficial as getting an extra 891 mg of calcium per day.

Mineral Metabolism

Although we've talked about the importance of calcium (along with vitamins D, B_6, B_{12}, folic acid, and estrogen), various other minerals also help keep your bones healthy.

Magnesium, which is so helpful against cardiovascular disease, also plays an integral role in protecting you from osteoporosis. This mineral helps with the absorption of calcium and the conversion of vitamin D into its active form. Women who have osteoporosis generally have lower levels of magnesium than women who don't.

I usually suggest 200 to 400 mg of magnesium per day; also increase your intake of almonds, spinach, wheat germ, and other whole grains. Other minerals such as boron, manganese, and silicon help to strengthen bones as well. Supplementing with 3 mg of boron per day can reduce calcium loss from the urine by 44 percent. Boron also seems to help increase natural estrogen production and make it more biologically active. Be sure you increase your intake of dark-green leafy vegetables, peas, apples, and grapes to enhance your boron intake, but, even so, a supplement may be necessary.

The mineral silicon helps strengthen your collagen, which contributes to the strength of the connective tissue that provides the framework for strong bones. Vitamin C also plays an integral role with the manufacture of collagen, so bone up on those oranges, strawberries, peppers, grapefruits, and kiwi.

Note from Your Doctor

It has been estimated that if the elderly increased their intake of calcium and vitamin D, they would see a 20 percent reduction in the rate of hip fractures. This would translate to 40,000 to 50,000 fewer hip fractures per day in the United States, saving between $1.5 billion and $2 billion per year.

Don't Forget the K

No, vitamin K isn't potassium; it's actually a vitamin. Recent research has pointed to the importance of increasing your intake of foods containing vitamin K to prevent osteoporosis. Post-menopausal women, in fact, have a greater likelihood of being deficient in this important vitamin. Vitamin K is helpful in the formation of a substance known as osteocalcin, a protein involved in bone mineralization. Blood levels of vitamin K in women with osteoporosis are 74 percent lower than in women without this problem. Vitamin K can also help you retain more calcium in your bones, and it decreases calcium loss from the urine.

Vitamin K can be ingested by consuming dark-green leafy vegetables, such as kale, collard greens, cabbage, broccoli, turnips, and spinach. If you're taking blood-thinners such as Coumadin, talk to your physician before ingesting extra vitamin K.

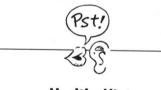

Dietary Delights

There's no question that diet also plays an important role in improving your bone density and preventing osteoporosis. If you're eating a high-meat diet, you are likely to lose urinary calcium at a more rapid rate. You may think that vegetarians are at a higher risk for osteoporosis, but that's not really the case. The bone mass for meat-eaters and vegetarians in their 20s, 30s, and 40s is roughly the same. From age 50 on, vegetarians generally have stronger bones and are at less risk for osteoporosis than meat-eaters.

Healthy Hints

In countries where meat is the primary source for protein, people face a much higher rate of hip fractures. Try to incorporate more beans, lentils, peas, soybeans, and whole grains into your diet, in place of beef, steak, and hamburger.

The type of protein you eat is also important. Try to lean toward vegetarian sources of protein, as opposed to meat, several days per week.

Make sure you're not consuming an abundance of the mineral phosphorus, which can also rob your body of calcium. Phosphorus is generally found in sodas and refined processed foods. Even though the amount of phosphorus in the diet should approximately equal the intake of calcium, the phosphorus intake is generally much greater in the average diet. A high-phosphorus, low-calcium diet is associated with osteoporosis.

Increase your intake of dark greens, soy milk, rice milk, nuts, and seeds—including sesame seeds and sesame tahini. While these foods may not be quite as high in calcium as dairy products, they are still good sources of calcium and other bone-building nutrients.

Limit your caffeine to no more than two cups per day, especially if your diet is low in calcium. Those of you who have a high caffeine intake and low calcium intake are particularly susceptible to weak and brittle bones.

As mentioned in the previous two chapters, soy is an important component in the fight against the diseases of aging, and osteoporosis is no exception. Soybeans, which are particularly high in isoflavones, have been shown to enhance bone density and thereby prevent osteoporosis. Simply eating 30 to 50 mg of isoflavones per day can help prevent bone loss, similar to the effect of estrogen-replacement therapy. Remember that a one-half cup of tofu contains approximately 35 mg of isoflavones, and one-quarter cup of roasted soy nuts contains 60 mg. Try using soy milk in place of regular cow's milk. The taste and calcium content are similar, and you will also get the benefits of the extra isoflavones.

Exercise Essentials

Exercise should be a part of any osteoporosis prevention and treatment program. Start early in life, as activity helps build up bone density and prevents bone loss in later years. It's best to do weight-bearing exercise, such as walking, jogging, tennis, or dancing, for 30 minutes at least four days per week. Try to do this on a regular basis because, if you stop for a long period of time (such as six months), you may lose the benefit you've previously gained.

A combination of exercise and sufficient calcium intake has a stronger effect than either therapy alone. It seems that exercise is more beneficial for building strong bones when your calcium intake is high. Also consider strength training and resistance exercises, both important for maintaining strong bones.

If you're inactive and live a sedentary lifestyle, you're more likely to lose excess calcium through the urine.

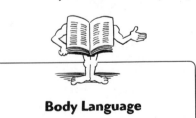

Body Language

Weight-bearing exercises include walking, jogging, tennis, volleyball, and basketball. These activities require your legs to bear the weight of your body, in contrast to swimming, rowing, or bicycling.

Remember, the goal is to absorb more calcium into your bones than you are losing. As the Director of Prevention, keep in mind that a regular exercise program is part of osteoporosis prevention.

Drug Therapy

After menopause, bone loss actually accelerates because you are no longer producing as much estrogen to maintain strong bones.

Several new drugs on the market are useful in the treatment of osteoporosis. These include alendronate (Fosamax) and calcitonin (Miacalcin and Calcimar). These medications slow the loss of minerals, help build strong bones, and prevent bone fractures. Some people, however, have gastrointestinal distress or upset stomach and are unable to take these medications. If this occurs, talk to your physician about other options and alternatives.

New screening techniques also can help assess whether you have osteoporosis—and, if you do, to what degree. The most common technique is the DEXA scan, a rather expensive X-ray procedure. However, some newer techniques examine your heel or hand and generate a computer-analyzed bone density report. These techniques are less expensive and expose you to less radiation than the DEXA scan. Some argue that the DEXA scan is more accurate. My own view is that the latter techniques are relatively new and the final word is still pending.

Osteoporosis remains a significant problem for the aging population. It's best to start in your early adult years on a prevention program. Try to incorporate calcium-rich foods, along with vitamin D, trace minerals, and regular exercise. Hold your head up high and take an active approach to keep your bones strong. And hopefully, you'll be as tall when you're 65 as when you were 20.

The Least You Need to Know

➤ Osteoporosis involves the loss of bone density.

➤ Osteoporosis affects millions of people, both women and men, and increases the likelihood of bone fracture.

➤ Dietary steps to prevention include taking calcium and vitamin D, and restricting sodium and alcohol intake.

➤ Exercise is also beneficial in the fight against osteoporosis.

Chapter 15

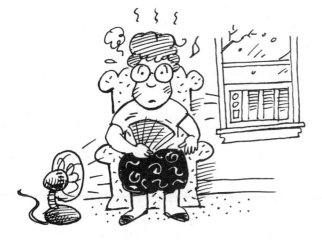

Menopause: Get Out of the Heat

In This Chapter

➤ Menopause and its symptoms

➤ Is synthetic hormone therapy for you?

➤ Natural hormone therapies

➤ Supplements and foods to help ease the transition

You just hit the big 5-0. You can't believe you made it to a half a century. Moreover, those wrinkles around the eyes have gotten a little bit more pronounced, you need to color those gray roots a little bit more frequently, you're having trouble losing those extra 5 pounds you picked up during vacation, and now, to make matters worse, you're starting to get sweats at night, hot flashes, mood swings, and you have difficulty falling asleep. What's going on? You probably thought that reaching 50 was supposed to be the start of your golden years. All of a sudden your sex drive has gone down, you are becoming more forgetful, and your periods are becoming more irregular.

But don't despair; there is hope—and there's a lot you can do during your perimenopausal and menopausal years. I'm talking to all you women, of course. However, you men should not skip this chapter: You need to know how to deal with your wife, girlfriend, or simply people of the opposite sex.

Are Hot Flashes Inevitable?

Menopause occurs when your ovaries are no longer functioning up to par and you no longer get your monthly menstrual period. This occurs at an average age of 52, but it can affect women ages 45 to 55. The time leading up to menopause, known as perimenopause, usually begins around age 45. During this time, your periods generally become more erratic and irregular. Your cycles may either shorten or lengthen, and your menstrual flow usually diminishes. You begin to notice hot flashes, flushes, or night sweats. Your hormone levels, especially estrogen and progesterone, begin to decline.

Today, at least 20 million American women are experiencing menopause. By the year 2010, that number is expected to grow to 60 million.

Is menopause a disease? Not at all. It is a natural transition that all women experience; it's a natural part of the aging process.

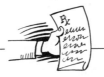

Note from Your Doctor

Menopause develops before the age of 40 in only 1 percent of women and after the age of 53 in 5 percent. Frequently, menopause occurs at a similar age as one's mother. Women who have had total hysterectomies—removal of the uterus, Fallopian tubes, and ovaries—experience what is known as surgical menopause at that time. If this occurs at an early age, you're at greater risk for developing heart disease and osteoporosis.

Menopausal Symptoms

As you approach your menopausal years, you probably notice that your menstrual periods become more irregular. Hormone levels fluctuate and your ovaries begin to produce less of the female hormone, estrogen. Another female hormone, follicle stimulating hormone (FSH), begins to rise as estrogen levels fall. Hot flashes are probably the most predominant and most annoying symptom that occurs as you approach menopause. You may feel a sudden rise in temperature, intense heat or perspiration, and flushing of the skin. The hot flashes may be related to fluctuations in your estrogen production. Levels of other hormones also change around menopause: Progesterone production from the ovaries usually declines, and luteinizing hormone (LH) levels rise.

Let's take a look at some of the most common symptoms that occur during menopause:

➤ Hot flashes and night sweats

➤ Irregular or absent menstrual periods

➤ Decreased vaginal lubrication

➤ Elevated FSH and LH levels

➤ Thinning of the lining of the vagina, which may cause painful intercourse

➤ Mood swings

➤ Insomnia

➤ Depression

➤ Forgetfulness and difficult concentration

➤ Urinary irritation and incontinence

➤ Loss of sex drive due to declining testosterone levels

➤ Fatigue and weakness

➤ Diminished moisture to your skin

➤ Loss of bone mass and risk for osteoporosis

As you can see, menopausal symptoms are quite varied and can affect almost any and every part of your body. Many of these symptoms, however, are preventable and can be dealt with or at least lessened with some simple dietary and lifestyle changes.

> **WARNING**
>
> **Totally Toxic**
>
> Heavy cigarette smokers tend to go through menopause 5 to 10 years earlier than non-smoking women. This also puts them at greater risk for weakening of the bones and osteoporosis.

Hormone Replacement Therapy: Help or Hindrance?

Two of the most prevalent problems that arise during the menopausal years are heart disease and osteoporosis. Both diseases have been associated with a fall in the estrogen level, as well as diet, exercise, nutrients, and lifestyle habits.

The most popular treatment to control the symptoms of menopause is hormone replacement therapy. This involves taking medications, including extra estrogen and progesterone, in an effort to replace what your body is no longer producing. However, hormone replacement therapy does carry potential risks and side effects. As you approach menopause, your decision to take hormone replacement therapy can be confusing, and many questions are usually raised. There's little doubt that estrogen and progesterone can benefit both the cardiovascular and skeletal symptoms and alleviate some of the uncomfortable symptoms associated with menopause.

But there's a dilemma: Many women xperience side effects when taking synthetic forms of these hormones. These can include fluid retention, headaches, weight gain, elevated blood pressure, depression, acne, and breast-swelling. More importantly, there is still a lot of debate as to whether taking estrogen puts you at increased risk for uterine and breast cancer. Although conflicting evidence points to different conclusions, women who have had a prior history of breast cancer or uterine cancer are often cautioned to avoid hormone-replacement therapy.

The most commonly prescribed form of estrogen is Premarin, which is the most prescribed drug in the United States. Because synthetic estrogen may cause a thickening of the lining of the uterus—which may then lead to uterine cancer—most physicians also prescribe a progesterone derivative (such as Provera) to offset this effect. For women who have had a hysterectomy and have no uterus, estrogen alone may be sufficient.

The debate continues regarding the risk of breast cancer and hormone-replacement therapy. Some studies indicate that there is no increased risk of breast cancer; others, a decreased risk; still others, an increased risk. Of great concern is a *New England Journal of Medicine* study performed at Harvard University on 122,000 nurses, which found that women of ages 50 to 64 who used hormone-replacement therapy for five to nine years had a 46 percent greater risk of developing breast cancer. On the other hand, a University of Washington study one month later found no increase in breast cancer in women taking estrogen alone or with progesterone.

So what's the bottom line? First, not every woman needs to be on hormone-replacement therapy. The next section addresses some of the options that are available. If you've had only brief episodes of menopausal symptoms, or perhaps if you're not at high risk for developing heart disease or osteoporosis, you may do just as well not to take extra hormones.

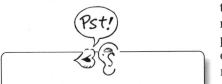

Healthy Hints

If you've previously had breast cancer or uterine cancer, I recommend staying away from hormone replacement therapy.

Medical conditions that may put you at risk if you are taking extra hormones include the following:

➤ Active liver disease

➤ Active thrombophlebitis (blood clots in the legs)

➤ History of pulmonary embolism (a blood clot in the lung)

➤ Gall bladder disease

➤ Uncontrolled blood pressure

If you choose to take hormone-replacement therapy, you should be monitored on a regular basis by your physician; try to make an appointment every six months for a routine pelvic and breast examination, and schedule a yearly Pap smear and mammogram.

My Doctor Never Told Me I Had Options

As you may have noticed, the above section mentioned "synthetic" hormone-replacement therapy. This implies that a "nonsynthetic" form of hormone-replacement therapy is available. Well, actually, there is—and, unfortunately, it is still being kept a secret.

When women do experience adverse symptoms from hormone-replacement therapy, they frequently stop taking the hormones or assume that the treatment simply does not work for them. Unfortunately, they are unaware that natural hormone-replacement therapy options are available to them.

What are natural hormones? They still consist of estrogen and progesterone, but there's a major difference. Natural hormones are chemically identical to the hormones that you produce in your body. On the other hand, synthetic hormones, such as those found in Premarin and Provera, are structurally different from what your body makes. They act differently and produce very different effects because those forms of hormone-replacement therapy are produced in a pharmaceutical laboratory. Doctors who pre-scribed natural hormone-replacement hormone therapy generally individualize the treatment for each patient. It's not a "one-size-fits-all" mentality you typically find with synthetic hormone-replacement.

To tell you a bit about natural hormone-replacement therapy, I first need to tell you that your body actually makes three different forms of estrogen: estriol, estrone, and estradiol. Most of the prescribed estrogens are converted in your gastrointestinal tract to estrone, the type of estrogen thought to be linked with an increased risk of breast cancer. On the other hand, estriol, the weakest form of estrogen, may actually help to protect you against breast cancer.

Note from Your Doctor

Estriol is produced in large amounts during pregnancy and is thought to protect against breast cancer. It is also found in high quantities in vegetarians and Asian women, which may account for their low incidence of breast cancer.

Natural estriol has been very effective in alleviating the symptoms of menopause and still providing most of the protection against osteoporosis and heart disease. It can also be used as a vaginal cream to help prevent recurrent urinary tract infections in meno-pausal women, according to a recent report in the *New England Journal of Medicine*.

As another advantage, estriol does not stimulate the growth of uterine tissue and therefore can be used without progesterone. However, I usually recommend taking natural progesterone along with estriol, because progesterone has bone-enhancing effects and can reduce many of your menopausal symptoms.

Because your body makes all three forms of estrogen—estriol, estrone, and estradiol—some physicians elect to use a percentage of all three forms when treating menopausal symptoms. This formula can be custom-compounded by a pharmacist with a prescription from your doctor. Even though estrogen appears to protect you from osteoporosis, you should consider progesterone as well because it has been associated with decreased bone loss. Furthermore, some debate still exists regarding the isolated use of estrogen; although estrogen appears to decrease the rate of bone breakdown in the first five years of usage, bone loss may continue after that point at the same rate as that in women who are not using estrogen.

Rather than using synthetic progestins, as is commonly prescribed, a natural form of progesterone is also available. This is known as natural micronized progesterone, which can be readily absorbed through your gastrointestinal tract or applied as a topical skin cream. Progesterone has been effective in women with premenstrual syndrome, which frequently involves anxiety, cravings, mood swings, and irritability before menstrual periods.

Interestingly, the combination of estrogen and natural micronized progesterone can improve your blood cholesterol profile and reduce your cardiovascular risk more efficiently than a combination of estrogen and synthetic progestin. In a 1995 *Journal of American Medical Association* trial, the use of synthetic progestins partially negated some of the beneficial cholesterol-lowering effects noted upon taking estrogen. On the other hand, natural progesterone maintained all the cholesterol-lowering benefits afforded by estrogen without the side effects associated with progestins.

Deciding whether to take hormone-replacement therapy—and determining which type—is certainly a complicated question and a complex issue. You should discuss this matter with your physician in more detail.

Dietary Decisions During Menopause

Before you decide to take hormone-replacement therapy, let's talk about some of the ways to deal with the symptoms and minimize the effects of menopause itself. Dietary guidelines and suggestions can certainly help protect you as you go through the menopausal years. Let's take a look at some of the most important factors.

➤ Try to minimize your intake of hot coffee, spices, chocolate, and alcohol. All these foods can make your hot flashes a little worse.

➤ Minimize your intake of salt, as it can lead to increased water retention.

➤ Try to use more spices, seasonings, or mustard to flavor your foods.

➤ Eat small, frequent meals throughout the day; large meals may increase your body temperature and make your hot flashes worse. It's also easier to metabolize smaller meals and maintain normal blood sugar levels.

➤ Limit your intake of high-fat foods and sweets. Optimize your intake of foods high in fiber, phytonutrients, and fruits and vegetables. This can help protect you against cancer, heart disease, osteoporosis, and menopausal symptoms.

➤ Try sprinkling freshly ground flax seed on your cereals and salads. It contains the all-important phytonutrients—isoflavones—that have a mild estrogen-balancing affect on your body.

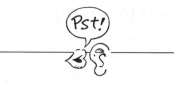

Healthy Hints

Fresh flax seed is a wonderful source of beneficial Omega-3 oils, which help maintain moisture and luster in your skin and scalp. You can purchase this in a health food store, grind it yourself, and keep it in the refrigerator to be sprinkled on your food. Flax seed contains isoflavones and lignans, which may protect you against breast cancer and other hormone-dependent cancers.

➤ Increase the intake of soy in your daily diet to increase your isoflavone intake. Remember, these are the estrogen-balancing phytonutrients that are derived from tofu, tempeh, soybeans, and soy milk. The next section discusses more of these foods.

Soy to the Rescue

Hopefully you're not soy-ed out by now, because I have more soy news for you. As mentioned previously, soy contains isoflavones, which are naturally occurring, plant-derived, estrogen-like compounds to help protect you against a variety of cancers and heart disease. Studies have shown that eating 4 ounces of soy per day can help reduce menopausal symptoms, such as hot flashes and vaginal dryness. Try to incorporate 30 to 50 mg of isoflavones into your diet on a daily basis.

Phytoestrogens found in food can act like estrogens by binding to your estrogen receptor sites and thus enhance the effect of naturally occurring estrogen. Interestingly enough, in China and Japan—where soy intake is far greater than in the United States—hot flashes during the menopausal years are quite rare. You may be able to reduce your hot flashes by 40 percent simply by adding more soy to your diet. Try drinking 16 ounces of soy milk or eating 2 ounces of tofu. You can also try switching from those fatty hamburgers to veggie burgers; they make great meat substitutes.

Vital Vitamins for Menopause

I certainly recommend eating a wholesome diet and minimizing your intake of sweets and refined, processed foods. Those foods are low in trace minerals, vitamins, and key antioxidants, all of which protect you from diseases that typically arise during the menopausal years. Even if you've cleaned up your diet, nutritional supplementation may also put the fire out under those hot flashes. Let's take a look at some of the more important nutrients:

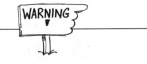

Totally Toxic

Generally speaking, vitamin E is very safe and has almost no side effects. However, if you are taking anti-coagulant medication, or if you recently had a stroke or have been diagnosed with a bleeding disorder, you should consult your physician before taking vitamin E supplements.

➤ Even though vitamin E is best known for its antioxidant effect and ability to cut down your risk of heart disease, many women find that it also can help relieve hot flashes and vaginal dryness. In fact, I frequently prescribe vitamin E suppositories to be used intravaginally for patients complaining of vaginal irritation, vaginal dryness, or painful intercourse.

➤ Vitamin C is helpful in relieving some of the physical and emotional stress associated with menopause. It also functions as an antioxidant and can help protect you from heart disease and cancer, which is more prominent during the menopausal years.

➤ Some of you will find that calcium and magnesium can help reduce some of the symptoms associated with menopause, especially hot flashes and night sweats. These two minerals are also extremely valuable in preventing bone loss and reducing your risk of osteoporosis.

➤ Bioflavonoids, which help in the absorption of vitamin C and have their own antioxidant and anti-inflammatory properties, can also be valuable in relieving menopausal hot flashes. You can ingest more bioflavonoids by increasing your intake of citrus fruits.

➤ You may want to consider a variety of other nutrients during menopause as well, as they help protect you against many diseases that are associated with advancing age, including heart disease and cancer. These vitamins include vitamin D, B-complex vitamins, and folic acid. Unfortunately, many of the elderly simply do not consume even two-thirds of the recommended amounts for these nutrients, which often leads to deficiencies. A shortage of any of these nutrients can make your mood swings, insomnia, irritability, and memory loss even worse.

Exercise for Everyone

A regular regimen of exercise should be a part of your menopausal program. A combination of both aerobic training, such as walking or tennis, and strength training or weight-lifting can help prevent menopausal bone loss and improve your sense of well-being. Start by walking at least 20 minutes three days per week, and gradually increase your time and frequency as the weeks go on. To add more interest to your program, vary the activity. Try bicycling, swimming, or taking an aerobic dance class. No doubt exercise also can reduce your risk for heart disease, combat weight gain, help you sleep better, and reduce your risk for osteoporosis.

If you haven't worked out in a while, it may be a good idea to consult with a knowledgeable instructor to get you back on pace. Take a friend with you—and don't be intimidated by those 23-year-old, muscle-bound weight-lifting specimens working out on the machines next to you.

Herbal Remedies

Numerous herbal formulas on the market have been formulated to help with menopausal symptoms. Some of these are quite effective and can even take the place of hormone-replacement therapy at times. Most of these herbal products contain a combination of various herbs, including black cohosh (Cimicifuga racemosa), dong quai, chasteberry (Vitex agnus castus), and perhaps ginseng and licorice root (Glycyrrhizaglabra), and red clover. All these herbs possess sources that have hormone-like activities.

Perhaps the most well-known of the herbal therapies used in Europe for menopausal symptoms is black cohosh. Interestingly enough, this is actually a native North American herb that was widely used by Native Americans to relieve female complaints. In a recent study completed in Germany, 80 percent of the more than 600 women who were given black cohosh reported improvement in menopausal symptoms, such as hot flashes, palpitations, depression, and headaches, after only three to four weeks. Even more impressive, after six to eight weeks, many of these women reported complete remission of their symptoms.

The evidence is still unclear as to whether Black Cohosh may have the ability to protect you against osteoporosis and heart disease, as estrogen does. However, if you are uncomfortable taking estrogen-replacement therapy, or if you have experienced side effects or previously had breast cancer, black cohosh and other herbal therapies may provide a valuable option for you.

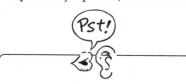

Healthy Hints

Whereas estrogens may cause high blood pressure, weight gain, and vaginal bleeding, black cohosh does not seem to induce any of these side effects.

The Least You Need to Know

➤ Menopause is not a disease; it is a natural part of a woman's life.

➤ Symptoms of menopause include irregular periods, hot flashes, and a decline in hormone levels produced by the body.

➤ Synthetic hormone therapy may be beneficial to you, but be aware that there are other choices.

➤ Natural hormones include estriol and progesterone.

➤ Exercise and diet can help alleviate certain symptoms. Be sure to remember vitamin and mineral supplements, and consider taking black cohosh.

Chapter 16

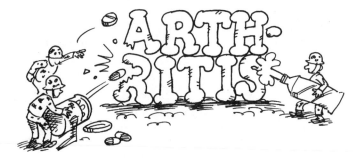

An Arsenal Against Arthritis

In This Chapter

➤ The main kinds of arthritis

➤ Are anti-inflammatories the answer?

➤ The role of diet

➤ Dietary supplements you may not know about

Think back to those achy, breaky back days we talked about way back in Chapter 1. You know, the ones that you hope you don't have too many of as you get older. And maybe it's not your back but perhaps your sore hips or knees, or maybe you're having trouble getting started in the morning. Perhaps even getting out of bed is an effort. If you do have painful and aching joints, there's a good chance that you might be developing arthritis.

Oh, Those Aching Joints

Arthritis is a general term for conditions characterized by discomfort and pain in the joints. Numerous forms of arthritis exist, but the most common two are osteoarthritis and rheumatoid arthritis. Both forms can cause noticeable disfigurement in the joints.

Osteoarthritis is by far the most common form of arthritis and is generally caused by wear and tear on your joints. The cartilage that lines the surfaces of the joints wears away, and you're left with rough surfaces. As a result, your joints become stiff and painful. Almost any joint can be affected by osteoarthritis, although it primarily affects the weight-bearing joints—such as the hips, knees, and back—as well as the hands and wrists.

On the other hand, rheumatoid arthritis more commonly involves inflammation and swelling of the joints rather than a wearing away of the cartilage. In either case, you can experience pain and stiffness. Rheumatoid arthritis is generally more crippling and can affect your entire body.

Note from Your Doctor

People with rheumatoid arthritis are at greater risk for developing lung and kidney diseases, infections, and gastrointestinal bleeding. Unfortunately, their average life expectancy is reduced by about 4 years in men and by 10 years in women.

Let's take a look at the raw numbers as they relate to arthritis:

➤ Osteoarthritis, also known as degenerative joint disease (DJD), affects approximately 16 million people in the United States.

➤ Rheumatoid arthritis affects approximately 2.5 million people in the United States and more commonly occurs in women in their 30s, 40s, and 50s.

➤ Women are three times more likely than men to develop rheumatoid arthritis.

➤ Nearly 50 percent of all people suffering from rheumatoid arthritis are disabled from it within five years.

➤ Nearly half the population over age 65 can expect to develop at least a touch of osteoarthritis.

➤ The incidence of osteoarthritis increases as you get older. It occurs in one of eight people under age 50 and in one of four over age 50.

Osteoarthritis develops much more slow and can progress for years without noticeable symptoms. Rheumatoid arthritis is thought to be an autoimmune disease. In this case, the body's immune system reacts against itself and the fluid that lubricates the joints becomes inflamed. This inflammation damages the cartilage and bone, leading to pain, swelling, redness, and warmth in the joints.

It has been estimated that 40 million Americans are affected by it. That number is expected to rise to nearly 60 million by the year 2020.

Are Anti-Inflammatories the Answer?

While most physicians feel that no cure exists for arthritis and that not a lot can be done for this problem, most of the treatment focuses on reducing the symptoms of painful and aching joints. The most frequent conventional treatments to help control the symptoms of arthritis involve the use of nonsteroidal anti-inflammatory drugs (NSAIDs). These medications help reduce the inflammation and pain associated with arthritis. NSAIDs, however, do not stop the progression of arthritis; they simply alleviate the symptoms.

You may have tried either ibuprofen or naproxen and noticed stomach inflammation. Unfortunately, NSAIDs have been associated with significant side effects—frequently quite serious. Be careful with these, as they can cause stomach ulcers, bleeding in the digestive tract, liver damage, or kidney impairment—especially in the elderly population. Because they became available on the "over-the-counter market" and are no longer "prescription-only," more people are running into serious side effects from nonsteroidals. In higher strengths, many are still available only by prescription, but even so, it seems that many people who take several NSAIDs per day face a much greater risk of serious problems.

Totally Toxic

Whenever taking NSAIDs, make sure you take them with food and never on an empty stomach. Furthermore, never combine aspirin and NSAIDs. The combined use of these two medications can put you at extremely high risk for ulcers and intestinal bleeding.

Another potential risk in taking NSAIDs bears mentioning. By irritating and inflaming the lining of the GI tract, the medications may make your intestinal lining more permeable to food allergens and different bacteria. If this occurs, these food allergens and bacteria are more likely to gain access into the blood stream and further worsen your arthritic symptoms. These medicines are obviously not cure-alls and, in some instances, have actually been associated with worsening of symptoms.

For many years, aspirin has been the old standby used in the treatment of arthritis. Even though it works well as an anti-inflammatory and pain-relieving substance, aspirin, too, has been associated with gastrointestinal irritation, inflammation, and possible intestinal bleeding. The most recent recommendation by The American College of Rheumatology suggests that acetaminophen (commonly know as Tylenol) should be the first choice in treating osteoarthritis. I recommend using up to 4,000 mg per day to help control the pain.

Once again, acetaminophen provides only symptomatic relief and does not improve joint function or repair the degenerative process. High doses of acetaminophen also may cause kidney and liver impairment, especially if you're drinking alcohol as well. If acetaminophen is unsuccessful, try either aspirin or anti-inflammatories, such as ibuprofen or naproxen.

189

Note from Your Doctor

People who use NSAIDs have three times the risk of gastrointestinal bleeds than non-users. Up to 3 percent of the users may experience a significant GI bleed, and up to 25 percent of NSAID users may require medications to treat ulcers. I strongly urge you to look at other options in dealing with your arthritis.

I hope you get the point by now. NSAIDs and other medications certainly do not provide the whole answer for arthritis. They may reduce some of your symptoms, but the longer you use them, the greater risk you face of suffering from their side effects. The best solution is to put on that all-important Director of Prevention hat and do your best to prevent this disease in the first place.

Diet and Arthritis

Just as diet plays an important role in heart disease, cancer, and osteoporosis prevention, we can't neglect the importance of diet in the prevention and control of arthritis. First of all, maintaining your ideal body weight is absolutely essential in the development and progression of this disease. Can you imagine what it would be like to put a 30 pound bag of books or bricks in a backpack and carry that around with you all day? Over time, added weight puts extra stress on your joints, damages the cartilage, and worsens your symptoms.

Recently, The Centers for Disease Control found that men or women who are overweight are 30 percent more likely to develop arthritis than their lean counterparts. Weight loss can take some of the load off your joints—especially your knees and hips—and help reduce pain, stiffness, and other arthritic symptoms.

Some arthritic patients have been found to be deficient in certain vitamins and minerals. Generally speaking, people with arthritis tend to have lower intake of B vitamins, vitamin C, vitamin E, and beta carotene. They also tend to eat higher amounts of dietary fat and fewer carbohydrates, less fiber, and fewer fresh fruits and vegetables.

Some people have found that fasting may help relieve the pain of acute rheumatoid arthritis. I don't recommend this for a long period of time because it would mean drinking only water for one to three days. (Obviously, it would be impractical to fast for longer than that.) Some experts postulate that food allergies may also aggravate arthritis, which may explain the advantage that some people have had upon fasting. Although your specific food allergens may vary, the most common foods to contribute to arthritis include milk, wheat, eggs, corn, citrus, and pork.

You may also find that you're able to reduce your arthritic symptoms by leaning more toward a vegetarian diet. Plant-based foods are high in naturally occurring flavonoids, which have strong anti-inflammatory properties. Fruits and vegetables may also be valuable because they contain many of the vitamins and minerals that so much of the population lacks.

However, one word of caution: Even though veggies are generally healthy for you, some foods belonging to the nightshade family can worsen arthritic pain and stiffness. Dr. Norman Childers, professor of Horticultural Sciences at The University of Florida, believes that potatoes, tomatoes, eggplant, peppers, cayenne, and paprika should be avoided. These foods put out a small amount of a naturally occurring substance known as solanine that Dr. Childers has found to be troublesome to the joints. While many experts disagree with his theory, I see nothing wrong with a three-month nightshade-free diet. In my experience, a small minority of patients have found this to be quite helpful.

Totally Toxic

Fasting is certainly not for everyone. If you are pregnant or lactating, or if you're taking heart medications, fasting is a real no-no. And if you've had problems with liver damage, kidney troubles, anemia, diabetes, cancer, or AIDS, fasting would not be advisable.

While diet alone is probably not the cause or the cure for arthritis, sensible dietary guidelines are certainly advisable. The following may help you reduce your symptoms:

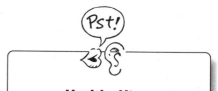

Healthy Hints

Tobacco is also a member of the nightshade family. If you're still smoking cigarettes and have arthritis, this is another good reason to kick the habit.

➤ Increase your intake of fresh fish, especially cold-water fatty fish such as salmon, tuna, sardines, swordfish, sea bass, and anchovies. Try to eat at least three to four servings of fish per week that are high in Omega-3 fatty acids. These types of fats reduce the production of hormone-like prostaglandins.

➤ Optimize your intake of fresh fruit, vegetables, whole grains, and fiber-containing beans. Switching to a vegetarian-like diet may help reduce morning stiffness, joint pain, and swollen joints.

➤ Eat plenty of foods rich in vitamin C, which aids in the formation of collagen, the connective tissue that helps repair cartilage. Furthermore, vitamin C is an antioxidant and has a mild anti-inflammatory effect.

➤ Avoid foods that you may be allergic to and that might worsen your symptoms. Try to eliminate these foods for two weeks, and then reintroduce one every other day to see if they aggravate your symptoms.

➤ Drink a cup or two of ginger tea per day. Ginger has natural anti-inflammatory effects and can help reduce swelling, morning stiffness, and pain, as well as improve your joint mobility.

When selecting fish, try to find those that are highest in the Omega-3 oils. Remember, these kinds of fats have anti-inflammatory effects and may help reduce your symptoms of arthritis.

Fish (3 ounces)	Omega-3 Fats (grams)
Anchovies, canned	1.76
Pink salmon, canned	1.45
Blue fin tuna, broiled	1.28
Atlantic sardines, canned	1.26
Swordfish, broiled	0.90
Oysters, steamed	0.81
Muscles, steamed	0.70
Salmon, smoked	0.38

Supplements You Should Reach For

Because arthritis increases the amount of free radicals produced in your body (which can then damage your joints and other tissues), antioxidants should be an important part of arthritis treatment. Not only can they help counteract free radical damage, but they also may slow the progression of the disease.

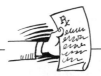

Note from Your Doctor

For Niacinamide to be helpful in the treatment of osteoarthritis, Dr. Kaufman found the necessary dose to be rather large, at anywhere from 500 mg to 1,000 mg three times per day. At this dose, some potential for liver problems exists, and I would recommend that you have your blood checked for liver enzymes every three months for one year, and then annually thereafter.

Let's take a look at some of the more important antioxidants and their role in arthritis:

➤ Boosting your intake of vitamin E has been found to reduce pain. A dose of 600 IU twice per day was particularly helpful in people with rheumatoid arthritis. Vitamin E may also lessen the inflammation associated with osteoarthritis. Taking 600 IU per day for 10 days provides significant reduction in pain, compared to people who do not take vitamin E. I frequently recommend taking 100 to 200 micrograms of selenium along with vitamin E because it enhances its effectiveness. Furthermore, selenium has an antioxidant effect of its own and has been found to be low in many people with arthritis.

➤ The B vitamin pantothenic acid, also known as B_5, has been found to be deficient in people with rheumatoid arthritis. Taking anywhere from 250 mg to 500 mg per day may provide marked improvement in morning stiffness and reduce the pain associated with arthritis.

➤ As mentioned earlier, vitamin C is helpful in the formation of collagen, which forms the protein network that's the foundation for many tissues, including cartilage, bone, tendons, and muscles. Vitamin C has an anti-inflammatory affect, can gobble up those free radicals, and might encourage the growth of new cartilage. It also works together with vitamin E to protect cartilage from breaking down.

➤ Niacinamide, a form of vitamin B_3, has been very useful in reducing symptoms of osteoarthritis. It is particularly helpful in relieving joint swelling and pain, as well as improving muscle strength, mobility, and range of motion. No one knows exactly why this treatment works, but it's thought to improve the metabolism of cartilage. Pioneering work on the relationship between niacinamide and osteoarthritis was conducted by Dr. William Kaufman, who found this therapy to be effective in more than 1,000 patients.

➤ One of the promising herbs for rheumatoid arthritis is curcumin, the yellow pigment that gives turmeric its color. Curcumin is a wonderful anti-inflammatory that can improve mobility and decrease morning stiffness and joint swelling. I usually recommend 400 mg three times per day with meals.

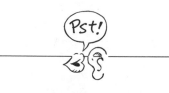

Healthy Hints

Applying capsaicin cream, a chili pepper extract, can help reduce pain associated with arthritis by depleting a chemical in the nerves known as substance P. Substance P is responsible for sending pain messages to the brain. Capsaicin may initially cause a burning sensation on the skin, but this is usually short-lived. Make sure you wash your hands thoroughly soon after applying it.

Taking a well-balanced multivitamin with minerals is certainly advisable because people with arthritis are frequently deficient in vitamin C, vitamin E, beta carotene, and B-vitamins.

The Glucosamine Sulfate Secret

One of the more popular therapies in the treatment of arthritis in recent years has been the use of glucosamine sulfate. This substance is an essential component of cartilage, and supplements can help reduce the pain associated with osteoarthritis and improve joint mobility. In fact, its pain-killing effect may be as good or better than ibuprofen. However, most people find that it takes at least eight weeks before its beneficial effects kick in.

Another component to cartilage is known as chondroitin sulfate. This compound, too, can help stimulate the production of new cartilage, and it has been shown to also reduce pain and improve joint mobility associated with arthritis. Both chondroitin and glucosamine sulfate work well together and serve as a dynamic duo to improve the symptoms of arthritis. Both are very safe but must be taken on a regular basis. I frequently recommend 500 mg of glucosamine sulfate three times per day, along with 250 mg three times per day of chondroitin sulfate.

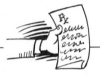

Note from Your Doctor

Glucosamine sulfate is not the only form of glucosamine. In a health food store you can also find glucosamine hydrochloride and N-acetyl-glucosamine. Although it may be slightly more expensive, glucosamine sulfate appears to be more effective and is more readily absorbed into the body than the other forms.

Funky Fish Oils

As previously mentioned, eating fish containing Omega-3 fatty acids has been of great value in reducing the symptoms of rheumatoid arthritis. Fish oil is high in fatty acids known as eicosapentaenoic acid (EPA) and docosahexaenoic acid (DHA). Both substances have strong anti-inflammatory effects and have been helpful in reducing the joint pain associated with rheumatoid arthritis. When used in conjunction with standard antiarthritic medications, fish oil seems to have an additional benefit. In fact, most people have been able to reduce their dosage of NSAIDs when they also concurrently take Omega-3 fish oils.

Even though EPA and DHA capsules are very effective in reducing pain and stiffness associated with rheumatoid arthritis, some of you may have difficulty tolerating them; as such, it's best to take these capsules with meals and not on an empty stomach. Other unpleasant side effects can include belching, indigestion, and diarrhea. A newer form, known as enteric-coated fish oil capsules (delayed-release), seems to be tolerated better. This form also is very efficient in reducing inflammation and alleviating the symptoms of arthritis. As another side benefit, Omega-3 oils reduce your triglyceride level, thus decreasing your risks of heart disease.

One of the more exciting anti-inflammatories that has worked quite impressively in both osteoarthritis and rheumatoid arthritis is derived from an ancient Indian traditional form of healing known as ayurvedic medicine. This substance, known as boswellia, inhibits some of the inflammatory pathways responsible for the pain and swelling of arthritis. A standardized extract of boswellia is now available in dietary supplements, and numerous studies have shown that it's capable of reducing joint swelling, increasing joint mobility, and lessening morning stiffness. More importantly, perhaps, boswellia can improve the overall quality of life and activity in people affected with arthritis.

Boswellia can be taken in capsule form or applied topically. It can be used along with other nutritional therapies and is tolerated quite well.

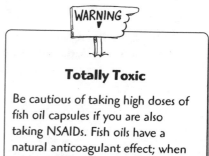

Totally Toxic

Be cautious of taking high doses of fish oil capsules if you are also taking NSAIDs. Fish oils have a natural anticoagulant effect; when taken in combination with NSAIDs, fish oil could increase your risk for gastrointestinal ulcers and bleeding.

Arthritis and Exercise

Keeping fit and staying physically active are certainly assets to anyone suffering from arthritis. If your joints are swollen and painful, you're probably not going to be in the mood to exercise. But keep in mind that, overall, physical activity can help prevent swelling, stiffness, and pain in the joints. It can also help build muscle tone and strength, which can take some of the stress and pressure off the joints. Generally speaking, people who exercise are at lower risk for developing arthritis in the first place. So get used to doing regular exercise to prevent arthritis later in life.

Even if you've already developed some early arthritis, it's not too late. Starting an exercise program can still help get the disease under control. Be sure to stretch each day, especially before exercise, to stretch the joints, reduce stiffness, improve flexibility, and make you feel more limber. A recent study indicated that regular walking, stretching, and weight-lifting could help people with arthritis reduce pain in the knees and improve their range of motion by nearly 30 percent.

To begin a joint friendly exercise program, follow these guidelines:

➤ Get in the habit of walking, swimming, cycling, and stretching at least three days per week. Try to do at least 30 minutes per session. If you notice you're too stiff in the morning, do your exercise later in the afternoon. (Chapter 22 discusses exercise in greater detail.)

➤ It's a good idea to stretch before going to sleep. This may help reduce some of the morning stiffness and make you more flexible when you wake up.

➤ Get involved in either Tai Chi or yoga. Correctly done, both activities are wonderful for your joints and do not put stress or pressure on your bones. They help increase flexibility and range of motion, and can even help build strength. Better yet, you'll feel better, seem more relaxed, and probably get a better night's sleep.

➤ If you have arthritis in the hands or wrists, it's a good idea to buy a sponge ball or putty and exercise your fingers while watching TV or simply taking it easy. You may want to soak your hands in warm water after getting up in the morning.

Note from Your Doctor

If you have arthritis, you might find that working with a physical therapist is helpful in starting and maintaining a good stretching and exercise program. It's important not to force your movements, motions, or stretches. Consult with a physical therapist to start on a healthy exercise program.

The Least You Need to Know

➤ *Arthritis* is a general term covering various conditions causing joint pain. The most common forms are osteoarthritis and rheumatoid arthritis.

➤ Even though NSAIDs (anti–inflammatories) might alleviate the symptoms of arthritis, their potential dangers may far outweigh their benefits.

➤ Dietary changes to help fight arthritis symptoms include eating more fresh fish and avoiding foods to which you're allergic.

➤ Important supplements include vitamins B_3, B_5, C, and E.

➤ Consider using glucosamine sulfate in conjunction with chondroitin.

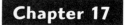

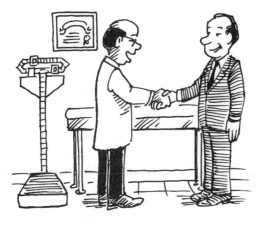

Chapter 17

Solving Prostate Symptoms

In This Chapter

➤ What is the prostate?

➤ What are the symptoms of an enlarged prostate?

➤ Is prescription medication or surgery for you?

➤ The advantages of proper diet and dietary supplements

You're now waking up two to three times in the middle of the night to urinate. Soon after urinating, you feel like you have to go again. Furthermore, your stream is not as strong as it once was. What's going on here? As you proceed into your middle ages, chances are your prostate gland begins to enlarge. Whereas you used to sleep like a baby, now you're troubled with interrupted sleep. This scenario is almost as common as developing those strands of gray hair or wrinkles around your eyes that we discussed in Chapter 2.

Where Is That Thing Anyway?

The prostate gland is a chestnut-shaped organ located just below the bladder and in front of the rectum. It surrounds a portion of the urethra, the tube that transports urine from the bladder to outside the body. It's responsible for producing a portion of the semen, which it secretes into the urethra during ejaculation. The prostate also secretes a fluid that the sperm cells need for nourishment as they exit the body.

From birth to puberty, very little growth of the prostate gland takes place; however, during puberty the gland begins to enlarge, at which time it may double in size and weight. The average weight of the adult prostate gland is approximately 20 grams—that's about two-thirds of a ounce. However, as you proceed into your 40s, 50s, and 60s, your prostate gland frequently begins to enlarge. This condition is known as benign prostatic hyperplasia (BPH).

Is Prostate Enlargement Inevitable?

Even though the prostate gland enlarges as you get older, it may be possible to slow the growth enough to avoid surgery or drugs. BPH creates a significant problem for men as they proceed into their middle and older ages. As the prostate gland enlarges, it can put pressure on the urethra, causing urine to back up into the ureters. The ureters, which normally carry urine from the kidneys to the bladder, may then become dilated, which can lead to kidney disease and eventually kidney failure. Also, as the prostate enlarges, you notice that you have to urinate much more frequently because the bladder may not fully empty each time. This can become a significant problem, especially at night, and can interrupt your sleep pattern.

Note from Your Doctor

In light of the magnitude of prostate cancer, research dollars are greatly neglected. The U.S. government spends only about $13 million per year to research prostate cancer, compared to $77 million on breast cancer, and $750 million dollars on AIDS research.

Take a look at these statistics:

➤ More than half of all men over age 50 have an enlarged prostate. By age 80, that percentage increases to nearly 80 percent.

➤ Half of the men with BPH have symptoms, and about a quarter of these people undergo surgery to alleviate their symptoms.

➤ Nearly 10 percent of all men in the United States will undergo a prostate procedure during their lifetime.

➤ The annual medical cost for managing prostate enlargement exceeds $3 billion per year in the United States.

➤ Prostate surgery is the second most common surgery for men over age 65, with more than 400,000 surgeries being performed each year (cataract surgery is number one).

➤ The prostate gland accounts for more than five million doctor's visits, 950,000 hospitalizations, and 44,000 prostate-related deaths each year in the United States.

Symptoms of Enlargement

It seems that the main risk factor for developing prostate enlargement is simply getting older. Most men begin to notice symptoms after the age of 50. Some of the more common symptoms include the following:

➤ Decrease in the force and magnitude of urinary flow.

➤ Trouble initiating urine flow (known as hesitancy).

➤ Trouble shutting off the urine flow. This is known as dribbling.

➤ Feeling of fullness in the bladder, even after urinating.

➤ As BPH worsens, you may notice having to wake up in the middle of the night to urinate (known as nocturia) and being unable to voluntarily control your urine flow (known as incontinence).

Diagnosing BPH

The first part of diagnosing BPH is experiencing the symptoms just discussed. If you suspect that your prostate may be enlarging, your doctor may begin by performing a digital rectal exam (DRE). Because the prostate gland rests in front of the rectum, your doctor will be able to feel if the gland is swollen or enlarged, or if it has growths or nodules. If he suspects that there may be a problem, he might suggest a blood test known as prostate specific antigen (PSA).

PSA is a protein that's produced by the prostate gland, and it begins to rise whether you have simple enlargement, inflammation, or a cancerous growth of the prostate gland. The normal level for PSA is 0 to 4 nanograms (ng). A level above 10 is thought to be highly suggestive of prostate cancer. If your PSA is 4 to 10 ng, this frequently serves as more of an indicator of either BPH or prostatitis, inflammation of the prostate gland.

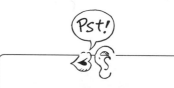

Healthy Hints

The PSA can be abnormally elevated after a long bicycle ride or after engaging in sexual activity. Refrain from either of these activities for at least 24 hours prior to having this blood test performed.

Some doctors also elect to perform a urinary flow study to help diagnose BPH. They use an instrument called a urinary flow meter to measure the speed of urine as it is eliminated through the urethra during urination. As the prostate gland begins to enlarge, the velocity of urine flow begins to decline. As you advance in age, the rate of urinary flow begins to decline.

What Causes BPH?

At least two necessary factors contribute to enlargement of the prostate gland. The first is aging. While prostate enlargement might not occur in your 20s or 30s, it might occur in your 40s and continue as you proceed into your later years.

The second factor that seems to be necessary is the production of a substance known as dihydro-testosterone (DHT). DHT is formed within the prostate from the production of testosterone, secreted by the testes. Most authorities agree that the production of excessive amounts of DHT in the prostate gland can cause enlargement. Most of the current pharmaceutical therapies available have therefore focused on reducing DHT levels by inhibiting a specific enzyme known as 5-Alpha Reductase. This enzyme stimulates the conversion of testosterone to DHT; if it's inhibited, DHT cannot accumulate.

By now, I think you get the point. Although the prostate is a small gland, it can lead to big problems.

Is Proscar Your Only Option?

As mentioned, most pharmaceuticals have focused on shutting off the production of the enzyme that causes the buildup of DHT, the naturally-occurring substance thought to be responsible for BPH. A few years ago, the FDA approved a new drug to help treat benign prostatic hyperplasia. This drug is known as finasteride (Proscar), which quickly reached sales of $1 billion per year. This medication is thought to improve the symptoms of BPH and reduce the risks associated with urinary retention. Although some men have found it to be very useful, more than 50 percent have found it to be no better than a placebo after taking it for a full year. Proscar is relatively expensive and has some unpleasant side effects associated with it. You might find a decrease in your libido, problems with ejaculation, or impotency. Many men have had to discontinue the use of this medicine due to the unpleasant side effects.

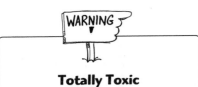

Totally Toxic

Proscar has profound detrimental effects in pregnant women. Women who are planning to become pregnant or who are pregnant should not even handle this drug or expose themselves to the semen of men who are taking it. Proscar has been shown to cause birth defects.

Besides Proscar, a few other medications have also been approved for BPH. These include Cardura, Flomax, and Hytrin. All have similar side effects and a limited degree of efficacy. Quite simply, the clinical improvement that most men notice has been very minimal and disappointing.

Avoiding Surgery

If all else fails, have surgery. Right? Wrong. Before you opt to have surgery, try your hand at numerous lifestyle changes, nutritional modifications, and a variety of supplements, all of which may do the trick and prevent further enlargement of the prostate gland. Moreover, in evaluating five studies on the natural course of BPH in men who were followed for five years, the following was found: 40 percent will improve, 45 percent will show no change, and only 15 percent will worsen. This is one of the reasons why watchful waiting when you're first diagnosed with BPH should be strongly considered as one of your options. Even in light of the new drugs on the market and the surgical procedures, it seems that only 15 percent will get worse. The problem is, however, there is still no way of telling who might get better, who may stay the same, and who may deteriorate.

The most common surgical procedure performed to reduce the size of the prostate gland is known as a transurethral resection of the prostate (TURP). During this procedure, a urologist inserts an instrument known as a cystoscope into the penis and through the urethra. He then advances the scope and trims the portion of the prostate tissue that is impinging on the urethra. This helps relieve pressure around the urethra and the bladder so that you're once again able to urinate more freely, with better force, and with less frequency.

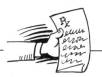

Note from Your Doctor

In addition to TURP, urologists are also using some newer techniques to treat BPH: 1) laser prostatectomy; 2) microwave therapy; 3) prostatic stents; 4) transurethral incision of the prostate (TUIP). TUIP seems to have fewer complications and a shorter recovery time. All these procedures have their pluses and minuses. Before opting for any surgery, discuss these with your surgeon.

This procedure can be of great benefit to many men as they age. Most note that their symptoms are greatly reduced and that urine flow improves. At least 75 percent who have had a TURP report being satisfied and are better able to urinate. Sounds good doesn't it? But here are some of the problems associated with this procedure:

➤ Up to 25 percent of the men who have had a TURP do not have satisfactory results. In fact, 15 to 20 percent require second surgeries.

➤ Up to 75 percent begin to experience what's known as retrograde ejaculation, which means that the semen is discharged backward into the bladder instead of going out of the body.

➤ About 5 to 10 percent report becoming sexually impotent.

➤ Urinary incontinence occurs in 2 to 4 percent.

➤ Post-operatively, urinary tract infections are quite frequent and occur in 5 to 10 percent of the cases.

So a TURP has its inherent problems. Although many of you may have had successful outcomes, I hear the ones with the complaints each and every week. For these reasons, more of you are probably going to be looking for alternative options to help cope with your prostate problems. Fortunately, some natural therapies may be able to "come to the rescue."

Food Factors for Prostate Power

As with all your body parts, giving them proper nutrition helps make them healthier. You can't expect your engine to run well without providing the key ingredients for preventing it from deteriorating and keeping it in top condition. Unfortunately, most conventional therapies for prostate disorders focus solely on reducing symptoms by using either drugs or surgery. But it's quite possible that dietary manipulation, lifestyle changes, and natural, non-prescription therapies can do wonders to prevent and treat BPH.

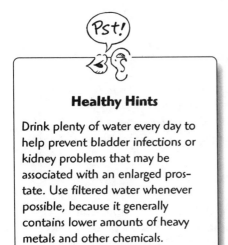

Healthy Hints

Drink plenty of water every day to help prevent bladder infections or kidney problems that may be associated with an enlarged prostate. Use filtered water whenever possible, because it generally contains lower amounts of heavy metals and other chemicals.

Follow a healthful, low-fat, high-fiber diet, and prevent yourself from becoming overweight. Wholesome foods emphasizing fruits, vegetables, whole grains, modest amounts of nuts and seeds, lean meats, fish, and modest amounts of eggs and dairy products are advisable. Try to minimize your intake of cake, pies, donuts, candy, and fast foods high in sugar and saturated fat. Also minimize your intake of alcohol and white flour products, such as white bread, white pasta, and white rice.

Keeping your waistline svelte can help improve your symptoms of prostate enlargement. Men who have a waistline of 43 inches or greater are 50 percent more likely to complain of symptoms of BPH or to require surgery for this condition, compared to men of normal weight. Losing about 35 pounds and bringing down your waistline by about 7 inches may help prevent and treat prostate enlargement. That's why it's so important to eat a whole-foods diet that restricts alcohol, sugar, and saturated fat. Doing some regular exercise at least 20 to 30 minutes three days per week should be helpful. Try walking, swimming, biking, or jogging.

Botanical Solutions

As mentioned earlier, medications such as Proscar are becoming a popular treatment for prostate enlargement. Unfortunately, this treatment has not been as effective as many patients would like. An herbal therapy, however, has been extremely helpful in managing BPH. Saw-palmetto berry extract, also known as Serenoa repens, has been used quite successfully in thousands of patients. It's been shown to reduce the symptoms of moderate BPH, including poor blood flow, urinary frequency, and prostate swelling. The dosage that seems most helpful is 160 mg two times per day. Most men notice an improvement in your symptoms within 8 to 10 weeks.

Saw-palmetto is thought to work by inhibiting the enzyme 5-Alpha Reductase, which inhibits the conversion of testosterone to DHT. Numerous well-controlled scientific studies all confirm the positive effects of saw-palmetto. Many report improvement in the velocity of urine flow, night urination, frequent urination, and the amount of urine left in the bladder after voiding. In fact, when tested against the drug Proscar, saw-palmetto extract was found to be superior. Furthermore, it costs only one-fourth the price and produces no known side effects. It sounds to me that this herb should perhaps be tried first before taking other prescription medications.

Another herb that seems beneficial for the prostate is pygeum africanum. Pygeum is actually an evergreen tree that grows as high as 100 feet tall in central and southern Africa. It has been used since the early 1980s in Germany for the treatment of BPH. Additional benefits result when pygeum africanum is combined with saw-palmetto, and the two together can help relieve BPH symptoms. A dose of 100 mg of the standardized pygeum africanum extract may help to improve your symptoms of urinary frequency, urgency, and painful urination, as well as enhance your urinary flow. A small number of men may experience some gastrointestinal symptoms upon taking pygeum, but the benefits greatly outweigh this small inconvenience. In France, nearly 80 percent of the prescriptions for prostate enlargement include this herb.

As mentioned in Chapter 10, stinging nettles (urtica dioica) is frequently used to help reduce symptoms of allergies and sinusitis. But there's another very important use for this herb as well. When stinging nettles is combined with pygeum africanum, it improves urinary flow and results in less residual urine left in the bladder. Both of these herbs also seem to inhibit the 5-alpha reductase enzyme, similar to the action of saw-palmetto.

Note from Your Doctor

The helpful dosage of stinging nettles is one 300 mg capsule of the standardized extract twice per day, combined with 50 to 100 mg of the standardized extract of the bark of pygeum africanum. Combine these with saw-palmetto for a greater effect. Some supplements in the health food stores contain all three of these herbs.

Nutrients Not to Be Missed

Along with the herbal therapies to reduce symptoms of BPH, specific nutrients should also be a part of the prostate power team. Because zinc is found in high concentrations in the prostate gland, it is thought that this mineral might play an important role in nourishing and maintaining the health of the gland. The normal prostate gland contains almost 10 times the amount of zinc than any other organ in the body. In one small study, in fact, 14 of 19 men experienced shrinkage of the prostate gland when they took zinc every day. Furthermore, high doses of zinc seems to inhibit the activity of the enzyme 5-alpha reductase so that the conversion of testosterone to DHT is less efficient.

Not all doctors feel that zinc is of value in treating enlarged prostate. When using large doses (in the 80 to 120 mg per day range), you need to be cautious about gastrointestinal upset or depleting your body of another mineral, copper. If you're considering taking more than 50 mg of zinc per day, you should consult with your physician first.

We've also recently learned about the benefits of vitamin E in protecting against prostate cancer. A recent study in Finland examined 27,000 male smokers taking just over 50 IU of vitamin E each day. Compared to those who were taking a placebo (dummy pill), those men taking vitamin E supplements had 32 percent fewer cases of prostate cancer. More impressively, 41 percent fewer prostate cancer deaths occurred among these men.

That's pretty powerful statistics, especially considering that these men were smokers. It's quite conceivable that the benefits could have even been better had the study tested nonsmokers. Also, keep in mind that the dosage of vitamin E was quite low—much lower than the typical dose used to treat and prevent cardiovascular disease and immune system weakness. It's quite possible that different dosages of the same vitamin may be more helpful in one disease than another. This is why individualizing the treatment in nutritional therapy and preventive medicine is so important; as you can see, one size doesn't fit all.

You may also find that amino acids provide some relief of BPH symptoms. Three, in particular—glycine, alanine, and glutamic acid—showed a 95 percent improvement in night urination, 81 percent improvement in urinary urgency, and 73 percent improvement in urinary frequency in a study examining 45 men. Even though not many scientific studies support the use of these amino acids, you might find them clinically helpful in reducing your symptoms. They can frequently be purchased along with the other vitamins and herbs in a "multiple prostate formula."

The prostate gland also concentrates some of the important essential fatty acids in its tissue, namely the Omega-3 and Omega-6 fatty acids. For this reason, it's a good idea to incorporate some flax seed oil, which is high in the Omega-3 fats, into your diet. Evening primrose oil capsules contain high amounts of Omega-6 oils, which can also play an important role in reducing BPH symptoms. Whenever taking fatty acids, take small amounts of vitamin E and selenium as well to prevent the oil from turning rancid. Other oils can be obtained eating pumpkin seeds or sunflower seeds, and they also contain a bit of zinc to support your prostate.

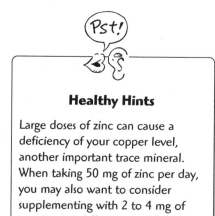

Healthy Hints

Large doses of zinc can cause a deficiency of your copper level, another important trace mineral. When taking 50 mg of zinc per day, you may also want to consider supplementing with 2 to 4 mg of copper at a different time during the day.

Note from Your Doctor

Tomatoes contain a "miracle nutrient," lycopene, an antioxidant that can significantly reduce your risk of developing prostate cancer, perhaps by as much as 35 percent. Cooking tomatoes, or cooking tomato sauce with oil, can also raise lycopene levels. So having that slice or two of pizza once in a while may not be so bad after all.

Following a wholesome food diet, keeping your weight down, and taking the appropriate vitamins, minerals, and herbs can go a long way toward keeping your prostate healthy.

The Least You Need to Know

➤ The prostate is a gland located below a man's bladder.

➤ When the prostate enlarges, it can interfere with various bodily functions.

➤ Although some men benefit from it, the prescription medication Proscar (Finasteride) is expensive and often ineffective.

➤ Surgery is not the cure-all for prostate problems; it can create a host of undesirable side effects.

➤ The best ways to fight prostate problems with diet include taking vitamin E and zinc—and don't forget Saw-Palmetto berry extract and Pygeum Africanum.

Chapter 18

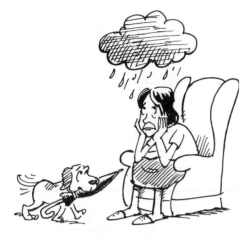

Depression Is Not a Prozac Deficiency

In This Chapter

➤ Why depression is such a feared condition

➤ Biochemistry's role in causing depression

➤ Does Prozac merit its popularity?

➤ Seasonal affective disorder

➤ The importance of diet and supplements in fighting depression

---

Ever had those days when you feel down in the dumps, you just can't get going, and life seems gloomy? Virtually everyone has had days when they wish that the sun would shine for just a little bit longer and that someone or something would bring them out of their doldrums. We've all had days like that—and, fortunately, we usually get over it. We know there's some good news not too far ahead and that when that week of rain has passed, the sun will come back out, the clouds will clear, and we'll see happier, more pleasurable days.

Unfortunately, not everyone comes out of their funk; some of you probably continue feeling blue. Things just aren't right, and you can't seem to climb out of those doldrums. While a little bit of ice cream or chocolate may pick you up for a short period of time, it's only temporary and doesn't offer lasting effects. Let's talk about ways of battling depression and what you can do to ensure that you look forward to a full and happy life every day.

Singing the Blues

If you're feeling more than a little blue, the scenario might go something like this: You go to your doctor and complain of feeling down or depressed. You're not sleeping as well anymore, and you've lost your zest for life. Your appetite may have decreased, you've lost interest in activities that you once thought were enjoyable, and you no longer feel a sense of worth. You may have experienced a loss in sexual drive, and now you're having difficulty concentrating. You may even have thoughts of death or suicide. These obviously are signs of classical depression. Most people report at least four or five of these symptoms for at least one month before they're diagnosed with depression.

Depression can happen to anyone, although it's more common with advancing age. Experts estimate that nearly 25 percent of us may experience some type of depression or mood disorder during our lifetime that requires medical attention. We're all familiar with the kind of depression that occurs after a significant emotional upset, such as a divorce, loss of a job, or the death of a loved one. Life is certainly full of its ups and downs, and depression can affect anyone of any age. It's much more common, however, if someone else in your family has had depression. Depression also may surface in teenagers as they move through adolescence, in people experiencing a mid-life crisis and in recent retirees. Hormonal fluctuations that may occur premenstrually, soon after the delivery of a baby, and during menopause also tend to make women more susceptible to depression.

Note from Your Doctor

An estimated 12 million Americans suffer from depression and do not even know it. Depression is frequently a condition that people prefer to hide because they dread being labeled as having depression. Symptoms usually come on slowly and can range from mild to very severe.

It's Not All in Your Head

Until recently, if you were troubled with depression, you were probably told, "It's all in your head." You may have been instructed to sit down on the psychologist's couch and were asked, "What happened during your childhood that caused depression as an adult? Did your baby-sitter spank you? Did you have an argument with your father?

Or did you not like the cod liver oil that your mother was forcing down your throat when you had that terrible cold at age 8?"

While your earlier years may play an important role in developing depression, it's now recognized that numerous factors should also be considered, such as dietary, physical, biochemical, psychosocial, and other lifestyle-induced factors.

Increasingly, depression is thought to be caused more by physiological factors than psychological matters. It's now believed that brain biochemistry plays an important role in why you may develop depression. As it turns out, your brain has millions of cells that transmit information and messages. These cells communicate through substances known as *neurotransmitters* produced by the brain cells, known as neurons.

More than 40 different neurotransmitters exist, and each has specific functions. For example, some are responsible for carrying the messages for memory, hunger, alertness, sleepiness, or movement. If an imbalance or deficiency in any of these brain messengers occurs, you may experience depression, anxiety, panic, obsessive-compulsive behavior, or memory loss.

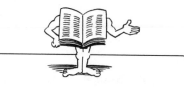

Body Language

Neurotransmitters are substances produced by the brain that send chemical messages from one cell to another. After carrying their messages, these neurotransmitters are either broken down or taken back up by the brain cells.

This new biochemical model has led to the development of a wide range of antidepressant drugs for the treatment of depression. As a result, many physicians today rely solely on the use of medications to treat this condition. In fact, the most common antidepressant, Prozac, has become the most widely prescribed psychiatric drug in the United States, with more than a million prescriptions written for it each month.

Prozac is a member of the new category of antidepressants known as selective serotonin reuptake inhibitors (SSRIs). Researchers report that the drug is effective in disorders ranging from anxiety to depression to obsessive-compulsive behaviors. Even though it has been extremely valuable for millions of people, Prozac also has a high degree of side effects. A high percentage of people experience nausea, headaches, anxiety, nervousness, insomnia, diarrhea, dry mouth, loss of appetite, sweating, tremors, or rashes. In addition, Prozac may inhibit ejaculation in men and orgasms in women. As a result of these side effects, many people have had to discontinue it.

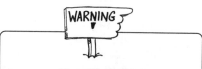

Totally Toxic

People taking Prozac may experience side effects that are actually some of the symptoms it was designed to alleviate. For example, 15 percent have experienced anxiety, 14 percent report insomnia, and 9 percent may lose their appetite.

Prozac is not the only medical therapy offered to treat depression. However, all drugs merely cover up the symptoms and do not truly address the causes of the problem. Let's take a look at some of the other available medications used to treat depression and their potential side effects.

Antidepressant	Side Effects
Tricyclic antidepressant (Tofranil, Elavil, Sinequan)	Headaches, dry mouth, nausea, jittery feelings, constipation, sweating, blurred vision, dizziness, sun sensitivity
Monoamine oxidase (MAO) inhibitors (Nardil, Parnate)	High or low blood pressure, weight gain, insomnia, sexual dysfunction
Selective serotonin reuptake inhibitors (SSRIs) (Prozac, Zoloft, Paxil)	Anxiety, nausea, insomnia, jittery feelings, dry mouth, loss of appetite, sexual dysfunction

The SSRIs have become the most popular drug therapy for treating depression. These medications work by elevating blood levels of the neurotransmitter serotonin, which can then improve your mood, sleep pattern, appetite, and sense of well-being. Fortunately, some dietary measures can be taken along with some natural supplements to combat depression. Why take an expensive and potent medication before trying safer, less expensive, and frequently more effective natural therapy?

Many doctors prescribe antidepressants to their patients because they are told they have a "chemical imbalance." Yet, the doctor does nothing to help find or diagnose this apparent imbalance. I've seen hundreds of patients who were placed on antidepressants by their physicians but never had their levels of neurotransmitters checked. If a deficiency of serotonin exists, for example, shouldn't that show up in the lab work? And if doctors treat patients with Prozac or related antidepressants, shouldn't they monitor the serotonin level to see that it's going up? That sounds rather logical to me.

Another strange treatment phenomenon presents something of a paradox. Many conventional doctors often are not willing to suggest or recommend a vitamin or mineral unless they find that you are deficient in it. For example, if you're not found to be deficient in B_{12}, they rarely suggest this B vitamin for depression. Yet, on the other hand, they are more than willing to prescribe drugs such as SSRIs without any knowledge of deficiency, excessive, or imbalance of the neurotransmitters, the substances they're purporting to treat. However, this viewpoint is slowly changing as more physicians are becoming more open-minded and are gaining interest in alternative and complementary medicine.

Note from Your Doctor

Quite a bit of controversy surrounds Prozac's ability to cause suicidal tendencies or violent behavior. Although this is highly controversial, the use of Prozac and other related medications should be reserved for only the most severe cases of depression, or only after other more natural therapies have been exhausted.

Overcoming Depression

You have a variety of options and alternatives to help you overcome depression. Changes in your diet can dramatically affect your levels of neurotransmitters and how you feel. We will discuss the specific nutrients to help you get rid of those blues, but first let's take a look at some of the dietary guidelines.

As mentioned earlier, raising your blood serotonin levels may help alleviate depression. As it turns out, serotonin is derived from the amino acid tryptophan, which is found in high-protein foods such as chicken, turkey, tuna, and tofu. But that's still not enough. It's necessary to also eat carbohydrate-rich foods, which prompt your pancreas to release the hormone insulin. Insulin then attracts other amino acids to be absorbed into your cells and allows for tryptophan to enter your brain to increase serotonin levels. So eating some tuna and a potato is not such as bad idea. Certainly stick to the complex carbohydrates, such as pasta and whole grains, and limit your intake of simple carbs, such as table sugar, sodas, and candy.

Another amino acid derived from protein-rich foods is tyrosine. Interestingly, tyrosine also helps elevate two additional neurotransmitters in your brain: dopamine and norepinephrine. Low levels of these two neurotransmitters have also been associated with depression, and increasing your levels can make you feel a whole lot better.

Try to decrease your intake of coffee, tea, chocolate, and sodas as well. They may initially boost your mood and give you a pick-up, but you may face a lull in your energy a few hours later.

Nearly 25 percent of people with depression are deficient in some of the B vitamins, most notably vitamins B_2, B_6, B_{12}, and folic acid. On top of this, many medications, including birth control pills and anti-inflammatories, can lower your blood level of vitamin B_6, which is so necessary for the production of serotonin and other brain chemicals. Having even marginal deficiencies of B vitamins may make you more susceptible to insomnia, irritability, depression, mood swings, and nervousness. In fact, one study showed that 79 percent of the patients with depression were deficient in vitamin B_6, compared to 29 percent of people without depression.

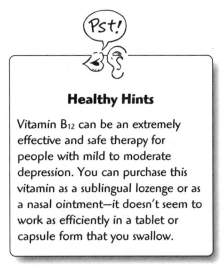

Healthy Hints

Vitamin B_{12} can be an extremely effective and safe therapy for people with mild to moderate depression. You can purchase this vitamin as a sublingual lozenge or as a nasal ointment—it doesn't seem to work as efficiently in a tablet or capsule form that you swallow.

B-complex supplements are probably important for almost anyone suffering from depression. These supplements can help elevate your mood, reduce insomnia, and increase appetite. Vitamin B_{12} is extremely helpful in combating symptoms of depression. Most commonly I administer this by intramuscular injection because it seems more efficient than taking B_{12} orally. I will frequently combine B_{12} with folic acid because a lack of folic acid has also been linked to depression.

Eating a low-fat diet may also help stabilize your mood and reverse depression. This may work because a low-fat diet generally is higher in nutrient-rich fiber containing foods packed with more vitamins and minerals. Try to avoid fried foods, remove the skin from chicken, and cut the fat off your meat. Switch from whole milk to 1 percent or skim milk, and choose low-fat cheeses.

Sugar Snacks

Perhaps one of the most effective dietary suggestions to combat depression is to remove as much sugar from your diet as possible. For many of you, simply removing sugar and caffeine may be all you need to do. You might at first think that eating sugary foods may give you a lift and pick you up, but most of the time the depression quickly returns after the sweets have been metabolized. Then what happens? You reach for another chocolate bar and repeat the cycle. You're not really addressing the problem, and your blood-sugar levels drop after a few hours, causing more depression. Furthermore, eating large amounts of refined, processed, sweet foods means that you're not eating the all-important vitamins and minerals to combat the problem in the first place.

Dietary Decisions for Depression

When trying to eat your way out of a depression, don't just reach for the cookie jar. Reach for healthy carbohydrates and lean proteins that can help boost your serotonin level. Here are some simple guidelines:

➤ Eat a wide variety of fresh fruit, vegetables, whole grains, beans, fish, chicken, and lean meats.

➤ Try not to overeat (something even I am guilty of once in a while). Spread your meals out throughout the day, and eat healthy snacks.

➤ Try to eat some complex carbohydrates at almost every meal. For example, at breakfast try some whole-grain waffles, pancakes, cereal, or French toast with fruit. At lunch and dinner, include some brown rice, millet, beans, pasta, potatoes, or vegetable soup along with the rest of your food. Snack on fresh fruit, yogurt, whole-grain crackers, almond or cashew butter, or baked tortilla chips and salsa.

➤ Limit your intake of sugar-filled desserts, such as cake, pie, donuts, ice cream, chocolate, or candy. Replace these foods with fresh fruit, dried fruit, or a granola bar.

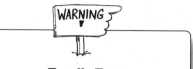

Totally Toxic

Try not to drink too much alcohol or caffeine. If you avoid these completely, be aware that at first you might experience headaches, fatigue, or dizziness due to withdrawal symptoms. However, after a week or so, your energy level and mood should improve.

➤ Try not to skip meals, because your blood-sugar level may fall, triggering depression. And chances are, if you skip a meal, you'll end up grabbing some fast food loaded with sweets or fried foods low in nutritional value.

➤ Drink plenty of water throughout the day.

➤ Make sure you're eating foods high in the B vitamins, such as fish, bananas, potatoes, sunflower seeds, lentils, broccoli, oranges, tofu, collard greens, avocado, chicken, brown rice, barley, and green, leafy vegetables. Keep in mind that it's preferable to avoid refined processed grains because more than 70 percent of the B vitamins have been removed.

Boost Your Energy with Exercise

Even if you're feeling down in the dumps, don't forget about regular exercise: It's actually a wonderful antidepressant. Taking a brisk walk for 30 minutes three times a week can be a powerful mood enhancer. Exercise helps stimulate the production of a brain substance known as *endorphins*, which can elevate your mood. The more consistent you are with exercise, and the more you do, the higher your endorphin levels will become.

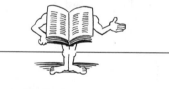

Body Language

Endorphins are pain-relieving and mood-elevating substances naturally produced by the brain in response to exercise. By increasing your brain endorphin production with brisk walking, biking, or jogging, you may be able to reduce your symptoms of depression.

Turning SAD into Glad

Have you ever woken up and driven off to work when it's still dark? And then, after working a long, hard day, get back into your car and drive home also in the dark? This is particularly prominent for some people living in the northern climates—especially in the winter, when the days grow progressively shorter. Many of you may notice that you don't feel quite as well between October and March when you're not getting exposed to natural sunlight much of the day or when it's too cold to go outside. Some of you may feel irritable, fatigued, desperate, and depressed, and you may struggle to maintain your weight. If these symptoms primarily occur during the winter, you may be troubled with seasonal affective disorder (SAD).

If you think you're troubled by SAD, you may notice intense cravings for carbohydrates—and a corresponding weight gain. Most of the time, these people aren't satisfied by eating the complex carbohydrates found in brown rice or potatoes; instead, they crave sweets found in chocolate, ice cream, and cake. Even though sweets may temporarily elevate your serotonin level, in the long run they worsen your symptoms. And remember, they don't supply the all-important essential vitamins and minerals needed to combat this problem.

One of the therapies you might want to try if you're suffering from a seasonal affective disorder is what's known as a full-spectrum light. This form of light has a wider range of wavelengths than your regular incandescent or fluorescent light bulbs. You can easily purchase these full-spectrum lights from a health food store or a mail-order catalog specializing in environmental products or nutrients. Try sitting in a room where the full-spectrum light is on for at least one to two hours per day. Even if you're cooking in the kitchen or watching television in the evening, simply having exposure to this light may be very helpful. Light therapy can help combat your depression because the light entering into your nervous system through your eyes modulates the release of your brain neurotransmitters.

Full-spectrum light therapy really presents no disadvantages, and it's worth a try. In fact, when I built my medical office and thought I might be spending 10 to 12 hours per day there, I outfitted the entire office with full-spectrum lights in place of the more standard fluorescent light bulbs. Considering that I'm now spending 14 to 16 hours per day in my office in an effort to complete this book, I think it was a good idea!

I Never Really Did Drugs

Even though drugs are still the mainstays of treatment for depression, a variety of other options are available. Try a more natural approach first, utilizing dietary changes, vitamins, minerals, herbs, amino acids, and any other safer and less-expensive modalities. Let's talk about some of the more popular and effective supplements now available.

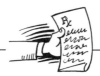

Note from Your Doctor

According to the *Journal of the American Medical Associates,* nearly 35 million Americans may suffer from seasonal affective disorder (SAD). It's particularly prevalent in the northern climates, such as Alaska, where up to 10 percent of the population may be affected. In Florida, where the sun shines brightly most of the day and people are more apt to engage in outdoor activities, only 1 percent of the population is affected.

St. John's Wort: Nature's Antidepressant

Perhaps the most popular herbal therapy for depression over the last three to five years is St. John's wort, also known as hypericum perforatum. This is the most frequently prescribed substance to treat mild to moderate depression in many European countries, including Germany. More than 25 well-controlled trials published in the scientific medical literature support the use of this herb for depression. The usual effective dose is 300 mg of the standardized 0.3 percent hypericin, two or three times per day. In fact, in head-to-head trials comparing St. John's wort to other standard antidepressant drugs, this herb has been found as effective and without the common side effects associated with standard antidepressants.

Although the exact mechanism that may account for St. John's wort's benefits are not completely understood, most evidence now indicates that it raises serotonin levels. St. John's wort can also come to the rescue if you're suffering from seasonal affective disorder (SAD). In a recent study of 20 people with SAD, four weeks' worth of St. John's wort significantly alleviated feelings of depression. Those people who added full-spectrum lights to the treatment program gained an even greater benefit.

Note from Your Doctor

It was initially thought that people taking St. John's wort should avoid excessive sun exposure because it would cause photosensitization (skin rashes when exposed to the sun). However, it now appears that photosensitivity from St. John's wort occurs only in animals, not in humans.

Although St. John's wort has almost no side effects, you should discuss it with your doctor if you are taking other antidepressants. He may consider tapering your prescription medication while slowly increasing your dose of St. John's wort.

5-HTP: The Mood Enhancer

One of the hottest treatments to enhance mood and alleviate depression has been the use of 5-HTP. (The full name is known as hydroxytryptophan, but it's certainly a lot easier calling it 5-HTP.) This medication is actually a brain chemical that is metabolized from tryptophan into serotonin. Because low serotonin levels have been associated with depression, and because many of the current pharmaceutical agents increase serotonin blood levels in the brain, scientists are looking for other effective ways to enhance serotonin status. 5-HTP may be the answer.

Tryptophan, which is naturally found in chicken, turkey, and milk, can be taken up by the brain cells. It is then transformed into 5-HTP before it is eventually converted into serotonin. Until 1989, tryptophan was available as a dietary supplement. However, a batch of it became contaminated by a bacteria during the manufacturing process; several people died, and more than 1,000 became ill. Tryptophan was then banned due to an outbreak of a condition known as eosinophilia-myalgia syndrome and has not been brought back into the market since then. However, 5-HTP is now available from your local health food store or pharmacy. To date, no suggestion of ill effects from 5-HTP has been reported.

Not only might 5-HTP help reduce symptoms of depression, but it also has been useful in curbing carbohydrate cravings, maintaining weight, improving sleep, relieving muscle aches and pains associated with fibromyalgia, and alleviating chronic headaches.

One of the more impressive studies supporting the efficacy of 5-HTP for depression evaluated 100 patients who had previously failed any conventional antidepressant therapy. Forty-three of these patients reported a complete recovery, and eight showed significant improvement. Even though that may look like only 50 percent of these patients improved, keep in mind that every one of these had previously tried conventional antidepressants—and, in fact, some had even undergone electric shock therapy.

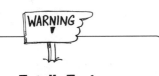

Totally Toxic

If you're already taking a prescription drug to treat your depression, be extremely cautious about taking 5-HTP because both can elevate your serotonin levels. Discuss this with your physician and continue under his supervision.

What happens if 5-HTP is tested against an SSRI, such as Prozac, Paxil, or Zoloft? Believe it or not, in those people taking 150 mg of a standard SSRI versus 100 mg of 5-HTP three times per day, the people taking 5-HTP showed a slightly better response. More importantly, whereas 20 to 65 percent of those taking the standard antidepressant reported significant side effects, only a handful of those taking 5-HTP had complaints.

The most common side effect from 5-HTP is mild nausea, which may occur only initially during the first few weeks of taking this substance.

The recommended starting dose for 5-HTP is 50 mg three times per day for mild to moderate depression. If you're not noticing any particular benefits after two to three weeks, consider increasing the dosage to 100 mg three times per day. Doses in the 900 mg per day range, however, reportedly caused nausea during the first six weeks in 70 percent of patients. The nausea, however, did not continue into the second six weeks.

Inositol: The Forgotten B Vitamin

Inositol is a little-known B vitamin that offers several benefits for your body: It may help lower cholesterol levels, reduce the accumulation of toxins in the liver, and improve the communication between nerve cells in the brain. Perhaps the most exciting recent news is inositol's ability to relieve symptoms of depression. Recent work out of Israel has shown that doses in the range of 6 to 12 grams per day could significantly improve your mood, anxiety, depression, insomnia, hopelessness, and agitation, all within four to eight weeks. Inositol doesn't seem to produce any significant side effects at all and should be considered as part of your depression treatment program.

NADH for Brain Energy

NADH is actually a newcomer to the field of nutritional supplements and natural healing. It's been proven to improve brain energy and shows great promise in treating conditions such as Alzheimer's disease, Parkinson's disease, chronic fatigue, and depression. It may help improve your energy, mood, stamina, and concentration as well.

NADH is actually a metabolite of vitamin B_3 that enhances the production of some important brain neurotransmitters, including dopamine, noradrenaline, and serotonin. In a recent clinical trial, nearly all patients given NADH for depression reported improvement in their symptoms and the absence of side effects or adverse reactions. NADH also may decrease your appetite and assist you in weight loss.

If you're considering taking NADH tablets or capsules, try finding those that are enteric-coated, a form that's not broken down by the stomach acid and thus can be more readily absorbed. The usual dosage of NADH if you're over age 50 is 2.5 to 5.0 mg per day; if you're younger, you may want to consider taking it every other day.

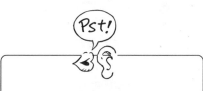

Healthy Hints

We're still learning a lot about the properties of NADH, but it may increase the production of your neurotransmitters in the brain by more than 40 percent.

Alternative Aminos

Tyrosine is an amino acid similar to tryptophan. You might find that taking tyrosine supplements can also pull you out of that depression. Many people with depression seem to have low levels of tyrosine circulating in the brain. Taking 500 mg three times per day between meals or with a carbohydrate, such as a glass of juice or a piece of fruit, can be an effective antidepressant.

Tyrosine works by stimulating your body's production of several neurotransmitters, including dopamine and norepinephrine. Another amino acid, phenylalanine, is also part of the building blocks to manufacture more neurotransmitters to improve alertness and decrease pain. You might find that 500 to 2,000 mg per day of this amino acid can greatly reduce your depression.

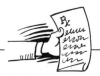

Note from Your Doctor

The form of phenylalanine that is more efficient for depression appears to be DL phenylalanine (DLPA). This can help you produce a substance in your body known as phenylethylamine (PEA), which helps you focus and, at the same time, has a mellowing effect. Incidentally, PEA is also found in chocolate. People with depression generally have low levels of PEA, which tells us that the phenylalanine is not being metabolized effectively. DLPA often works when all else fails.

A Freudian Slip

If no other treatments work, there's always counseling. I'm actually being a little facetious here: Counseling should probably be incorporated into any treatment program for depression. Various types of counseling and therapy may actually reduce your symptoms, and the key is to find the modality that works for you. Don't hesitate to call several therapists, and speak to them first to find out what techniques they commonly use. Talk to your friends, colleagues, physicians, neighbors, pharmacists, or health food store operators for suggestions.

Also try to find a therapist who does not suggest medications as a first line of treatment, but rather one who uses more subtle, gentle, and health-enhancing techniques. But don't expect miracles after one counseling session: That wouldn't be realistic. It may take several weeks, or perhaps even months, before you start to notice improvement.

It's Never Too Late to Make a Friend

If you're feeling down in the dumps and still singing the blues, get involved in a volunteer group, a church or synagogue group, or some other social function. Socializing is extremely important in combating depression. Don't lock yourself in your house, turn on the TV, turn down the lights, and eat. Find a friend who can encourage you, who is positive, and who can help you deal with your negative thoughts. In fact, consider purchasing a pet, perhaps a dog or a cat. You've heard that expression: A dog is man's best friend. He can also be a woman's best friend as well. This gives you a companion and a chance to go outside, take a walk, meet your neighbors, and take your mind off some of your problems.

Busy as a Bee

Get involved in community activities: Volunteering at a hospital or library gives you the opportunity to meet friendly people, to partake in activities, and to improve your physical well-being. If you have grandchildren, get involved in their activities and watch them play that afternoon little league game. Think about getting active in a book reading group, or perhaps playing cards with your friends on a weekly basis.

And there's always that all-encompassing Internet. If you haven't had a chance to learn about computers, take an adult class and find out how to surf the Web. There's a wealth of information on the Internet you can explore to learn new things or discover new areas of knowledge. In fact, you can communicate with other people as if you had a pen pal. If you're interested in sports, you can check out the latest scores. If you want to trade stocks, you can do that as well on the Internet. Thinking about taking a trip to a sunny island to get rid of those mid-winter blues; you can read about your destinations on the Internet as well.

The Least You Need to Know

➤ Although many people choose to ignore depression, more than 25 percent of all Americans have experienced depression serious enough to warrant medical treatment.

➤ Depression is largely "in your head"—in your brain chemistry, that is. It is not merely psychological.

➤ Prescription medicines such as Prozac can mask the symptoms of depression, but they do not address the causes.

➤ Specific dietary changes, such as decreasing sugar intake and eating a variety of foods, can help you overcome depression.

➤ Supplements helpful for fighting depression include 5-HTP, St. John's wort, inositol, and amino acids.

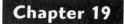

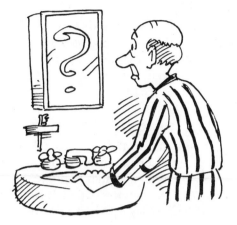

Chapter 19

Alzheimer's Disease

In This Chapter

➤ What is Alzheimer's disease?

➤ The symptoms of Alzheimer's

➤ General diet suggestions

➤ Supplements for avoiding Alzheimer's

You've just walked into your home, you put your keys down, and an hour later they're not there. In reality, you probably didn't put them on the counter, but you can't recall where you actually did put them. Or what about the times when you can't remember what you ate for dinner the night before? Or you can't recall whether your doctor's appointment is on Tuesday or Wednesday, just an hour after you've confirmed your appointment on Monday.

I'm sure you've had those types of experiences. We all forget different details about our life from day to day. But relax, that's not so abnormal. Just the very fact that you know you can't remember as well as you used to is actually a good sign. Even though you've probably had fears about developing Alzheimer's disease, I doubt you have it if you're actually worried about it. People with Alzheimer's disease generally deny having a memory problem in the first place.

Was I Always Like This?

You've all had those days when you don't seem to be able to remember your kid's name, your friend's phone number, or whether you took your medication. As you get older, chances are you don't feel as mentally sharp. You can't recall things as quickly as you used to. You're more easily confused. Simple tasks that you used to do with such fluidity are now becoming a real chore. As you get older, it seems that your memory begins to fail. You and your family members are starting to hope that you're not developing Alzheimer's disease.

Alzheimer's disease develops exceedingly slowly, perhaps over 6 to 10 years. You may have difficulty remembering events that occurred just yesterday or the day before. You may have trouble with names, dates, and places, and your personality may change. This is one of the most feared diseases to deal with because as it continues to progress, most people have difficulty taking care of themselves. You are then forced to rely on family members or health care professionals to help with everyday activities you once took for granted.

There's no question that Alzheimer's disease creeps up as you get older. It is currently the fourth-leading cause of death in the United States, just behind heart disease, cancer, and strokes. Approximately four million Americans are affected, and that number is expected to double by the year 2020—and perhaps triple by 2040—due to the rapid increase in the number of senior citizens. But unless you carry certain specific genes, you don't have to be one of them.

Alzheimer's Disease

Alzheimer's disease was discovered in 1906 when Dr. Alois Alzheimer, a German neurologist, performed an autopsy on the brain of a woman who had died after several years of progressive mental deterioration, including confusion and memory loss. He noted an unusual disorganization of the cells of the brain that were responsible for reasoning and memory. Some cells were bunched in rope-like knots, which he called neurofibrillary tangles. Alzheimer also saw an accumulation of debris around the nerve bundles, which he called senile plaques. He then speculated that the nerve tangles and plaques were responsible for the progressive dementia in this woman. When other similar findings were found in other patients after autopsies were also performed, this disease process was later named Alzheimer's disease.

The Dreaded Diagnosis

Unfortunately no simple technique exists by which to diagnose Alzheimer's disease with 100 percent certainty. The real diagnosis can be found at autopsy, when the brain tissue is investigated and found to have abnormal nerve cells bunched up like a knotted rope. These are known as *neurofibrillary tangles*. At autopsy, these tangles are usually accompanied by an accumulation of cellular debris, known as *senile plaques*.

When these two conditions are met, the patient is then said to have had Alzheimer's disease.

Obviously a lot of distress and anxiety can arise over whether your loved one really has Alzheimer's disease. But, unfortunately, no simple, quick, reliable, non-invasive test can accurately diagnose this disease. It's usually diagnosed based on a physical examination by a physician and the signs and symptoms exhibited.

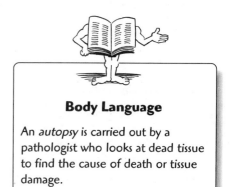

Body Language

An *autopsy* is carried out by a pathologist who looks at dead tissue to find the cause of death or tissue damage.

Although no simple test can diagnose whether you or your loved one suffers from Alzheimer's disease, your doctor may suggest some routine laboratory blood studies or a special x-ray imaging of the brain, such as a computed tomography (CT) scan or magnetic resonance imaging (MRI). Even though these studies are far from conclusive, they're the best we have at this point, especially in the early stages of the disease.

Alzheimer's disease is very uncommon in young people and rare in the middle ages, but as you advance through the years, it becomes increasingly more prevalent. An estimated 20 percent of people over the age of 80 may be affected.

Signs of Concern

However, Alzheimer's is certainly not an inevitable part of the aging process. We all know many elderly people who remain as sharp as a tack into their 80s and 90s. The symptoms of early Alzheimer's disease are quite varied and slow in onset. Some of the things to look out for include the following:

➤ Difficulty answering simple questions

➤ A loss of interest in hobbies or socializing with friends or acquaintances

➤ Problems with memory, especially involving more recent events

➤ Difficulty learning new information

➤ Trouble remembering names and appointments

As the disease progresses, these symptoms become more evident and more debilitating. Some people have difficulty taking care of themselves and getting dressed, lose interest in their appearance, and neglect personal hygiene.

What causes Alzheimer's disease? We're not quite sure yet. It appears that these tangles and knots that occur in the brain do play an important role, but some other partners in crime probably also contribute to this dreaded disease. One of the more recent theories centers on the formation of a blood protein known as Apo E. This protein, which normally carries cholesterol through the blood, also appears to carry the amyloid plaques, which are then deposited into the brain, where they then harden.

225

Totally Toxic

Recently, cigarette smoking has been shown to double the risk of Alzheimer's and other dementias. Smoking for only two years seems to double the risk of developing Alzheimer's, compared to those who have never smoked. However, smoking seems to increase the risk only in those people who do not have the gene for Alzheimer's disease, Apo E-4.

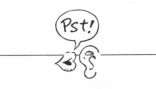

Healthy Hints

Aluminum may also be found in up to 50 percent of the municipal water supplies in the United States in an effort to help remove contaminants. Baking powder and some brands of table salt also contain small amounts of aluminum. To help prevent Alzheimer's, it's best to avoid sources of aluminum whenever possible.

One particular form of this protein, Apo E-4, has been implicated as a major risk factor for development of Alzheimer's disease. People with two copies of the Apo E-4 gene have been found to be eight times more likely to develop Alzheimer's, compared to those who did not inherit this gene. In one study that examined 46 people with Alzheimer's disease, 21.4 percent were found to have two Apo E-4 genes, compared to just 2.9 percent who were free of Apo E-4.

In addition to this new theory, researchers have found that this same gene carries LDL cholesterol (the bad cholesterol). Many now feel that when LDL is deposited into the brain tissue, it is highly susceptible to free radical damage. The brain is primarily composed of fatty tissue and is particularly prone to the damage inflicted by free radicals.

But don't lose all hope. Just as antioxidants help protect against free radical damage that may contribute to heart disease or cancer, antioxidants may also help protect against developing Alzheimer's disease—or at least delay its onset and progression.

A debate continues over whether aluminum found in your pots or pans or your antacids may contribute to Alzheimer's disease. High aluminum levels have been found in the brain of many Alzheimer's victims, but we're not sure if this toxic metal causes the disease. In the meantime, play it safe. It's best to avoid the use of aluminum-containing pots and pans, canned soft drinks, and aluminum-containing antacids and antiperspirants.

Tell Me Again About Diet

While there's no clear dietary cure for Alzheimer's, some logical and simple measures certainly improve your odds.

➤ Do your best to avoid sodas and excessive amounts of sweets. These foods are virtually devoid of important vitamins and trace minerals that are so helpful in improving brain transmission and memory.

➤ Do your best to avoid fried foods because the frying process causes more free radicals to form—and you certainly don't need that.

➤ Bolster your intake of fresh fruits, vegetables, and phytonutrient-containing beans and grains. These foods have high amounts of naturally occurring antioxidants to protect your brain from free radical damage.

➤ Control your alcohol intake, as it may deplete your stores of B vitamins and can contribute to memory loss.

➤ Limit your fat intake to no more than 25 percent of your total calories. Excessive fat can cause cholesterol to be deposited in the brain and lead to hardening of the arteries in the brain.

B Wise

There's no question that B-vitamins are important in maintaining healthy brain function. Vitamin B_1, also known as thiamine, is an important component of the neurotransmitter acetylcholine, which is involved in memory. In general, acetylcholine has been found to be low in people with Alzheimer's, and up to 37 percent of these patients may be deficient in vitamin B_1. One recent study showed that taking 3,000 to 8,000 mg of thiamine per day mildly improved memory. It certainly didn't cure the disease, but it may provide some hope. This dosage of thiamine is quite high, however, so take this amount only under the supervision of your physician.

You should also consider trying B_6, B_{12}, and folic acid if you're noticing signs of early Alzheimer's. All three B-vitamins have been shown to improve cognitive function tests in people with Alzheimer's. In addition, B_{12} deficiency is not too uncommon in the elderly population, the largest segment affected by Alzheimer's disease. B_{12} is important in maintaining healthy nerve tissue, which can account for why a deficiency may contribute to the progression of Alzheimer's.

Low levels of folic acid and B_6 have also been associated with Alzheimer's disease. It's thought that a deficiency of these B-vitamins can result in elevated levels of the blood protein homocysteine, which, when it accumulates in the brain, can function as a nerve toxin and impair memory and mental alertness. Again, all these B vitamins are very safe and are worth a try.

Healthy Hints

Simply trying a therapeutic trial of B_{12} injections may be a good idea for someone who has early Alzheimer's disease. This means receiving 1,000 mcg of B_{12} once or twice per week for a few months. This can be extremely helpful, especially because a deficiency of B_{12} in the brain may not show up in the standard laboratory tests. It's very safe, and you may even notice more energy and improved mental functioning.

Grab the Ginkgo

Of all the available herbs with a strong history of reducing Alzheimer's symptoms, ginkgo certainly ranks as my first choice. In fact, in Germany, it's the number-one agent prescribed for memory loss and symptoms that suggest Alzheimer's disease. As you may recall from earlier chapters, ginkgo is a potent antioxidant that can help protect the brain and circulatory system against the damage of free radicals.

Recently, the *Journal of The American Medical Association* published a study that found that 40 mg of ginkgo biloba extract taken three times per day could significantly improve the cognitive performance and social functioning of Alzheimer's patients. After six months, those who took ginkgo showed much less deterioration—and many actually improved. This is certainly not what you would expect to find with the natural course of this progressive disease. You would typically expect virtually everyone to get worse. Ginkgo has been shown to be not only an antioxidant but also an anti-inflammatory, and it may improve blood flow to the brain. It's certainly worth a try, as it is very well-tolerated and has no known side effects.

E and Me

Perhaps one of the most exciting areas in regard to Alzheimer's treatment is the use of vitamin E. As you know, this all-important fat-soluble vitamin helps boost your immune system, can cut your risk of heart disease, and helps you fight cancer. But now, we find that it might slow the progression of Alzheimer's disease. A few years ago, vitamin E was shown to protect brain cells from the damage caused by the destructive amyloid protein discussed earlier. However, that was found to occur in a test tube, and up until recently we didn't know whether vitamin E would have that protective effect in the human brain.

As it turns out, the answer is yes. Recently, a Columbia University College of Physicians and Surgeons researcher found that a combination of a Parkinson's drug and vitamin E could significantly slow the progression of Alzheimer's. A total of 341 patients who were moderately impaired with Alzheimer's were given daily doses of a Parkinson's drug known as selegiline hydrochloride, along with 200 IU daily of vitamin E. After two years, the patients who were given placebo progressed to severe Alzheimer's disease after about $14^1/_2$ months; however, those who took vitamin E supplements did not progress as rapidly—and didn't develop severe Alzheimer's until 22 months later, delaying the inevitable deterioration by $7^1/_2$ months. The drug selegiline also produced a similar effect.

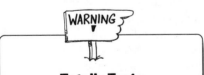

Totally Toxic

Vitamin E supplements are generally very safe and don't seem to have many side effects. However, if you're taking aspirin or blood-thinner drugs, you should probably talk to your doctor about your vitamin E dosage.

What might be going on here? It has been suggested that the strong antioxidant properties of vitamin E trap the free radicals that may damage brain cells. Selegiline may also act as an antioxidant. Both substances reduce damage to the neurons of the brain and may delay further deterioration in people with Alzheimer's.

Promising Possibilities

You also may want to try a little-known nutrient known as acetyl-L-carnitine. One recent study found that taking 3 gm of this substance daily for one year slowed the progression of Alzheimer's disease in people under the age of 65, though it didn't seem to do a whole lot for those who were older. One of the old standbys that has been used for many years to help with declining memory has been the use of lecithin, which is frequently used as a food additive in ice cream, margarine, mayonnaise, and chocolate bars. Lecithin contains choline and inositol, important building blocks for the neuro-transmitter acetylcholine. You might find that using lecithin granules, liquid, or capsules may sharpen your mind and improve your memory. You can simply add the granules to food such as applesauce, yogurt, or cereal.

Another dietary supplement related to lecithin, phosphatidyl serine (PS), is the newest guy on the block to assist brain function. It's absorbed very rapidly into the brain and has been shown to improve cognitive function, including the abilities to think clearly, to reason, and to remember. Several studies indicate that 300 mg of PS per day can help with a wide range of memory parameters. For example, you might be able to recall names, places, or faces more easily. Other people have reported that they can concentrate better while reading, conversing, or performing a variety of tasks.

No dangers appear to arise from long-term use of PS. A few people, however, experience nausea, which can be greatly reduced if you take it at mealtime. A very small number of people report that taking it before bedtime sometimes delays their ability to fall asleep. Try taking PS with breakfast in the morning to minimize this side effect.

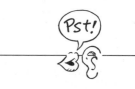

Healthy Hints

Phosphatidyl serine is derived from soy, and very small amounts are found in lecithin. PS is not found in foods and may be a valuable addition in the fight against Alzheimer's.

Helpful Hormones

We previously spoke about some of the important aspects of estrogen and other hormones in fighting menopause and osteoporosis. It appears that this all-important hormone may protect you from more than weakened bones and heart disease: The latest evidence also supports the use of estrogen against Alzheimer's disease. We now find that estrogen may also be a brain tonic and improve brain function, make you happier, cut down on mood swings, and improve your memory. In one study, it was able to cut the risk of developing Alzheimer's by 30 percent.

Another naturally occurring hormone produced by the adrenal gland that may help with brain function is DHEA (dehydroepiandrosterone). DHEA is found in extremely high concentrations in the brain and in the blood stream. Although the use of this substance in supplement form has been highly controversial, it nonetheless produces important physiological effects. Chapter 23 discusses these effects in greater detail. But for now, it's important to mention that low levels of DHEA in the blood and brain are thought to contribute to many symptoms of aging, including poor memory. People with Alzheimer's disease may have low blood levels of DHEA, and it may help improve your brain function and reverse many of the aspects of the aging process.

Although the use of hormones in the prevention and treatment of Alzheimer's disease is currently in its infancy, this is probably an area that shows great promise.

The Least You Need to Know

➤ Alzheimer's disease is characterized by memory loss, difficulty in learning, and a loss of interest in hobbies or socializing.

➤ Though many people fear Alzheimer's disease as they get older, it is not inevitable, and steps can be taken to avoid it.

➤ Dietary steps to avoiding Alzheimer's include reducing free radicals and moderating the intake of alcohol.

➤ Effective supplements include acetyl-L-carnitine, phosphatidyl serine, ginkgo biloba (which has few or no known side effects), and E.

➤ Useful hormones include estrogen and DHEA.

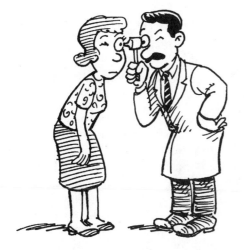

Chapter 20

Seeing Eye to Eye

In This Chapter

➤ Cataracts and antioxidants

➤ Preventing macular degeneration

➤ Helpful herbs

➤ Nutrients to use

Don't you hate it when you have to hold that book or magazine either closer to your face or farther from your eyes? If you're approaching perhaps your 45th or 50th birthday, you know what I mean. You can no longer see as well as you could when you were in your teenage years. In fact, you probably need glasses to read this book.

On the other hand, if you're still in your 20s or 30s, chances are that your vision is still sharp and you take it for granted. You wake up in the morning each day and just go about your way.

But unfortunately, with advancing age, eye disorders occur far too frequently. Whereas you may have had no difficulty reading those street signs several years ago, now they may just be a big blur. Let's talk about some of the most common eye problems that arise as you get older—and what you can do to prevent them and treat them more naturally.

20/20 on Prevention

Whether your eyes are blue, brown, green, or gray, they provide perhaps the most important sources of information you need in going about your daily life.

They allow you to read or watch TV. They allow you to watch your son's Little League game or your daughter's dance recital. We receive constant information consciously and subconsciously through the windows of our eyes.

That's why it's so important to take care of your eyes. You're only given two, and they're supposed to last your entire life. That's why I stress to my patients that they should have a full eye examination every year. Try to make it a point to see an ophthalmologist or a skilled optometrist on a routine basis. She will probably ask you to read an eye chart and then will look into your eyes with a small instrument known as an ophthalmoscope. In doing so, an eye doctor can pick up abnormalities in the eye sometimes even before a disease is obvious. For example, she may note changes in the retina of the eye that indicate high blood pressure, diabetes, or hardening of the arteries. On the other hand, it's important to control your blood pressure or diabetes so that you can prevent degeneration of the retina and abnormal changes of the blood vessels leading to the back of the eye.

In regard to eye disorders, one thing is fairly clear: More complications arise as you get older. For example, it was long believed that with advancing age, you gradually lose your sight. However, more evidence shows that slowing visual loss may be possible with lifestyle changes, diet modifications, and taking key nutritional supplements and herbs. Even though this is certainly not foolproof, it can go a long way in maintaining the health of your eyes.

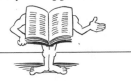

Body Language

An *ophthalmologist* is a medical doctor who first completed medical school and then completed a residency specifically dedicated to the eye and visual problems. She is allowed to prescribe medications and perform surgery. An *optometrist*, on the other hand, has not attended medical school but has completed her optometry training, where she, too, has learned about the eye. She is able to examine the eye and prescribe glasses or contact lenses, but she is not permitted to perform surgery.

Ophthalmology Options

After seeing your eye doctor, hopefully everything is copacetic. And, hopefully, your eyes appear healthy and she tells you to come back in another year. However, some of you won't be as fortunate, and some form of medical treatment might be necessary. The most common problems that affect the eyes are listed here:

➤ Infections that can be caused by viruses or bacteria. These are frequently treated with warm compresses, eye drops, or ointments for a short period of time. You have probably seen people who have a "red eye." This is known as conjunctivitis, and is commonly seen in children during the school year.

➤ Glaucoma, which is caused by a buildup of pressure within the eyeball. If this continues untreated, it can damage the optic nerve and cause gradual vision loss, even leading to blindness. Glaucoma can commonly be treated and controlled with eye drops. If it progresses uncontrollably, however, surgery may be necessary.

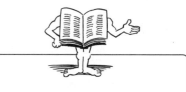

Body Language

Conjunctivitis is a common infection of the conjunctiva, the outer layer of the eye, that can cause irritation, inflammation, tearing, or even thick secretions coming from the eye.

➤ Cataracts, caused by a clouding of the proteins in the lens of the eye, resulting in gradually blurred vision. Cataract formation is much more common in people who smoke, who have diabetes, or who have been exposed to sunlight for prolonged periods of time. When a cataract has advanced enough and caused enough clouding of your vision, your eye doctor might have it surgically removed.

➤ Macular degeneration, the number-one cause of age-related blindness. In this condition, the area of the retina called the macula becomes damaged, and gradual vision loss ensues. In this condition, you may notice a blind spot or blurriness in the center of your vision. This condition is frequently treated with lasers or surgery.

If you've been told that you have any of these conditions, it is certainly best to prevent the damage from getting any worse. Better yet, let's talk about ways prevent these problems in the first place.

Antioxidants and the Cataract Connection

Cataract formation is the second-leading cause of blindness in the United States, just behind macular degeneration. Cataracts usually develop with advancing age. Though they were once thought to be a natural consequence of the aging process, more recent findings show that aging alone does not cause cataracts. It's now believed that long-term exposure to free radicals may damage the proteins within the lens of the eye. These damaged proteins begin to clump together and cloud vision.

It's a good idea to wear sunglasses with UV filtering when you're outdoors, especially if you're exposed to sunlight for prolonged periods of time. I would also certainly recommend that you boost your intake of antioxidant-rich foods, such as fresh fruits and vegetables high in flavonoids, carotenes, and other antioxidants.

Note from Your Doctor

Cataracts affect only 4.5 percent of people under age 45. However, the incidence begins to rise to almost one in two individuals over 75 years of age. More than 400,000 new patients of cataracts are reported each year, and more than a million cataract surgeries are performed each year in the United States, making this surgery the most commonly performed in people over the age of 65.

Quite possibly, maintaining a high intake of antioxidant nutrients, vitamin C, vitamin E, and carotenes could counteract the sun-induced damage to the lens of the eye and prevent the development of cataracts and vision loss. People with cataracts generally have low blood levels of antioxidants, so taking an antioxidant supplement may actually reduce your risk of developing cataracts by more than 25 percent.

Seeing with C

The lens can be protected from free radical damage with higher intakes of antioxidants, especially vitamins C and E. Recently, the Nurses Health Study found that vitamin C supplements could significantly reduce the development of cataracts. Those women who consumed extra vitamin C for 10 years had about an 80 percent lower incidence of cataracts. Those who took vitamin C supplements for fewer than 10 years did not show any reduction in their occurrence of early cataracts. How much vitamin C did the trick? The average was 400 to 700 mg per day, with a few taking more than 700 mg daily.

As it turns out, the lens of the eye is very rich in vitamin C. In fact, it contains anywhere from 10 to 30 times the concentration of vitamin C compared to other parts of the body. Vitamin C is a water-soluble supplement, and taking it in extra quantities may be a simple, safe, and inexpensive way of reducing cataract formation—and possibly cardiovascular disease and cancer, as previously discussed. When it comes to preventing cataracts, it seems that the average person simply does not get enough vitamin C in their diets alone. Another study found that nurses who took 250 to 500 mg of vitamin C supplements per day were 45 percent less likely to develop cataracts serious enough to require surgery.

How much should you take? Once you get into the 500 mg per day range, the concentration of vitamin C begins to increase in the lens. This is the minimum dose to take on a regular basis, although I frequently recommend twice that for many patients. Of course, you should still eat plenty of foods rich in vitamin C, such as peppers, oranges, grapefruits, and kiwi.

Eyeing Vitamin E

There's also good news about vitamin E as an antioxidant that prevents free radicals from damaging the lens of the eye. One study showed that simply taking 400 IU of vitamin E per day could cut the risk of developing cataracts in half, compared to those who didn't take vitamin E. People who have high levels of vitamin E in their blood are about half as likely to develop cataracts, compared to those who have low blood levels. This also demonstrates the importance of obtaining high blood levels of most antioxidants, not just levels in the low or normal range.

Vitamin E also appears to slow the progression of cataracts. Recently, it was found that older people who take vitamin E supplements or who have higher blood levels were half as likely to have their cataracts worsen over a 4^1/$_2$ year period. Evidence also indicates that simply taking vitamin E on a preventive basis could make your chance of developing cataracts in the first place much less likely.

How much vitamin E do you need? Probably about 400 IU per day—and it is virtually impossible to get this amount through your diet alone. Most people obtain about 10 IU of vitamin E per day from their food. Here's an example of what you'd have to eat to provide 400 IU of vitamin E through your diet:

Totally Toxic

Alcohol and smoking may increase your risk of developing cataracts. Those who drink on a daily basis increase their odds of developing cataracts by 33 percent, compared to people who rarely drink. And men who smoke at least one pack a day are more than twice as likely to develop cataracts as non-smoking men.

Vegetables	Amount	Vitamin E (IU)	Calories	Fat (grams)
Spinach	1 lb	21	127	1
Mung bean sprouts	1 lb	14	140	1
Green peas	1 lb	18	315	1.5
Black-eyed peas	1 lb	18	492	3.6
Sweet potatoes	1 lb	31	460	0.5
Total	5 lbs	102 IU	1534	7.6

Nuts, Seeds, Oils	Amount	Vitamin E (IU)	Calories	Fat (grams)
Almonds	1 cup	42	677	115
Cashews	1 cup	22	787	64
Mayonnaise	^{1}/$_2$ cup	98	320	32
Peanuts	1 cup	25	840	71
Sunflower seeds	1 cup	114	821	144
Total	4^1/$_2$ cups	301 IU	3445 cal	426 g
TOTAL		403 IU	4979 cal	434 g

235

Obviously, this is more than you could—or should—eat. You'd have to eat 4 pounds of vegetables, 4 cups of nuts and seeds, and one-half cup of mayonnaise! And even though you'd be getting 403 IU of vitamin E, it would be accompanied by 4,979 calories and 434 grams of fat.

Note from Your Doctor

Suffering from dry eyes? Try chamomile tea. To make the tea, steep 1 teaspoon of the dry herb or one tea bag in boiling water, and then strain the leaves. Refrigerate the tea until you're ready to use it. When your eyes are burning or dry, soak a piece of cotton gauze in the tea and apply the compress to your closed eyes for 10 minutes.

Macular Degeneration: The Mac Attack

As mentioned earlier, the condition known as macular degeneration is the leading cause of blindness in the United States in people over the age of 50. People who have macular degeneration have a blind spot in the center of their vision. In the early stages, they may still see shapes but have difficulty reading the newspaper or small print in a magazine. They may have difficulty seeing over long distances and therefore have probably stopped driving.

The small blood vessels supplying the back part of the eye, known as the macula, begins to leak, swell, and cause a scarring that leads to blurred vision. Treatment is geared toward sealing off the leaking blood vessels, usually with the use of lasers. The problem here, however, is that the laser also destroys some of the healthy retinal cells. That's why prevention of macular degeneration is so important.

Some evidence now indicates that antioxidants can help protect against macular degeneration. Free radicals seem to contribute to this condition, just as is the case with the formation of cataracts. Generally speaking, people who have high levels of antioxidants, vitamin E, vitamin C, beta carotene, zinc, and selenium are at much lower risk of developing this condition. Eating a diet rich in phytochemicals found in fruits and vegetables also can help you maintain healthy eyes. People with age-related macular degeneration generally consume fewer fresh fruits and vegetables. Phyto-nutrients such as lycopene, lutein, and zeaxanthin are particularly helpful in retarding macular degeneration. In fact, consuming 30 mg of lutein will not only increase your blood level by tenfold, but it also can help prevent the development of macular degeneration.

Perhaps one of the most important nutrients to ward off macular degeneration is beta carotene. This functions as a strong antioxidant, and people who eat foods rich in this vitamin seem to be less likely to develop this condition. Simply taking 8,700 IU of beta carotene per day can cut your risk by 50 percent. Good sources of beta carotene include carrots, broccoli, spinach, and apricots, which should be included as part of your Director of Prevention program. For preventive purposes, or to slow the progression of macular degeneration, I usually recommend approximately 25,000 IU of beta carotene. Frequently combine this with other antioxidants, such as vitamins C and E, both of which may also play a protective role.

One study showed that simply taking 80 mg of vitamin C per day could reduce the risk of macular degeneration by 30 percent. Vitamin E can also protect the retina from those damaging free radicals. A study at Johns Hopkins University School of Medicine found that people with high blood levels of vitamin E were half as likely to develop macular degeneration when compared to people with low blood levels. I usually recommend at least 1,000 mg of vitamin C and 400 IU of vitamin E, along with beta carotene, for a patient faced with macular degeneration.

Two trace minerals have been found to have powerful antioxidant effects. Zinc shows up in high concentrations in the retina and is an important aspect of keeping your vision sharp. Zinc supplements can slow vision loss in people with progressive macular degeneration. On the other hand, the mineral selenium may also be protective as a part of the antioxidant known as glutathione peroxidase; recently, low levels of this enzyme were associated with macular degeneration. A recent study found that selenium levels are much lower in patients with macular degeneration, compared to those with healthy eyes.

Note from Your Doctor

Two common forms of selenium supplements exist: sodium selenite and selenomethionine, the organic form. Interestingly enough, sodium selenite had no effect in raising blood selenium levels in a group of elderly people with macular degeneration. On the other hand, selenomethionine was better absorbed and actually raised the selenium level. As you can see, the form of selenium that you supplement may have a major impact in the prevention and treatment of age-related macular degeneration.

Consuming generous amounts of fresh fruits and vegetables, stopping smoking, and avoiding excessive exposure to sunlight are all important factors in reducing your risk of macular degeneration. Increasing your risk of antioxidants—especially those found in caratonoids such as carrots, spinach, and collard greens—is good advice in reducing your risk for macular degeneration.

Nutrients.NET

We discussed quite a bit about the important antioxidants to protect you from both cataracts and macular degeneration. Recently, researchers found that taking supplements of vitamins C and E could help prevent or postpone the development of 50 to 70 percent of cataracts. Obviously, this would be of great benefit to our overall health—and certainly to our pocketbook. Most antioxidants work together and produce an additive effect. In fact, simply taking a multivitamin with minerals may cut your risk of developing cataracts. Doctors who regularly took a multivitamin supplement were able to decrease their risk of cataracts by 27 percent and lower the risk of having a cataract operation by 21 percent, according to a Harvard University study. A Canadian study found that a multivitamin supplement could reduce the risk of cataracts by up to 40 percent.

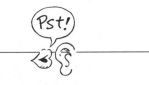

Healthy Hints

As far as I can see, Popeye should never develop cataracts. A Harvard University study found that women who ate five servings of spinach per week were 47 percent less likely to need cataract surgery, compared to those who ate spinach only once per month.

In addition to the antioxidants vitamins C and E, beta carotene, zinc, and selenium, growing evidence suggests that the amino acid taurine also helps prevent eye disorders.

First, the retina is particularly high in taurine, which may protect against harmful effects of sunlight. Taurine also has an antioxidant effect and can be used intravenously with zinc, selenium, and glutathione to produce remarkable improvement in some patients with macular degeneration. In fact, one particular patient was initially unable to read the newspaper or magazine when he first came to my office. After six treatments, this 84-year-old farmer was able to go back to work, read his morning newspaper, and even drive his car. Surprisingly, this is not an isolated incident: Numerous patients have experienced similar results.

In striving to prevent age-related vision loss, start with a prevention program right away. Here are some general guidelines:

➤ Minimize your intake of saturated fat from red meat, whole milk, and cheese products because fat seems to have a negative impact on vision health.

➤ Load up on those fresh fruits, vegetables, and phytonutrients, which are high in crucial antioxidants, such as vitamin C, E, and beta carotene.

➤ Consider taking a well-rounded multivitamin with minerals and extra antioxidant supplements, especially including vitamins C and E.

➤ Wear sunglasses when exposed to the sun to help filter the ultraviolet rays.

➤ Minimize your intake of alcohol, and don't start smoking cigarettes. If you
already have, quit in a hurry.

A Host of Herbs

Two herbs are gaining wide popularity in regard to vision health: ginkgo biloba and
bilberry.

Bilberry is a member of the bioflavonoid family that gives foods such as blueberries
their deep pigment. Bilberry may be helpful in nourishing the retina, and may improve
circulation to the eye. Bilberry contains flavonoids known as anthocyanosides, which
are strong antioxidants that may be helpful in stopping cataract formation and even
improving nearsightedness. Try a standardized bilberry extract containing 25 percent
anthocyanosides. You can find this in a health food store, and I usually recommend
250 to 500 mg per day.

Bilberry may also help improve visual acuity at night and help you adjust quicker to
darkness. Some people have also found that it may help your eyes adjust quicker after
you're exposed to glare.

The second herb, ginkgo biloba, is an antioxidant that improves circulation throughout the body. It has been used to treat cataracts and macular degeneration. Look for an
extract standardized to contain a 24 percent concentration of flavonglycosides, the
active ingredient. Generally 180 to 240 mg per day suffices, along with the other
antioxidants.

Getting Some Shut Eye

Don't forget to give your eyes some rest. Just like
every other part of your body—including your
muscles and your brain—your eyes need to take a
break once in a while. Getting adequate sleep is
part of keeping your eyes healthy and feeling
vibrant. I know some of you probably only get five
hours of sleep each night, even though others may
require 10 to 12 hours per evening. It's a good idea
to try to get at least seven hours of sleep per night
so that your eyes can feel rejuvenated the next
morning. I don't know about you, but if I don't get
enough sleep, my eyes feel heavy and tired—and
the rest of my body does as well.

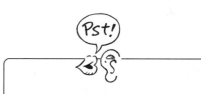

Healthy Hints

When buying sunglasses, try to find
those that block 99 to 100 percent
of the ultraviolet light to reduce
your risk of cataracts and macular
degeneration. Not all sunglasses
block UV light.

The Least You Need to Know

➤ A diet rich in vitamin C (at least 500 mg per day) helps promote the health of your eyes.

➤ Macular degeneration can be fought by antioxidants, zinc, and selenium.

➤ Vitamin E is especially important in slowing cataract growth and preventing free radical damage to the lenses of the eyes.

➤ Include ginkgo biloba and bilberry in your diet to fight cataract formation.

Part 4
Whole Body Fitness

This is where East meets West. Our Western medical thinking is mainly focused on medications and surgeries, looking for magic bullets instead of seeking answers from the world around us. We need to think of the mind and body as one, working together to ensure health and longevity.

In this section we explore a host of approaches, with both Eastern and Western origins, that have proven health benefits. This is an opportunity to be good to your body by working out both your physical being and your spiritual mind.

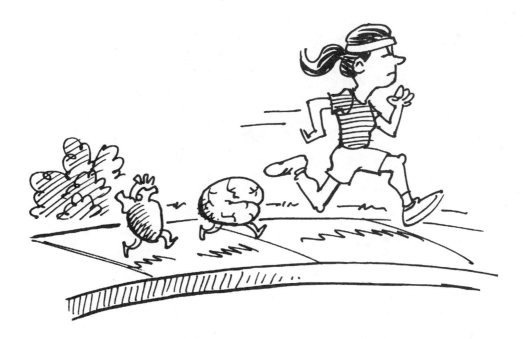

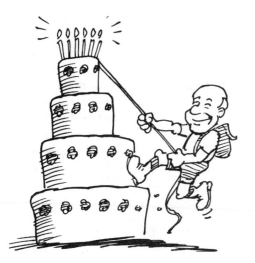

Adding Life to Your Years

In This Chapter

➤ How to get a new attitude

➤ How to stay on the cutting edge of youth

➤ How to add Eastern spirit to your Western life

➤ Simple strategies for survival

This chapter is about attitude: your attitude. If someone asks how old you are and you actually tell them the truth, then you need a new attitude. It is perfectly acceptable—and, in fact, the preferred response—to not answer that age-old question. Brush it off. You have no idea how old you are. Yes, in fact, you are aging, but you are not old. You have only a finite number of years, however you have an infinite number of opportunities available to enjoy. Don't fall into any stereotypes that define who you are by how old you are. It's a trap. From here on out, think Patti LaBelle and get a new attitude.

Aging Gracefully

Researchers at the University of Bonn, in Germany, studying longevity have concluded that the most important factors for living longer and healthier are your personality, your intelligence, and your behavior. I call this your attitude. What's really meaningful is the interaction between your mood, your level of activity, your ability to adjust and adapt, and your social skills.

This sounds a whole lot like everything you learned in kindergarten. And this makes complete sense: When you were young, you only knew how to be young. You loved what you were doing, you loved where you were doing it, and you played with anyone and everyone who would play with you.

Somewhere along the road you got bombarded with things like responsibility and maturity and work. You stopped thinking young, and you got old. So instead of getting older, let's try to age gracefully. Here's the difference in attitude between getting old and aging gracefully:

Getting Old	Aging Gracefully
I have little interest in life.	Every day is filled with wonder.
It's too late to change.	It's never too late to change.
The glass is half empty.	The glass is half full.
I've lost sight of any goals.	I make commitments.
Life is boring.	Life is fun.

While genetics certainly has a role in determining your lifespan, most experts agree that adopting a positive attitude and incorporating health-promoting behaviors both predispose you to a long life. We've spent the better part of this book on selecting the right behaviors for our body to maximize lifespan; now let's work on our head.

Keeping Your Mind Sharp

Scientists have shown that a direct correlation exists between a positive attitude about aging and memory performance and longevity. It's about optimism and believing you can do anything you set your mind to. To paraphrase Winston Churchill: "Never, never, never retire. Change careers, do something entirely different, but never retire." You have to keep your mind sharp. Education is high on the list of factors that promote longevity. So where do you go with your renewed optimism?

Back to school, of course.

Take a class to boost your memory performance, mental ability, and self-esteem. You are still in control of your future. What really excited you as a kid? Maybe you always wanted to be a photographer or a potter, a travel agent or a doctor. Get involved. Make your motto the immortal words of Robin Williams in *Dead Poets Society*: *Carpe diem*; make the most of today.

Take a class and learn a new skill. This is a great opportunity to meet others with your same interests. Engage in conversation, and keep on reading.

When you're done with this book, move on to the next. Switch between different types, perhaps fiction, an autobiography, and a how-to book. See what authors are coming to your local bookstore, and read their book before they arrive. I had a great-uncle who used to read the dictionary; he was sharp until his last day on earth. Make time to work on a hobby, develop a new skill, become a volunteer, or get another degree—or finish the first one that you have put off for all these years.

The Eight-Year Plan

This is the plan for college students who don't want to face the real world: They take eight years to finish a four-year degree. Jump on that plan. These kids think they can stay young forever, just by never leaving college. Now that we're getting older, it's not such a bad idea. In fact, I might try a 20-year plan.

Re-enroll in college. Maybe you're all ready for graduate school, or perhaps you'd prefer a Swiss finishing school. Or maybe you never finished grade school. Don't delay; you can't lose on this one. You will be the envy of your friends with your newfound knowledge. You will also be sought after by all your classmates who will want to work with you on group projects. These students will respect your years of experience. And you will always get a high mark from your professors, who will be so impressed with you just for having decided to return to the world of academia.

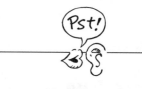

Healthy Hints

Look out for new "smart" centers, such as the Arizona Senior Academy in Tucson; the Chautauqua Institute near Buffalo, New York; and the Disney Institute in Orlando, Florida. There is a growing trend toward intellectual get-aways to educational institutions. Call your travel agent and book your next vacation to a smart community.

Note from Your Doctor

A recent study by clinicians at Duke University Medical Center revealed an improved quality of life for older adults who became computer literate and gained online capabilities. Learn to use email, and find a chat room. Make the computer your friend, and it will make you friends.

So check out the curriculum at a local college, or get in touch with your township to see whether it offers adult education programs. Community centers and libraries are good sources of information and opportunities. Go on a tour of your town, attend showings and lectures at a local museum, and seek out quality films and movies that interest you. Start your own group: a movie club, a book group, a bird-watching association, or a centenarians organization to do just about anything with other people who also want to be around a long time.

Smart Drugs

The kids you meet on the college campus could probably give you a better run-down of what's out there to keep you smart. (Just make sure it's legal advice!) A few supplements do have some mind-enhancing properties. Our brain is like a muscle: It needs to be used to keep it in top shape.

Remember that slogan "Use it or lose it"? So it goes with our brain. While we have become proficient at feeding our body, we also need to know how to feed our mind. As Director of Prevention, you know that your mind is responsible for carrying messages to the rest of your body. You also remember that the carriers of these messages are those neurotransmitters that we discussed in Chapter 19. Your neurotransmitters, when fed properly, keep your body happy; but when neglected, they wreak havoc on your health and lifespan. The following list of nutrients for your neurotransmitters highlights good food for thought.

➤ B-vitamins, especially choline, B_3, B_{12}, and folic acid

➤ Gingko biloba

➤ Gotu kola

➤ Pycnogenol

➤ Acetyl-L-carnitine

➤ Phosphatidyl serine

➤ Ginseng

These supplements will ensure that your brain is receiving a strong, essential blood flow and improved oxygen circulation. This circulation provides oxygen to the brain so that it can properly disperse neurotransmitters when needed by the rest of your body. These memory-sharpening supplements are not, however, a replacement for daily mental activity. The important thing is to exercise your mind every day with the three Rs: reading, writing, and arithmetic.

Now that you're fueling your mind, you may also want to include some spirituality in your life. In a past academic life or in your free time, you may have read some classic books on philosophy; now lets put those thoughts into practice.

Getting in Touch with Your Spiritual Side

For most of us, getting in touch with our spiritual being is a real challenge. We have been brought up to be analytical, methodical, and efficient. Spirituality can't always be easily explained, dissected, or understood. Tossing aside our preconceived notions of our role in the universe is not an easy task. Yet, those who are able to walk in the path of enlightenment are able to achieve an inner peace that is quite profound. Understanding this harmony between ourselves and our environment often brings with it improved health and longevity.

Our pragmatic Western philosophy keeps us grounded in the practical. Our scope of Eastern influences is often limited to our favorite Chinese restaurant and the epic made-for-TV classic, *Shogun*. In confronting Eastern spirituality, we are often lost in the esoteric world of Buddha, yoga, and meditation.

The ultimate goal of Eastern modalities is not learning a series of new tricks, but perfecting a series of techniques that will ultimately transform your attitude. It's about insight and finding your way along the path to a higher understanding of life. The best advice I can give you before embarking on your spiritual journey is to open up your mind and be willing to be yourself. You have nothing to fear and only health to gain, so let the transformation and rejuvenation begin.

Yoga: Practice Makes Perfect

The practice of yoga involves the unification of your spiritual, mental, and physical energies. Its underlying premise is that if your spirit is restless, so, too, will be the health of your body and mind. By practicing yoga, one can counter the ill effects of stress and toxins on the body, and maintain or restore mental and physical health.

Note from Your Doctor

In medical studies of yoga practitioners (or yogis) at the Menninger Foundation in Topeka, Kansas, researchers noted that the yogis had significant control of their body. By joining the mind and body through yoga, the disciples were able to control their body functions, ranging from thyroid output to heart rate.

The easiest recognizable form of yoga practice is Hatha yoga. This includes a variety of physical postures, or *asanas*, that can create immediate change in your body. At first glance, some of these poses may appear rather contortionist, and the immediate body change may appear somewhat frightening. However, with careful guidance and practice, these poses bring the spine and head into perfect alignment and promote proper blood flow throughout the body.

Most importantly, for the purposes of this book, yoga helps with the process of rejuvenation. Beginning with the Child pose, you are already feeling younger. Greet the

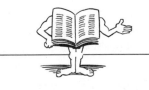

Body Language

Sanskrit for "ease," an *asana* is a yoga pose that, when done properly, brings the mind into a state of relaxation while energizing your glands, lungs, and heart. Two main types of asanas exist: therapeutic and meditative. Both create a balance between movement and stillness.

morning with the Sun Salutations as you energize, strengthen, and tone all your major muscles and organs.

With yoga you can learn to do the Twist, be a Warrior or a Half Fish, stretch like a Cobra, or elevate like a Locust. You can get in touch with your youth, pretending to be the Sun and Moon, a Tree, a Mountain and Lotus. It's like a great game of charades, with amazing health benefits.

Here's a list of some of the many benefits associated with yoga:

➤ Improves respiratory function

➤ Alleviates stress and anxiety

➤ Reduces blood pressure

➤ Enhances memory and intelligence

➤ Reduces cholesterol levels

➤ Heightens visual and auditory perception

➤ Diminishes frequency of asthma attacks

➤ Reduces insulin dependency

➤ Reduces heart rate

➤ Benefits cardiac arrhythmia

➤ Provides health, vitality, and peace of mind

There probably aren't too many benefits on this list that we would want to do without—and you are never too old to start getting the benefits that come from the practice of yoga. In fact, books and testimonials are available from older adults who began yoga late in life and experienced profound health benefits. Unlike many athletic activities, yoga is easy to start at any age, and with successful improvements (such as the ones noted in the Yoga Biomedical Trust Survey of 1983–1984), why not start today?

Health Conditions Benefited by Yoga

Ailment	% Claiming Benefit
Back pain	98
Arthritis	90
Anxiety	94
Migraines	80
Insomnia	82
Nerve/muscle disease	96

Ailment	% Claiming Benefit
Menstruation	68
Premenstrual syndrome	77
Menopause	83
Hypertension	84
Heart disease	94
Asthma/bronchitis	88
Ulcers	90
Hemorrhoids	88
Obesity	74
Diabetes	80
Cancer	90
Smoking	74
Alcoholism	100

Yoga Biomedical Trust Survey of 3,000 individuals with health conditions who utilized yoga as a treatment modality.

The best place to learn yoga is, of course, deep in the Himalayan Mountains. Don't have the time to make the pilgrimage? Take a class with a skilled yoga practitioner. Start asking around at health food stores, exercise clubs, and with other holistic care practitioners for recommendations of yoga teachers that can help you bend over backward better. Word-of-mouth referrals are invaluable. Many well-written and illustrated books also are available at your library or bookstore.

Another excellent source to help you learn yoga is videotapes. Many bang-up videos available provide you with a good program to follow—and some great footage of real flexibility. When you start to inquire, it is really amazing what your search may turn up.

Some national organizations can help you find a yoga teacher locally. Try the Iyengar Yoga National Association at (800) 889-YOGA, or tap into the group's Web site at http://www.iyoga. com/iynaus/. Also try Yoga International's Guide to Yoga Teachers and Classes, at (800) 821-YOGA, to find your guru.

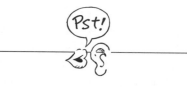

Healthy Hints

Many health insurance companies are recognizing the valuable health benefits of practicing yoga. Kaiser Permanente offers members yoga classes as part of its low-cost programs, and Oxford Health Plans and Blue Cross and Blue Shield of California are creating preferred provider networks of yoga instructors. Check with your insurance company to see whether it offers any special reimbursement plan for your yoga class.

Meditation Matters

Technically speaking, meditation is a state of focused concentration that should result in an increased sense of peace and awareness. Meditation has been shown to have a positive effect on immune system function and strengthens the body's natural defenses against infectious disease. So the next time you hear that "om" sound, don't run away: Sit down, cross your legs, close your eyes, and chant along . . . om . . . om . . . om.

You have just stimulated your hypothalamus, the amazing little gland in your brain that controls your breathing, brain waves, and blood flow.

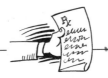

Note from Your Doctor

Meditation is so effective at reducing stress and tension that in 1984 the National Institutes of Health recommended meditation as the first line of treatment for mild hypertension, ahead of prescription pharmaceuticals.

As with yoga and so many other things in life, meditation improves with practice. The first step is to empty or fill your mind. Whether you empty your mind of thoughts and worries or fill it with worldly wisdom, the desired effect is to float freely toward nothing. You got it: You're going for nothing here, so you can't lose. Through meditation, you're seeking harmony and what is often described as a feeling of oneness with the universe.

Although there are many ways to meditate, most approaches can be grouped into either concentrative meditation or mindfulness meditation. With concentrative meditation, you focus on your breathing, a favorite place, or music to achieve calm. Mindfulness meditation involves awakening your senses to the full bouquet of life through a full range of sensations and feelings. Meditation can help you feel less anxious and more in control. It can help with the management of chronic pain, and it has long-lasting spiritual effects. Some of the conditions benefited by daily meditation include these:

➤ Immune function disorders, including cancer and AIDS

➤ Alcohol and drug addiction

➤ Anxiety and panic attacks

➤ Heart disease and hypertension

➤ Chronic illness

Meditation can be practiced just about anywhere—at home, surrounded by nature, while in the hospital (where I hope you're not), or on vacation. You can meditate alone or gain support and enlightenment from sharing your experience with others. For more information about meditation, try the Maharishi International University in Iowa, at (515) 472-5031; the Institute of Noetic Sciences in Sausalito, CA, at (415) 331-5650; or the Mind-Body Clinic at Harvard Medical School in Boston, at (617) 632-9530.

Biofeedback

Biofeedback is particularly effective for reducing the stress in your life, eliminating your headaches, controlling asthma attacks, relieving pain, and reconditioning any injured muscles. However, the positive effects can be realized only when you have accepted the idea that being hooked up to an apparatus that resembles a device from *One Flew Over the Cuckoo's Nest* can really benefit you. Through biofeedback training, you learn how to consciously regulate normal unconscious body functions. These functions can include your breathing, your heart rate, and your blood pressure. Biofeedback can enable you to take control of your health and prevent disorders that lead to costly degenerative conditions.

The biofeedback device is painless—honest. So are the electrodes that are placed on your skin to monitor your body's response. You run through various meditation exercises until you achieve your desired response, as evidenced by the blinking lights or beeps from the biofeedback machine. The lights and beeps are triggered by your body's ability to relax through a lowered heart rate or lower body temperature. By using computers to monitor the device's response, a rapid and detailed analysis of your activities assists the patient and practitioner in stabilizing your body's complex systems.

For additional information on biofeedback training and practitioners in your area, contact the Association for Applied Psychophysiology and Biofeedback in Wheatridge, CO, at (303) 422-8436.

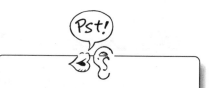

Healthy Hints

Doctors have noted that the self-regulation skills acquired through biofeedback training are retained even after treatments with the device have ceased. With practice, biofeedback skills actually continue to improve, ensuring steady improvement.

Planned Parenting

This is a double-edged sword, guaranteed to make you feel young and oh-so-old at the same time. Starting a second family—or your first—late in life will keep you hustling. Many famous celebrities have included planned parenting as part of their longevity plan, and it has its merits. Raising a child will keep you thinking young, will give you access to other young parents working on their first families, and will provide you with plenty of opportunity for running around—although that may not be the kind of exercise you were planning on.

251

Join the cast of Hugh Hefner, Jane Seymour, Susan Sarandon, Tony Randall, Madonna, Sandra Bernhardt, Roseanne, and Clint Eastwood.

Granted, men have certain biological advantages to enable them to father children much later in life than their female partners, but if your clock has stopped ticking, adoption is always an option.

According to research, having kids late in life should do the trick. Older parents with young children keep their minds sharp and increase their odds of living longer by engaging in these activities:

➤ Enjoying new experiences every day

➤ Adapting to challenges

➤ Taking on added responsibility

➤ Becoming involved in important projects

➤ Relishing the joy of meaningful relationships

➤ Participating in consistent routines

➤ Dispelling myths and stereotypes that relate to having children late in life

Live, Laugh, and Love

While stress management is a good buzz word around the office or in social settings today, we should really be striving toward a more optimistic attitude all the time. To get the most life out of your years, re-learn how to live—except, this time, really live. Enjoy every moment and find beauty in the magic that surrounds us. If you commit yourself to only one thing after reading this book, commit yourself to living life to its fullest, and everything else will fall into place.

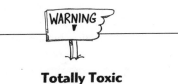

Totally Toxic

Depression is a risk factor for heart disease. A study at Johns Hopkins University followed a group of patients over 14 years and found that the depressed individuals in the group were four times more likely to suffer a heart attack than their optimistic counterparts.

So why did the chicken cross the road? To get to the other side. Okay, so everyone knows this joke. The point is to laugh at it anyway. When one person laughs, we all laugh along with him, as some saying goes. Laughter is contagious, so find someone laughing who can make you laugh, and go with it. Start laughing and make the next person laugh, too. Laugh until you cry; it's a great emotional detoxifier.

Laughter has been scientifically proven to boost your immune system and help your body fight off infection. A really good laugh speeds up your heart rate, improves your circulation, and works enough muscles to almost be considered exercise. So no matter how heavy you are, take yourself lightly.

Note from Your Doctor

A Canadian health study of attitudes in older patients suggests that doctors should focus their efforts on trying to improve satisfaction with outcomes rather than on making marginal improvements to their medical condition.

Finally, learn to love. Love yourself, love your family, love your neighbor, love your friends, love your pet. Seek companionship. Find a support group, ask for assistance, get a pet. Do anything just so you don't have to do it alone. The best way to reduce stress is to get support. This can be someone to help us when we need an extra hand. This can be someone to make us feel wanted, needed, attractive, and loved. This can be someone to relax and unwind with, and this can be someone who listens when we need to talk and gives advice when needed. Friendship is often the best medicine.

The Least You Need to Know

➤ Developing and keeping the right attitude is a critical element in staying young.

➤ Use it or lose it! Keep your mind engaged with intellectual pursuits.

➤ Spiritual exploration is personally rewarding and can bring about internal transformation.

➤ Yoga is both mentally and physically rewarding and has lasting benefits regardless of the age you begin to practice.

➤ Meditation is a great tool for reducing stress and can benefit the immune system, while alleviating symptoms associated with hypertension and heart disease.

Chapter 22

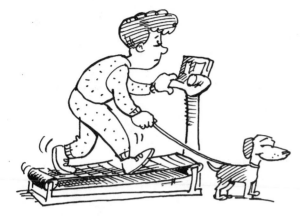

It's Your Bod, Baby!

In This Chapter

➤ Understanding the importance of physical fitness

➤ Enjoying exercise

➤ The benefits of walking

➤ Developing a personal program

It's your bod—and it's the only one you've got, so let's make the most of it. While it's true that what's on the inside is what really counts, that animal attraction thing is not based on your cellular function levels. Besides, when you look good, you feel great. And feeling great is really good medicine. Physical fitness will make you look better, feel healthier, and ultimately live longer.

According to the American Academy of Physical Education, physical fitness is defined as the ability to carry out daily tasks with vigor and alertness, without undue fatigue, and with ample energy to enjoy leisure pursuits and to meet the above average physical stresses encountered in emergency situations.

It's rather ironic that for a society going through a fitness craze, with exercise gurus and access to more gym apparatus than ever before, we are more unfit than we have ever been. What went wrong? Our ancestors never had to exercise to be fit; they had to be fit to survive. If our forefathers didn't work the fields, there was no food for dinner. And for our ancestors before that, if they didn't hunt for dinner . . . well, they were hunted for dinner.

Getting fit is fun and easy—it must be, or I would not keep doing it every day. Exercise does not have to be hard, it does not have to cost a lot of money, and it does not have to take a whole lot of effort. Of course, if you want the difficult, expensive, and laborious plan, we can accommodate you, too. Here's an easy-to-follow list with suggested physical fitness activities in each category. We'll call them "Cheap and Easy" and "High-Maintenance":

Cheap and Easy	High-Maintenance
Walking	Heli-skiing
Aerobics	Mountain climbing
Riding a bike	Golf
Stretching	Snowmobiling
Climbing stairs	Tennis
Skinny dipping	Parasailing

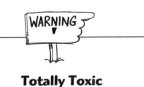

Totally Toxic

From 1962 to 1991, the rate of obesity in people ages 35 to 45 increased by 36 percent.

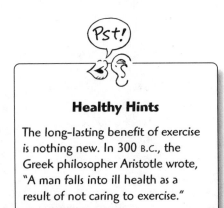

Healthy Hints

The long-lasting benefit of exercise is nothing new. In 300 B.C., the Greek philosopher Aristotle wrote, "A man falls into ill health as a result of not caring to exercise."

It is important to note that there are varying degrees to which you can participate in each of these activities, making them easier or harder. Tennis does not necessarily have to be a high-maintenance activity if you don't need a clay court and can forgo the fancy labels printed on an entire wardrobe of white clothes. Stretching can become a very expensive workout if you need a gym membership and a personal trainer instead of a video, a few free weights, and an exercise tube in your closet.

Let's take this one step farther. When deciding what physical activity you would like to do on a regular basis, remember, participation in even the most elite sports, such as polo and yachting, will involve much less money and effort than undergoing an angioplasty procedure because you failed to exercise in the first place. (If you forgot about that angioplasty procedure, be sure to double check Chapter 12.)

Who Said You Can't Teach an Old Dog a New Trick?

How many times have you said, "I'm just too old to do it?" That response is a mind maneuver. Don't be trapped by the numbers—how old you are, how much you weigh, or how long it will take. You're mentally stuck thinking that you should act a certain sedentary way because you have hit a certain birthday in your middle ages. The Middle Ages occurred sometime between the fall of the Byzantine Empire and the discovery of the New World. They have nothing to do with your current numerical age or passive lifestyle. Think about how many times you have also said, "I wish I were 18 again." Exercise is another way to get pretty darn close to that wishful thought.

For those of you ready to move on, let's go over some more advanced reasons for getting fit. Remember, no matter what shape you are in, there is always a benefit to working out:

➤ You will have a better attitude.

➤ You will have greater self-confidence.

➤ You will be better equipped to deal with stress.

➤ You will be smarter.

➤ You will increase your strength and endurance.

➤ You will have more stamina.

➤ You will have a stronger immune system.

➤ You will lower your blood pressure.

➤ You will reduce your risk of heart attacks.

➤ You will have better circulation.

➤ You will have stronger bones.

➤ You will slow the aging process and live longer.

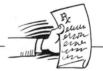

Note from Your Doctor

All the life-extending benefits of exercise can be yours for just walking 20 minutes a day. You can do this around your house, at the mall, or at your office. You can even do this while you are away on vacation, because your body doesn't really get to take a vacation, does it?

If any of those points have not fully convinced you of the merits of exercise, here are a few more reasons—these are the real clinchers:

➤ You will look better in a bathing suit.

➤ You will improve your sexual performance.

➤ You will sleep better after the performance.

I know you can't argue with any of those last points, so it's time to get moving. One more thing before we sweat together: Let's figure out our optimal level of exercise. This is the range of heavy breathing where our bodies can get the most benefit from working out.

Calculating Your Target Heart Rate

Calculating your target heart rate enables you to determine the effectiveness of your exercise. In other words, are you really exerting effort, or are you just going through the motions? Biologically speaking, when you are exercising in your target range, you increase the amount of blood your heart is capable of pumping with each beat and while at rest. There are a few different ways to determine the intensity of your exercise. While all of this is pretty straightforward, it will require a little mathematical calculation. Don't worry, I'll give you the formula.

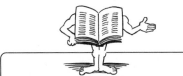

Body Language

Your *target heart rate* measures your level of exertion needed to produce measurable improvements in your cardiovascular system. Strive to maintain your heart rate at this level during exercise to get the most benefit for your effort.

The easiest formula is somewhat unscientific. Put simply, how do you feel while you are exercising? You want your level of effort to be somewhere between turning the pages of this book and working so hard that you are unable to hold a conversation. As you get more fit, your level of output should increase. You will actually be able to talk more during exercising as you become accustomed to your new levels of exertion.

The second way to measure effectiveness is the sweat test. If you were on a first date, sweating would not be attractive. However, if you are at the gym perspiring, it could be a real turn-on. Athletic sweat is a good thing: It means your body is working really well and pushing yourself to new levels of fitness. This is also a somewhat quasi-scientific yet reasonably accurate measure of health improvement.

Finally, the most exact measure of exertion involves your heart rate. This is where you might need a pencil or a calculator to help. To most precisely measure the benefit of your workout, you need to know two things: your resting heart rate and your target heart rate. Follow along in the box to get your target heart rate, and check out the sidebar if you forgot how to get your resting heart rate.

Just fill in the blanks to calculate your target heart rate and define your range of optimum cardiovascular benefit:

Worksheet for Calculating Target Heart Rate

(220 – [your age] _____) x .55= _____ (a)

This is the low end of your training range.

(220 – [your age] _____) x .85= _____ (b)

You do not want your heart rate to exceed this number; this is as high as your heart rate should go.

Your target heart range is between _____ (a) and _____ (b).

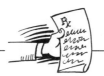

Note from Your Doctor

Certain medications can inhibit your heart rate. If you are taking any heart medications—especially beta-blockers or any antidepressants—check with your physician to ascertain your target heart rate before beginning an exercise program.

Here's my wife's strategy: She has a hard time finding her pulse, so she figures that as long as she is still breathing, then her heart is still beating and she is okay. So far this seems to have worked for her.

My wife would, however, like a heart-rate monitor for her birthday. These can be purchased at any sporting goods store and through many health clubs. It is a simple, painless gadget that wraps around your chest and monitors your heart rate. You get to wear another watch, and you watch the watch for your changing heart rate. (This is an easy way to monitor your work out pace, but it could also be added to the "High-Maintenance" category for some people.)

So now that you spent all this time figuring out your target heart rate and range of optimal benefit, what does it really mean as you sit reading this book, sedentary and snacking on the sofa?

Warming Up

Before you continue reading this chapter, sit up straight in your chair, with your feet flat on the floor. Look to the left, and follow with your torso to the same side. Take a deep breath, and repeat this twist on your right side. You've already started warming up. Now stretch out on the floor. Lie on your stomach, and gently use your arms to push your upper body off the floor while your hips and lower body stay on the floor. From this position, you could probably finish reading this section of the book and still be exercising.

The most important thing is to get up from the sofa and away from the table. Do some form of exercise every day. I don't care if you crawl, walk, jog, or run—just get at least 20 minutes a day of activity. Drag a friend to join you; misery loves company, and your friend will even thank you for it in the end.

You can even break down your 20 minutes of activity into two sets of 10 minutes. You can always find 10 minutes. Think of all the time you spend in the bathroom reading *People Magazine*. Ten minutes is probably the time it takes you to read the sports section in the daily paper. Read it on the treadmill, or catch the stats on CNN while you are stretching in front of the TV.

You Gotta Walk the Walk

Walking can be the most effective—as well as the most fun and inexpensive—fitness activity you can find. You don't need a class, a gym, or a whole lot of fancy stuff to really enjoy walking. As an added bonus, walking gets you outside, breathing fresh air and basking in sunlight. Walking can be a great quality-time family activity. You're never too young or too old to enjoy a walk. A brisk walk is best, but take it slowly at first and enjoy the benefits that come with physical fitness.

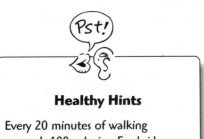

Healthy Hints

Every 20 minutes of walking expends 100 calories. For brisk walking, add 50 more calories for every 20 minutes of exercise.

If walking seems too mundane, try walking uphill or up stairs, or move to more rugged terrain. Walk faster, or make it a robust hike in the woods, up mountains, and back again. Swing your arms to add intensity, and breathe deeply. As your stamina increases, make it an active walk of at least an hour, or take along a backpack and keep on walking. Don't forget a walk into the sunset or, my favorite, a walk on the beach.

For those of you who find walking to be the answer, try to bring some company with you on your walk, such as a partner, a pet, or a walkman. I just started walking with my cellular phone so I can catch up with all my friends who claim they're too busy to walk with me but not to talk to me. And you know what the first thing they say is? You got it: "Wow, I wish I could be walking with you." They *should* be walking with me. It would better for both of us; they would be getting exercise, too, and I would be saving on my phone bill.

Other physical activities that can be enjoyed by anyone at any level include bicycle-riding, gardening, swimming, golf, dancing, and mall-walking—although that can get expensive. Pick your favorite activity, increase your output while participating in that activity, and have a great time while getting fit.

Shake, Rattle, and Roll

Let's talk about aerobic activity, primarily intended to improve your cardiovascular fitness. Aerobic activity is also the best way to burn calories and help you lose any extra weight quickly. Some great examples of aerobic activity are listed below:

Activity	Avg. Calories Burned in 30 minutes
Aerobic dance class	340
Basketball	300–400
Running	360–440
Swimming	200–260
Tennis, singles	250
Walking	150

In addition to losing weight, preventing heart disease, and lowering your blood pressure, aerobic activity in moderation can also have a profound effect on your immune system, reduce stress, aid in depression, and reduce your risk of osteoporosis.

Aerobic exercise challenges your heart and lungs through repetitive activity involving your larger muscles—your chest, legs, and tush. Aerobic activity requires your body to use oxygen efficiently while anaerobic activity, such as strenuous weightlifting, can lead to overexertion of your body. This is a high-intensity workout that can cause a burning sensation and force your body to stop working out.

Pump It Up

Weightlifting is not just for bodybuilders. It is for you and me, for energy, power, strength, and building better bones. Strong muscles and strong bones go hand in hand in preserving your body's physical abilities.

While aerobic activity burns calories, weightlifting builds, firms, and shapes your body. Don't be intimidated by weightlifters or the equipment they use. Ask for help, get a trainer, and follow directions. Pumping properly is very important. Good form and the ability to do a minimum number of reps is always more important than just loading up on weight.

Note from Your Doctor

By the age of 65, people who don't exercise lose 30 to 40 percent of their strength. By the age of 74, more than one quarter of American men and two-thirds of American women can't lift more than 10 pounds.

Setting Up a Personal Program

Why is it that when a doctor hands you a prescription for medication, you fill it and begin your treatment. Yet, if a doctor says, "George, you should get out a little bit more and exercise," it goes in one ear and right out the other. Maybe more doctors should write up a little slip of paper for you with an exercise prescription.

Based, of course, on your doctor's recommendations, let's begin setting up an individualized program for you. I certainly don't expect you to be on the Arnold Schwarzenegger plan; just find a perfect plan for you. While Arnold sure looks good, it is not what most of us strive for. We want health and longevity, and we can get that with an easy fitness program.

Body Language

Reps is gym lingo for the number of repetitions you do with weights or on a machine working a specific body part. Depending on your goal, you incorporate different numbers of reps into your routine. To tighten and tone like Miss America, you use low weights and high reps. If you'd rather bulk up like Mr. Universe, use heavy weights and fewer reps.

Your very first prescription should include something like this: "Walk 20 minutes a day for two weeks, increasing to 30 minutes a day thereafter." For those of you already moving, try walking 40 minutes a day. Remember, you can exercise your options: You don't have to just walk. You can shoot hoops with the kid next door, jump rope, ride on a stationary bicycle, or follow along with a fitness show on TV from the privacy of your own home. Just remember to close the blinds if you don't want your neighbors watching you.

To set up your personal program, you need to assess your current health and fitness status. By this, I mean determining which of the following best describes your current level of fitness:

A. I exercise my thumbs regularly on the TV remote.

B. I engage in cardiac activity three times a week.

C. I am a workout queen (or king), pushing my sweat glands to the limit four or more days a week.

If you answered B or C, the remainder of this section will not apply to you. You are already on the road to living longer and healthier. If you're a type A, here's the bottom line about your exercise program: Ten minutes a day is better than no minutes. And certainly 20 minutes a day is even better. Anything after that point might make you a B—and get you even closer to becoming a C.

And don't forget to reward yourself for meeting your goals. Your kids always get a prize for a job well done. So why shouldn't you? Treat yourself to a magazine subscription, a new tennis racquet, or a heart-rate monitor.

The Least You Need to Know

➤ Exercising can be fun, if you choose the exercise that's right for you.

➤ You're never too old to start exercising.

➤ Exercising has unbelievable life-extending benefits.

➤ Short walks go a long way.

➤ Develop a personal program that suits you. Start slowly and move up gradually.

Chapter 23

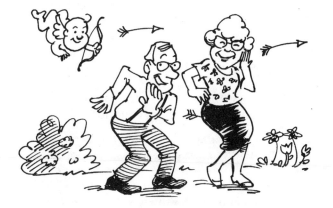

Oh, Those Raging Hormones

In This Chapter

➤ Declining hormone levels and aging

➤ Benefits of melatonin

➤ The potential of DHEA

➤ Anti-aging effects of estrogen, progesterone, and testosterone

You probably remember what it was like to go through your teenage years and proceed into your 20s and 30s. You felt strong and vibrant, as if you could "conquer the world." And now, as you proceed perhaps into middle age, your reflexes are no longer as quick, you're steadily gaining weight, and no matter how many times you go to the gym and exercise each week, weight loss seems like something of the past. Perhaps your memory is not quite as sharp, your skin is showing more wrinkles each year, and maybe your libido is fading as well.

What's going on here? You no longer feel like you're 20—and you certainly don't look like it either. Chances are, not only are you progressing in years, but you're aging along with it. Is there something more that you can do? Perhaps so. Getting your hormone levels up to levels that they were in earlier years may just provide you with one necessary answer.

Feeling 20 Again

Think about the following scenario. You're about to attend your 30th college reunion. You're 52 years old, but you are concerned about how you're going to look to your former classmates. You've gained 30 pounds since graduation, you've lost a lot of hair, and what little hair you have left has turned from black to silvery gray. Your belly protrudes far beyond your belt line. You've lost an inch of your height. And you're wearing glasses now, not only for reading, but all day long. Unfortunately, those wrinkles have formed along the sides of your eyes, and you've even begun to develop some age spots on the back of your hands and near the bridge of your nose.

As you walk into the facility housing your college reunion, you spot your two former roommates. One looks like he has aged at least 30 years as well. He has developed the same types of physical changes you have—in fact, he's probably gained at least 40 pounds since the last time you saw him. But your other roommate, Bill, looks different. He looks like he hasn't aged at all. He is still tall and slender, he hasn't put on any extra pounds, his skin is vibrant and full of life, he is not wearing glasses, and he doesn't have any age spots on his skin. In talking to him, he still seems as sharp as a tack. And, to top it off, he is accompanied by his wife, who also appears to be at least 20 years younger than you.

What's the difference? What's going on here? You sit down to dinner and talk to Bill. You find out that he and his wife have been taking natural hormone replacement therapy—not just estrogen and testosterone, but a whole alphabet soup of other substances that you've never heard of before, such as DHEA and melatonin. They also take a slew of different vitamins, minerals, and amino acids. Bill tells you that as a result of a program he's been following for 10 years now, he feels better than he has in years. He is still able to ski in the winter and bicycle in the summer. In fact, he has recently taken up mountain climbing. You, on the other hand, gave up snow skiing years ago, when your knees began to bother you and arthritis set in.

Oh, what it would feel like to be 20 again! To get those years back would be invaluable, you think. Could hormones really contribute to the fountain of youth? Let's take a look at some of the little known facts about your hormones.

Natural Versus Synthetic Hormones

All of us naturally produce hormones every minute of our lives because they support vital life functions. Production of many of your hormones peaks in your 20s or early 30s and then steadily declines as you get older. For example, DHEA (which is produced by the adrenal glands), reaches its peak in your mid-20s; by age 80, your DHEA level is probably only 20 percent of that level. As mentioned in Chapter 15, women's levels of estrogen and progesterone also start to decline after menopause, usually in the early 50s.

Could the high level of hormone production in your earlier years be one of the reasons why you generally feel stronger and healthier than you do in middle age or the elderly years? And could hormone supplementation reverse some of the aging process and help you find that fountain of youth? To some degree, the answer is yes, and yes. But taking extra hormones should be done with extreme caution: You should do this only after consulting with a physician who is familiar with their use benefits and potential risks.

Let's take a look at some of the most common hormones that are produced in the body and where they're found:

Site	Hormone
Brain	Pregnenolone/DHEA
Pineal gland	Melatonin
Pituitary gland	Growth hormone
Thyroid gland	Thyroid hormones
Adrenals	DHEA
Ovaries	Estrogen/Progesterone
Testes	Testosterone
Skin	DHEA

You probably know that if your thyroid gland is not functioning up to par, your doctor may prescribe a pill containing thyroid hormones. After menopause, when estrogen and progesterone levels begin to decline, a doctor might suggest that a woman take extra hormone replacement therapy. In fact, Premarin, which is prescribed for post-menopausal women for estrogen replacement therapy, is the most commonly prescribed drug in this country. As a society, we are all comfortable with these two examples. We also are comfortable with wearing reading glasses once we reach an age when we are no longer able to read the newspaper without them. But we are less comfortable with taking extra hormones that support the adrenal glands, pineal gland, or the brain. This is where the controversy begins.

All of us produce hormones naturally, and there's a lot of literature and clinical evidence now supporting the use of extra hormones to slow down or even reverse the aging process. These anti-aging potions are hitting the market at record speeds.

Most hormones can be subdivided into natural or synthetic forms. All hormones sold through a drug store or health food store are processed in some

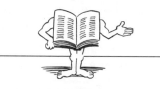

Body Language

Hormones are substances produced by specific glands of your body, such as the thyroid, adrenals, ovaries, or testicles. Hormones influence the way your organs, tissues, and cells respond. Extra hormones are also available in various forms, including pills, topical creams, and injections.

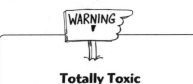

Totally Toxic

Anabolic steroids are used by body builders and weight lifters in an effort to "bulk up." These should *never* be used for this purpose, however. They can cause liver damage, testicular atrophy, heart disease, cancer, and even death.

way and placed in a tablet or capsule form. The term "natural," however, indicates that a hormone is structurally identical or fairly close to the chemical substance produced in your body.

On the other hand, the "synthetic" hormones differ structurally from what your body normally produces; these are typically manufactured by a drug company. One example is Premarin, a synthetic form of estrogen manufactured by Wyeth-Ayerst. A more natural form of estrogen, one that is chemically similar to what your body normally produces, can be made for you by a "compounding pharmacist." About 1,500 compounding pharmacies throughout the country can fill your natural hormone replacement with a physician's prescription. In this case, too, the actual dosage can be tailored for your specific needs. Take a look at Chapter 15 for further discussion of natural hormone replacement therapy.

Making Way for Melatonin

Melatonin is a hormone that's secreted by the pineal gland, a tiny gland within the brain. It helps regulate the body's time clock and influences sleep and wakefulness. It may also have an impact on how and when we age. The amount of melatonin produced by the pineal peaks around age 25 and then begins to decline. By the time you're 65, your level is usually about one-third to one-quarter of your peak amount.

This fact may partially explain why about one-third of people over age 65 are insomniac. Most experts agree that melatonin helps you achieve a restful night of sleep and can also fight jet lag. But more controversial are the claims that a decline in melatonin contributes to your susceptibility to age-related diseases and that taking this hormone in supplemental form can protect or even reverse aspects of the aging process.

At least in animal studies, melatonin seemed to have an anti-aging effect. For example, in mice who were given melatonin, researchers noted the following benefits:

➤ Improved muscle tone

➤ Improved digestion

➤ Less risk of cataracts

➤ Improvement in immune response

➤ Extended lifespan

➤ Greater energy

Sounds pretty good, but there's a problem. The last time I checked, I wasn't a mouse, and chances are neither are you. While there appears to be growing evidence of anti-aging affects in animal studies, there is less documentation for the use of melatonin in humans. It certainly does help as a sleep aid, but anti-aging claims are still being researched.

Among the possible effects of melatonin now being investigated are the following:

➤ It may protect against heart disease by lowering cholesterol levels and reducing the risk of atherosclerosis.

➤ It is a potent antioxidant that can help protect against damage caused by free radicals.

➤ It may play a role in the prevention of cancer, especially of the breast and prostate.

➤ It might help reduce the negative side effects of steroid medications because it seems to prevent the levels of corticosteroids from becoming too high. Because the adrenal glands put out more corticosteroids when we are stressed, restoring melatonin to our more youthful levels may help us cope better with stressful situations and avoid the immune-suppressant effects of corticosteroids.

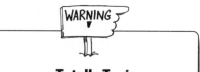

Totally Toxic

Melatonin should be taken with caution by anyone who has diabetes, major depression, autoimmune disorders, leukemia, or lymphoma. Immunosuppressing drugs such as corticosteroids and antidepressants can react adversely with melatonin.

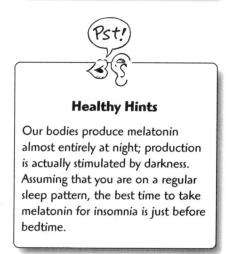

Healthy Hints

Our bodies produce melatonin almost entirely at night; production is actually stimulated by darkness. Assuming that you are on a regular sleep pattern, the best time to take melatonin for insomnia is just before bedtime.

People under the age of 40 should not take melatonin on a regular basis because they usually produce adequate amounts on their own. Pregnant and nursing moms and women trying to conceive should also stay away from it—they may transmit melatonin to their fetus or baby via the placenta or milk, and the effect of taking extra amounts is simply unknown.

We still don't have well-controlled long-term human studies evaluating the impact of taking melatonin supplements. Although this substance offers great promise as an anti-aging agent, it's still probably best for us to reserve judgment until more supportive evidence is in. Don't hesitate to discuss this substance further with your physician before considering taking it.

DHEA Does It All

DHEA (dehydroepiandrosterone) has probably received more recognition than any of the other anti-aging hormones, with the exception of estrogen and progesterone. This hormone is a naturally occurring steroid produced by the adrenal gland. Your body converts DHEA into testosterone and estrogen. The levels rise until about age 25 and then begin to decline. By the time you're 75, your level is probably only 25 percent of what it was during your more youthful years. It is speculated that the decline in DHEA, like that of melatonin, accounts for an increase in several age-related disorders.

What are the benefits of DHEA? According to its supporters, DHEA can help with the following:

➤ Improves your energy. When DHEA was given to men and women between ages 40 and 70, they noted increased energy, better sleep, a better ability to handle stress, and a more relaxed feeling.

➤ May be a predictor of heart disease. It appears that men with a history of heart disease generally have lower levels of DHEA in their blood. Conversely, people with high levels of DHEA are much less likely to die from heart disease. Furthermore, DHEA has been shown to reduce the level of bad LDL cholesterol (which is associated with heart disease) and to lower total blood cholesterol.

➤ Helps with sugar metabolism and assists the action of insulin. Insulin can then take up sugar from the bloodstream and store it in the liver, making you less likely to develop diabetes.

➤ Helps with obesity and weight loss. We know that weight seems to creep up on us as we get a little bit older. Furthermore, we tend to lose muscle mass and gain fat during our later years. DHEA may help increase muscle mass, reduce body fat, and assist with weight loss.

➤ May reduce your risk of developing osteoporosis. As you recall, after menopause, a woman's ovaries stop producing estrogen, progesterone, and testosterone. Those women who have the lowest levels of DHEA are at the highest risk for developing osteoporosis. After menopause, the DHEA level significantly declines, making women more susceptible to brittle bones.

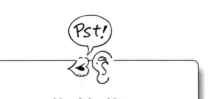

Healthy Hints

If you're hoping to lose weight with DHEA, you also need to combine supplementation with regular exercise, a low-fat diet, and a reduction in simple carbohydrates and excessive sweets.

➤ May rejuvenate the immune system by activating your white blood cells and increasing the number of cancer-fighting natural killer cells.

➤ May help combat lupus. In one study, people with lupus who took DHEA noted marked improvement and fewer of the kidney problems frequently associated with this disorder.

It sounds too good to be true, right? There's no question that the initial data look promising, but once again, I remind you that this research is still in its infancy. The long-term effects of DHEA are still largely unknown. I have frequently screened many patients for a deficiency of DHEA by running a blood test or saliva study, and an imbalance or deficiency is not uncommon. I use this hormone on many patients over the age of 50, usually starting them on a very low dose, in the 5 mg or 10 mg range. Anyone taking DHEA should be under a physician's care and supervised on a regular basis.

Some experts also believe that your level of DHEA could have an impact on your risk of developing cancer. The possibility of DHEA being an anti-cancer agent is extremely controversial, and some studies suggest that it may stimulate the growth of breast tumors or ovarian cancers in animal studies. Another concern in humans is the possibility that DHEA can enlarge the prostate gland because it is eventually metabolized into testosterone, which may worsen this condition. Although this risk has not been supported with hard data, the fear remains. On the other hand, certain animal studies have shown that DHEA may block the growth of breast tumors, colon cancer, and other cancers. As you can see, the evidence is contradictory—and far from conclusive. For this reason alone, my advice is to err on the side of caution unless your doctor feels that it's absolutely necessary for you to take it.

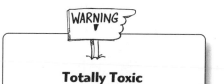

Totally Toxic

Some people, especially women, have noted that taking DHEA can stimulate facial hair growth or cause facial acne. If this occurs, it's best to reduce the dose or stop it completely. Fortunately, these symptoms subside soon after discontinuing the DHEA.

Well, Sex Is Still Good

Although you may be slowing down as you get older, it doesn't mean that everything has to decline. You know that old saying: "Like a fine wine, it gets better with age." With advancing age, your sex life can certainly continue—at least, in most cases. Some find it better than ever. The kids are probably out of the house now, you don't have to wait up for them to come in from their dates, and the two of you can just enjoy being with each other. If you're still in good physical health (and I hope you are, especially after you've read the advice in the first 22 chapters), there's no reason why you can't continue to have an active sex life.

However, some medical conditions might make performance more difficult, especially for men. For example, long-standing diabetes or hypertension can contribute to *impotency*. Certain medications, such as beta blockers, can also affect potency. On the other hand, many women need extra estrogen and testosterone to improve their libido or pep up their sex lives. In fact, whereas many years ago women were given only estrogen and progesterone after menopause, thousands are now given a combination of both estrogen and testosterone, a male hormone generally thought to increase libido.

The Answer to Your Prayers

With anywhere from 10 million to 20 million Americans suffering from impotency, men as well as drug manufacturers have been looking for "the magic bullet" to help with this problem. It's been estimated that nearly 25 percent of men over age 50 may be affected by some form of erectile dysfunction. Although at times the cause of this problem may be psychological, the majority of the cases are related to some kind of underlying physical condition. Hardening of the arteries and buildup of plaque is perhaps the most common cause. It sort of makes sense: If insufficient amounts of blood get to the penis, it's more difficult for a man to sustain an erection. As of March 1998, the FDA approved its first drug to treat male impotency: Viagra (sildenafil citrate). By now, almost everybody has heard of it, and more than one million prescriptions are written for it each month—that is expected to rise to nearly three million per month soon.

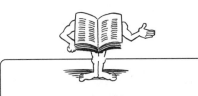

Body Language

Impotency is the condition defined as a man's inability to maintain an erection. This condition, which affects men usually as they grow older, is commonly seen as a result of diabetes or high blood pressure, or as a side effect of several medications.

Millions of men are now taking Viagra at a cost of approximately $10.00 per pill. Although this medication appears to be successful for most men, many are suffering from its side effects, and a few have not lived to tell about it. As it turns out, this drug may not be the magic bullet it was thought to be. During the first five months of its use, the FDA has confirmed 69 deaths among its users. Unfortunately, that number seems to be increasing with each passing month. To add to this concern, Viagra has recently been approved for use in Europe. Pfizer, the manufacturer, expects to receive marketing approval in at least 50 countries in the near future.

Even some women have been taking Viagra with the hope that it may help improve their libido. At this time, however, Viagra is only approved for men, and its effects on women are not truly known.

Although 70 percent of the men using this drug feel that Viagra is effective, it is associated with a number of side effects. The most common side effects include these:

➤ Headaches, which occur in about one out of eight men. Some of these are quite severe, especially when Viagra is taken in higher doses.

➤ Vision problems. About 3 percent of Viagra users report developing visual disturbances, ranging from blurred vision to seeing a bluish-green halo.

➤ Passing out. Viagra can lower blood pressure—when used in combination with nitroglycerin or other antihypertensive medications, there is a risk of fainting, blacking out, or even going into shock. Keep in mind that many of the people for whom Viagra is prescribed have high blood pressure and are taking blood pressure pills containing nitroglycerin.

Given these ongoing problems with Viagra, let's explore some of the perhaps wiser and more natural therapies that address the cause and treatment of sexual dysfunction.

Beyond Viagra

Atherosclerosis, high blood pressure, and diabetes are three of the major causes of impotency, so it makes a lot of sense to try to prevent these problems in the first place to protect against erectile dysfunction. Diet should be your highest priority: Here are my male potency power recommendations:

➤ Eat a diet rich in whole foods, including fresh fruits, vegetables, whole grains, and legumes. These foods are low in saturated fat and contain no cholesterol, thereby reducing your risk of plaque buildup.

➤ Get adequate protein from low-fat foods, such as legumes, tofu, lean meat, fish, and chicken. Try to avoid high-fat selections, such as hot dogs, hamburgers, ham, pork, and steak.

➤ Try to keep your blood cholesterol level below 200 mg/dl to prevent plaque buildup. Consider adding more garlic, oat bran, tomatoes, and blueberries to your diet.

➤ Maintain a good exercise program, and avoid obesity. This can help control your blood pressure and blood sugar.

➤ Limit or eliminate your intake of drugs that may contribute to impotency. These include blood pressure medications, antihistamines, antidepressants, tranquilizers, and antipsychotics, as well as alcohol.

➤ If you're a cigarette smoker, try to quit as soon as possible, because cigarette smoking has been associated with atherosclerosis and impotency.

In addition to a wholesome diet, nutritional supplements may play a role in improving sexual desire. Several years ago, the FDA approved the drug yohimbine, which is derived from the bark of a Yohimbe tree, a native plant in West Africa. Yohimbine seems to increase blood flow to the erectile tissue and may increase libido. But it's not 100 percent effective—it appears to be successful in about 40 percent of cases. Moreover, Yohimbine has potential risks, including elevated blood pressure and heart rate, dizziness, anxiety, headaches, and skin flushing.

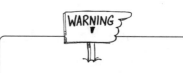

Totally Toxic

Viagra should absolutely *not* be taken if you're also taking any nitrates or medication containing nitroglycerin. This can result in serious side effects and possibly sudden death. You should also avoid the use of cimetidine, erythromycin, ketoconazole, or rifampin when taking Viagra.

Ginkgo biloba, an herb that increases blood flow and oxygen content to the brain and the rest of the body, should also be considered if you're troubled with erectile dysfunction. Try to find ginkgo that's standardized to 24 percent ginkgo flavonglycosides. I usually recommend about 80 mg three times per day.

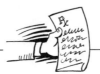

Note from Your Doctor

Although Panax ginseng has historically been thought to be a "sexual rejuvenator", the scientific evidence supporting this is quite weak. However, ginseng may help promote sperm formation and increase testosterone levels, so it may help improve libido if taken in a dose of 100 mg three times per day.

A third herb, known as muira puama (also known as potency wood), may be useful for erectile dysfunction and a lack of sex drive. A recent study found that this herb heightened the libido in 62 percent of the patients and reduced impotency in 51 percent. Although the mechanism for how this herb works is unknown, it appears that it boosts both the psychological and physical aspects of the sex drive. The dosage you might consider is 200 mg three times per day; some have reported improvement within one month.

Getting Your Hormones in Balance

For more than 30 years, women have been taking hormones after menopause to help keep their bones strong and their hearts healthy. In fact, more than 10 million women take estrogen on a regular basis, making it the number-one prescribed medication in the United States. Both estrogen and progesterone are generally regarded as female hormones, however, men actually produce a small amount as well, just as women produce the "male" hormone testosterone. However, a man's levels of estrogen and progesterone do not seem to decline as much as a women's might; therefore, men may not need extra amounts as they age.

In the past, these hormones were thought to treat menopausal problems, but now we're finding that they may have many more beneficial effects. All three of these may have anti-aging benefits and may protect you from chronic degenerative diseases and various aspects of the aging process.

Estrogen for Everyone

Estrogen has been prescribed by thousands of doctors for women who have undergone hysterectomies or who experience menopausal symptoms such as hot flashes, night sweats, insomnia, and mood swings. Lo and behold, while taking estrogen for these reasons, many women noted other improvements in their overall health and their sense of well-being. Here are some of the well-documented findings attributed to taking extra estrogen after menopause:

➤ Estrogen users do not suffer as much bone loss as those who do not take this hormone. They also seem to stand taller and straighter.

➤ Estrogen can protect women against heart disease. In fact, taking estrogen can reduce the incidence of heart disease by 50 percent, compared to women who do not take it. It has also been shown to improve cholesterol metabolism by lowering total cholesterol and increasing HDL cholesterol.

➤ Estrogen might reduce the overall death rate. A study at Kaiser Permantente Medical Care Program in Oakland, California, found that women taking estrogen lived not only longer lives but also healthier lives. A 46 percent overall reduction in the death rate resulted in the estrogen users.

➤ Estrogen may actually reduce your risk of tooth decay and tooth loss. Women who were taking estrogen for more than 15 years were half as likely to lose their teeth as those who never took estrogen.

➤ Estrogen may improve your brain function. Many women feel that it improves their mood, their energy, and their memory.

➤ Estrogen may have an impact on the development of Alzheimer's disease. As discussed in Chapter 19, this debilitating brain condition afflicts three times as many women as men. Women who take estrogen may be 30 percent less likely to develop Alzheimer's disease than those who have never taken this hormone. Even if you have Alzheimer's disease, those who take estrogen have shown improvement in their memory and social behavior.

Totally Toxic

Women who are pregnant or known to have breast cancer should not take extra hormones. Also avoid hormone replacement therapy if you've had a previous history of stroke, phlebitis in the legs, or liver disease.

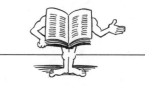

Body Language

Estrogen is an important female hormone produced primarily in the ovaries, and in smaller amounts in the adrenal glands. It is instrumental in regulating the menstrual period, fertility, and menopause.

➤ Estrogen can alleviate menopausal symptoms, relieving hot flashes, night sweats, vaginal dryness, and thinning of the vaginal wall.

There is a never-ending debate regarding the possibility that long-term estrogen use increases the risk of breast cancer. Most authorities do not agree that estrogen increases cancer risk, but some confusion and disagreement exists on this point. Recently, researchers found that women who take synthetic estrogen for more than 10 years may be at greater risk for developing breast cancer. On the other hand, estrogen has been shown to reduce the risk of developing colon cancer. The final word on this debate has yet to be written.

As mentioned earlier in Chapter 15, I generally recommend a natural form of estrogen replacement therapy that includes the three major types of estrogens: estradiol, estriol, and estrone. These are custom-compounded by a compounding pharmacy, according to your doctor's prescription. This form of estrogen is structurally the same as what your body naturally produces and therefore may differ from the common synthetic forms sold at most drug stores. The natural form of estrogen replacement does not seem to increase the risk of cancer—and, in fact, may actually help reduce your risk. It also provides all the other benefits similar to the more commonly prescribed synthetic estrogens.

The Power of Progesterone

As previously mentioned, progesterone is frequently taken along with its close relative, estrogen. It appears that estrogen is both more effective and safer when taken in combination with progesterone. Progesterone helps enhance the action of estrogen, but it, too, begins to decline after menopause. Although estrogen is primarily known for its capability of preparing the uterus for a fertilized egg and maintaining pregnancy, its most recent virtue is perhaps its anti-aging properties.

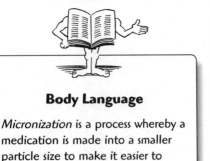

Body Language

Micronization is a process whereby a medication is made into a smaller particle size to make it easier to absorb and assimilate.

Although the most common form of progesterone prescribed today is a synthetic form known as progestin, more physicians are becoming knowledgeable and therefore prescribing natural progesterone. More women seem to feel better on this form of progesterone, and it may have a more potent anti-aging effect. Natural progesterone is structurally the same as what your body naturally produces and can be prepared by a compounding pharmacist, similar to natural estrogen. It can be well-absorbed orally after undergoing a process called micronization, which breaks it into very tiny particles that can be readily absorbed.

Natural progesterone can also be used topically, by applying it to your skin as a gel or cream. Many women prefer this means of administration if they don't tolerate pills well. Some women who take synthetic progesterone may complain of bloating, headaches, and moodiness, but these are much less common in women who take the natural form of progesterone. Furthermore, although some women complain of irritability and mood swings with the synthetic form, the natural form may actually have the opposite effect of reducing mood swings. Let's take a look at some of the beneficial aspects that have been attributed to progesterone:

➤ Natural progesterone actually works better than synthetic progestin in protecting against heart disease. It has a more powerful effect in raising the good HDL cholesterol and also protects against the development of uterine cancer.

➤ Natural progesterone can help build strong bones and reduce your risk of developing osteoporosis.

➤ Progesterone alone may ward off menopausal symptoms, most notably hot flashes. Progesterone cream has been the most effective for this purpose. Simply rub it into the skin on a daily basis. This is particularly advantageous to women who cannot take estrogen because of its side effects or who have a prior history of an estrogen-dependent tumor.

Some exciting benefits of progesterone could lie further out on the horizon. A French physician has found that progesterone may be an effective treatment against certain nerve disorders, including multiple sclerosis. Another researcher found that progesterone could promote the formation of the myelin sheath, the fatty substance surrounding and insulating nerve fibers: MS causes the loss of myelin and disrupts the normal nerve signaling in the body. This research is highly preliminary at this point, but the role of progesterone on progressive MS looks promising.

Touting Testosterone

Testosterone is a hormone produced primarily by a man's testes and in small amounts by the adrenal glands. However, women also produce small amounts of testosterone in the adrenal glands and the ovaries. This hormone helps regulate the sex drive in both men and women. Although we know that the level of testosterone begins to decline in men after age 20 or 30, it also declines in women after menopause, which can result in depression and loss of sex drive. About one-third of all men are affected by the drop in testosterone as they go through mid-life; this can contribute to both physical and emotional changes.

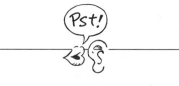

Healthy Hints

Low levels of testosterone have been associated with a higher risk for cardiovascular disease and an increased risk for heart attacks. One study showed great improvement in patients with angina pectoris when they were given extra testosterone.

Here are some of the most important aspects and new findings regarding testosterone in men:

➤ Testosterone may be an anti-aging hormone. Studies have found that men of any age with insufficient amounts of testosterone circulating in their blood stream do not feel well, look well, or function well. They seem to have a loss of muscle mass, loss of mobility and flexibility, loss of bone mass, loss of well-being, and diminished libido. Testosterone may decrease depression as well. Among men with depression who were given extra testosterone, 12 out of 13 reported improvement in their symptoms.

➤ Testosterone can improve muscle size and strength, along with bone strength. Men who are given testosterone are generally able to increase their muscle mass, even if they're not exercising. In addition, they generally show an increase in lean muscle mass and a decrease in their total body fat.

➤ Testosterone may help reduce risk factors associated with heart disease. In fact, it's been used for more than 50 years in Europe to help treat circulatory problems, including clogged arteries and diabetes. Men who have low circulating levels of testosterone generally are at greater risk for developing atherosclerosis or plaque buildup in the coronary vessels. On the other hand, men with the highest levels of testosterone seem to have higher amounts of the good HDL cholesterol, which protects against heart disease.

The concept of using testosterone for reasons other than increasing the sex drive is a relatively new idea. While we're familiar with the use of estrogen and progesterone for use in women during and after menopause, testosterone is now entering in the picture as well.

Just as women go through menopause, some men go through a phenomenon known as *andropause*. This condition involves the progressive decline in testosterone that occurs with advancing age (usually after age 60), usually resulting in erectile dysfunction or a loss in libido.

Note from Your Doctor

Pure natural testosterone is the preferred form of testosterone used today. It is commonly administered by intramuscular injections, suppositories, creams, patches, micronized capsules, or sublingual lozenges. This hormone should be taken only after you consult with your doctor and have diagnostic tests showing insufficient quantities of testosterone.

Great concern still circulates about the possibility that testosterone can stimulate the growth of a benign or malignant tumor in the prostate gland. Men should also be concerned that taking extra doses of testosterone may inhibit their own natural production of the hormone.

For women, the use of testosterone is showing promise. After menopause, the amount of testosterone produced by the ovaries diminishes by about 50 percent. Some women have found that taking extra testosterone with estrogen and (sometimes) progesterone has enhanced their sexual desire, relieved menopausal symptoms, improved their energy, decreased depression, and maybe even strengthened their bones.

Hormones on the Horizon

Three additional hormones are gaining wider popularity as well. Although the scientific documentation for these is not as strong as the previously discussed hormones, they merit a brief overview.

Pregnenolone Prowess

As mentioned in Chapter 4, cholesterol is derived both from your diet and your liver. A portion of this cholesterol is then broken down in the adrenal glands into a hormone known as pregnenolone. In turn, pregnenolone is metabolized into DHEA, progesterone, testosterone, cortisol, or estrogen. Hence, pregnenolone is the precursor for all other hormones we discussed in this chapter. Pregnenolone is thought to help improve your memory. When given to older men and women, an improvement in verbal recall and visual tasks occurred; both of these are markers indicating improved memory.

Interestingly enough, in the 1940s pregnenolone was used for the treatment of rheumatoid arthritis. Patients noted less pain and less fatigue, and felt much stronger after taking it. However, the drug cortisone was then discovered, and further research on pregnenolone fell by the wayside. Because cortisone may be associated with a litany of side effects—including osteoporosis, cataracts, liver inflammation, and immune suppression—pregnenolone might be a natural hormone to slow the aging process. This substance must be studied much further, however, before health claims can be made about it.

Homering with Androstenedione

Another adrenal steroid hormone that has gained some popularity of late is known as androstenedione. This substance is derived from DHEA and a progesterone metabolite (hydroxyprogesterone). Androstenedione is then broken down to form either testosterone or estrogen. Androstenedione became very popular during the summer and fall of 1998, when St. Louis Cardinals' first baseman, Mark McGwire, broke Roger Maris's Major League Baseball record for hitting the most home runs in a single season. As McGwire approached the record, it became public knowledge that he had been taking androstenedione. Because this hormone is broken down into testosterone, many feel that it may also provide some of the same benefits that testosterone does, such as building greater muscle strength and muscle size. We need more research on this substance, however, before we can know more about its long-term safety or overall effects.

Note from Your Doctor

Although it is illegal for professional football players to take any form of steroid hormones—including androstenedione—no such rule applied to pro baseball. Because androstenedione is available over-the-counter, and because it is not a prescription drug, Mark McGwire was allowed to continue using this substance during his record-breaking home run season in the summer of 1998.

Growing Younger with HGH

The pituitary gland, often called the master gland, is a tiny gland situated in the center of the brain. It controls the release of many of the body's hormones, including human growth hormone (HGH). This hormone has been used in conventional medicine in an effort to help children with growth failures reach normal adult development. HGH can trigger the onset of sexual maturity in adolescence, improve muscle strength and size, and stimulate bone growth. It's now being investigated and used in increasing numbers to help slow the aging process.

In one recent study, men who were found to have low levels of HGH were given injections of this hormone. After six months they noted an increase in lean muscle mass, a decrease in body fat, improvement in skin fullness and elasticity, and an increase in bone density. The researcher concluded that human growth hormone may be able to reverse 10 to 20 years of aging. This hormone also declines as both men and women proceed in their later years. For this reason, this substance is being investigated for other protective and beneficial uses.

In fact, HGH recently has been found to improve lung capacity, improve heart function, and improve kidney

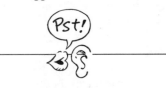

Healthy Hints

Most people who use human growth hormone will "cycle" it, meaning that they might take it for four to six weeks and then stop for about two weeks. This two-week rest period seems to help prevent the pituitary gland in the brain from naturally reducing its own natural growth hormone production.

function as well as immune system response. Some find that the skin is more resilient after taking this, and wrinkles may actually decrease. Some users of HGH report that this substance helps them feel happier, healthier, and stronger. Almost sounds too good to be true, doesn't it? In fact, one anti-aging specialist is predicting that by the year 2005, virtually everyone over the age of 50 will be taking a pill to help stimulate their body's own production of HGH. At the present time, this substance is usually administered by costly injections running more than $3,000 per year. However, some manufacturers are now claiming that other forms—such as pills, lozenges, or sublingual drops—may also be effective. The scientific data to support this is still quite sketchy, and most of the perceived benefits (other than that derived from the intramuscular injectable form) is merely anecdotal.

Because the use of HGH is so expensive, some physicians recommend a variety of amino acids to help your body produce more growth hormone on its own. The most commonly prescribed amino acids include arginine, ornithine, lysine, glycine, and glutamine. Most of these amino acids should be taken on an empty stomach, and the majority are taken at bedtime. However, we still need more clinical evidence that these amino acids can actually raise your growth hormone to levels close to those of your 20s or 30s. Moreover, we need further studies to evaluate the long-term effects on the stimulation of the pituitary and subsequent extra secretion of HGH.

The Least You Need to Know

➤ Hormone levels generally decline with advancing age. Restoring them to earlier levels may slow the aging process.

➤ Melatonin helps regulate the body's time clock and influences sleeping patterns.

➤ DHEA may improve energy, enhance your immune response, and prevent osteoporosis.

➤ Estrogen can help prevent osteoporosis, heart disease, Alzheimer's disease, and menopausal symptoms.

➤ Pregnenolone and androstenedione may have health benefits, but more research is needed.

Chapter 24

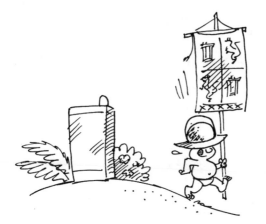

So, Is There Really a Fountain of Youth?

In This Chapter

➤ How to beat the clock

➤ The ins and outs of cosmetic surgery

➤ Beauty secrets to enhance your appearance

➤ Achieving real beauty from the inside out

So, are you still looking for the Fountain of Youth? Nobody has really found that magic water spring that will keep us going forever. For today, we still have to accept that death represents the culmination of our lifecycle. But new medical advances are making it possible to live a very long and healthy life. With the knowledge outlined in this book, it is entirely possible to be an agile and energetic centenarian. While we can't have immortality, we *can* turn back the clock and stay biologically young.

Note from Your Doctor

If you are already following the guidelines suggested in this book, you are probably already physically younger than your chronological age. However, if you have a sedentary lifestyle with poor eating habits and are in need of an overhaul, you can still beat the clock and feel like you've found your Fountain of Youth.

There's Always Cosmetic Surgery

The guys in the Bible lived hundreds and hundreds of years. But what about quality? Was it so great wandering alone in the desert for so many years? And did you ever notice that after their first 100 years of life, there were never any women with them? Maybe that's why women always feel so much pressure to maintain their youthful looks. After all, if the patriarchs were going to wander aimlessly without them, they should at least have fond memories. I suppose that is what cosmetic surgery is all about, creating fond memories. If we are doing everything right, we should all look as good as we can, for as long as we can.

If you want a more dramatic change, there is always cosmetic surgery. So are you a candidate for cosmetic surgery? If you answer yes to any of the following, then you might want to hire a good plastic surgeon who can turn you into the mythological god or goddess of your choice. Just remember, though, that these are cosmetic changes and not health-improving procedures.

1. You really eat a healthy, nutritional diet.
2. You supplement your diet with anti-aging nutrients.
3. You exercise regularly. (Once a month is good for consistency, but that's not regularly.)
4. As far as you know, you are disease-free.
5. You don't care that you'll never know what you would have looked like if you aged naturally.
6. Vanity is a big thing with you.
7. You have a huge stash of cash that is burning a hole in your pocket.
8. You would still like to enter the Miss America Pageant.

9. If your masculinity keeps you from entering the pageant, you would still like to date the contestants.

10. You don't care how much it will hurt because, after it's done, you'll look great.

Cosmetic surgery is immediate gratification to reward a lifetime of effort. If you have worked hard to get to this point, and if you can answer yes to five or more of these statements, then go for the big carrot.

The $6 Million Man

Remember Steve Austin? We can rebuild him; we have the technology. Name your part, and we can make it better. You may not have bionic powers, but you can sure look like it. Beauty is not just cosmetics and hair salons. Beauty involves taking care of your whole body, whether you're a man or a woman. So take a good look in the mirror and decide if you really like what you see. Is being rebuilt going to fix the problem, or does the problem need deeper attention?

Maybe it is just a full head of hair you're after. Maybe you have too much gut and not enough gusto, or maybe you want to do away with your Coke-bottle reading glasses. If permanently altering your physical features will help you develop a stronger and more positive attitude, then go for it.

The Bionic Woman

Here comes Jamie. It's amazing to me the number of women opting for elective cosmetic procedures. It almost seems harder to find a female who has *not* permanently changed her appearance in some way. If you include body-piercing (it's not just the ears anymore), you can include most of the female population of the world in this number.

Name your part—or parts. You can have your nose or your eyes or your chin and neck done, or you can have wrinkles removed with collagen injections and acid peels. There is liposuction and hip reduction and tummy tucks, too. There are implants and opportunities to move stuff from here to there and back again. You can go up a size in some areas and down a size in others. You can go in for the works and leave as a whole new you. Or you can just try to simplify your life by having your makeup permanently applied.

If you can dream it, you can look like it. Having not yet undergone any cosmetic procedures myself, I can only relay what I hear from my patients: "It hurts!" "I would never do this again!" "Will the pain ever go away?" "What about the itching?" "Why didn't they tell me about the scarring?" Nonetheless, those who do go under the knife say that the little bit of pain after the procedure is well worth the change. This is obviously a personal decision, and one not to be made without a fair amount of thought and research.

Should you opt for the surgical route to rejuvenation, make sure you check out your surgeon's credentials carefully. Of equal importance, look into the anesthesiologist's record, too. Before and after pictures in promotional material around the surgeon's office can be misleading, so ask for references—and follow up on them. And remember, the best facelift, boob job, and tushie tuck won't increase your lifespan unless you help your body heal itself.

Preserving Your Most Visible Asset

Some say beauty is only skin deep. You may say that's deep enough for you to do what you can to keep up a youthful appearance. After all, when you wake up in the morning and look in the mirror, what's the first thing you see? It's you and your attitude. So fool yourself into feeling good by looking good. The skin on your face, more than any other part of your body, reveals the most about how you feel mentally, emotionally, and physically. Here are some wonderful beauty secrets to help enhance your largest organ:

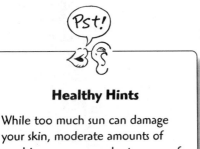

Healthy Hints

While too much sun can damage your skin, moderate amounts of sunshine serve as our best source of vitamin D to help prevent loss of bone density. Get your sun in the morning, before the sun's damaging rays do more harm than help.

Totally Toxic

Try not to put anything on your skin that you wouldn't put in your mouth. After all, what you put on your skin gets absorbed into your body through your pores.

➤ Stay out of the sun. The harmful rays of the sun can damage and age your complexion. Too much sun breaks down collagen and elastin, leaving you looking like a raisin.

➤ Eat lots of nuts and avocado. These contain naturally occurring fats that help enhance your complexion.

➤ Drink lots of water to moisturize you from the inside out. Coffee and soda do not count toward your eight glasses a day.

➤ Get plenty of sleep. You always look better when you are well rested, and you will have more energy to carry you through the rest of the day.

➤ Sweat it out through exercise or sauna; it's good to sweat out toxins and let your pores breathe.

➤ Dry-brush your skin with a natural bristle brush or a loofah. Do this before you shower. It hurts at first, but soon you'll be glowing from removing all your dead skin cells.

➤ Moisturize your skin with jojoba oil. Let your body soak it up for smooth, soft skin. Shampoo with it for added body and shine.

Helping Your Body Heal Itself

Real beauty comes from nurturing your whole self; that's inner beauty, and it radiates out to the world. When your mental, physical, and emotional components all work in sync, health and longevity are yours.

We know that there is no such thing as the Fountain of Youth, but don't neglect what we do know while you wait for the magical pill promising immortality.

Eat right, don't forget your vegetables, get lots of exercise, take your vitamins, and have a positive attitude—you've heard all this before, from your mother, from your doctor, from your spouse, and now from me. This time, start listening. You have come this far in the book, and now its time to turn back—the clock, that is.

Note from Your Doctor

In the last 70 years, our average life expectancy has increased from 47 years to nearly 80 years. Equally dramatic are the increases in rates of heart disease, cancer, and other degenerative diseases. If we can prevent these diseases from occurring, then we can surely boost our lifespan.

Finding a Like-Minded Health Care Practitioner

Where do you start? Now that your mind is going in the right direction, how do you find a diet specialist, a nutritionist, an herbal medicine consultant, a homeopath, a personal trainer, an acupuncturist, a chiropractor, a certified chelation doctor, and an environmental expert? What you really need is one-stop shopping: a knowledgeable physician who specializes in preventive medicine. Such a practitioner, while guiding you on your path to living longer and healthier, can also help you sort through the plethora of available traditional and not-so-traditional therapies.

It's not as hard as you might think to find a nutritionally oriented physician. Try getting in touch with the following organizations that can help you find a qualified and certified medical practitioner in your area.

➤ The American College for Advancement in Medicine (ACAM), 23121 Verdugo Drive, Suite 204, in Laguna Hills, CA 92653: (949) 583-7666.

➤ The American Preventive Medical Association, in Great Falls, VA: (703) 759-0662.

➤ The American Association for Naturopathic Physicians, in Seattle, WA: (206) 298-0126.

➤ American Academy of Environmental Medicine, in New Hope, PA: (215) 862-4544.

You Are What You Think

Over the next decade, science will give us a lot to think about, with cloning and reprogramming, neuron replacement, and more information on antioxidants, hormones, melatonin, and DHEA, to name a few. New advances make headlines in the newspaper every day. So read the paper, not just the sports section or the gossip column. Stay enlightened by keeping in touch with the world. Just as with exercising your body, work out your mind. Your mind, like your body, follows one simple rule: Use it or lose it.

Since the beginning of time, man has been looking for a miraculous elixir of youth. And, since the beginning of time, molecular processes have not changed. We know that everything in the universe ages, so why shouldn't you? But with advances in knowledge and science, we have also found ways to slow the molecular route to aging.

An entirely modern field of medicine has paved the way for new directions toward agelessness. This emerging science, known as psychoneuroimmunology, joins the different states of our mind and their effect on our brain response and our immune system function.

When put to practice, and put simply, psychoneuroimmunologists study how the mind affects the behavior of the rest of the body. Scientists are now confirming what we have known all along: that with the right attitude, we can do anything we set our minds to do—even slowing down our biological time clocks.

The Least You Need to Know

➤ It is possible to turn back your biological time clock.

➤ There are doctors out there who understand where you are coming from.

➤ Cosmetic surgery has cosmetic benefits.

➤ Use your mind to take control of your own destiny.

Additional Nutritional Information

Cholesterol and Fat Levels in Common Foods

Food	Cholesterol(mg)	Saturated Fat(g)	Total Fat(g)
Meat (3^1/$_2$ oz)			
Beef, top round, lean	84	2.2	6.2
Ground, lean	87	7.3	18.5
Beef, prime rib, lean	86	14.9	35.2
Processed Meats (3^1/$_2$ oz)			
Pork or beef	47	6.4	17.8
Sausage, smoked	71	10.6	30.3
Bologna, beef	56	11.7	28.4
Frankfurter, beef	48	12.0	29.4
Salami	79	12.2	34.4
Pork (3^1/$_2$ oz)			
Ham steak, lean	45	1.4	4.2
Pork, center loin	111	4.7	13.7
Pork, spare ribs	121	11.8	30.3
Poultry (3^1/$_2$ oz)			
Chicken broilers or fryers, roasted:			
Light meat without skin	85	1.3	4.5
Light meat with skin	84	3.1	10.9
Dark meat without skin	93	2.7	9.7
Dark meat with skin	91	4.4	15.8
Chicken skin	83	11.4	40.7

continues

continued

Food	Cholesterol(mg)	Saturated Fat(g)	Total Fat(g)
Fish (3¹/₂ oz)			
Cod	58	0.1	0.7
Lobster	72	0.1	0.6
Clam	67	0.2	2.0
Crab	100	0.2	1.8
Shrimp	195	0.3	1.1
Snapper	47	0.4	1.7
Oysters	109	1.3	5.0
Tuna	49	1.6	6.3
Mackerel	75	4.2	17.8
Eggs			
Egg white	0	0	trace
Egg, whole	272	1.7	5.6
Egg yolk	272	1.7	5.6
Nuts and seeds (3¹/₂ oz)			
Almonds	0	4.9	51.6
Sunflower seeds	0	5.2	49.8
Pecans	0	5.2	64.6
Walnuts	0	5.6	61.9
Cashews	0	9.2	46.4
Fruit (3¹/₂ oz)			
Peaches	0	0.01	0.09
Oranges	0	0.015	0.12
Strawberries	0	0.02	0.37
Apples	0	0.058	0.36
Vegetables (3¹/₂ oz)			
Cooked, boiled, drained:			
Potatoes, without skin	0	0.026	0.10
Carrots	0	0.034	0.18
Spinach	0	0.042	0.26
Broccoli	0	0.043	0.28

Food	Cholesterol(mg)	Saturated Fat(g)	Total Fat(g)
Squash	0	0.064	0.31
Corn	0	0.197	1.28
Avocados, Florida	0	1.74	8.86
Avocados, California	0	2.60	17.34
Milk and cream (8 oz)			
Skim milk	4	0.3	0.4
Low-fat milk	10	1.6	2.6
Whole milk	35	5.6	8.9
Light cream	159	28.8	46.3
Heavy whipping cream	326	54.8	88.1
Yogurt and sour cream (8 oz)			
Plain yogurt, skim milk	4	0.3	0.4
Plain yogurt, low fat	14	2.3	3.5
Plain yogurt, whole milk	29	2.8	7.4
Sour cream	102	30	48.2
Soft cheeses (8 oz)			
Cottage, low-fat	10	1.5	2.3
Cottage, creamed	31	6.0	9.5
Ricotta, part skim	76	12.1	19.5
Ricotta, whole milk	116	18.8	29.5
Cream cheese	250	49.9	79.2
Hard cheeses (8 oz)			
Mozzarella, whole milk	177	29.7	49.0
Provolone	157	38.8	60.4
Swiss	209	40.4	62.4
Muenster	218	43.4	68.1
American processed	213	44.7	71.1
Cheddar	238	47.9	75.1

Percent of Calories from Protein in Common Foods

Protein	Percent of Calories from Protein
Grains	
Wheat germ	31
Wheat	17
Oatmeal	15
Millet	12
Barley	11
Brown rice	8
Dairy products	
Cottage cheese	31
Cheddar cheese	24
Milk	18
Legumes	
Soybean sprouts	54
Mungbean sprouts	43
Tofu	43
Soybeans	35
Lentils	29
Split peas	28
Kidney beans	26
Navy beans	26
Lima beans	26
Garbanzo beans	23
Meat, fish, poultry	
Pork chop	82
Chicken with skin	78
Sirloin steak	71
White tuna	67
Ground beef	62
Flounder	51
Nuts and seeds	
Pumpkin seeds	21
Peanuts	18

Protein	Percent of Calories from Protein
Sunflower seeds	17
Sesame seeds	13
Almonds	12
Cashews	12
Fruit	
Honeydew melon	10
Cantaloupe	9
Strawberries	8
Oranges	8
Apricots	8
Grapes	8
Watermelon	8
Peaches	6
Bananas	5
Grapefruit	5
Pineapple	3
Apples	3
Vegetables	
Spinach	49
Kale	45
Broccoli	45
Brussels sprouts	44
Turnip greens	43
Collards	43
Cauliflower	40
Mushrooms	38
Parsley	34
Lettuce	34
Peas	30
Zucchini	28
Green beans	26
Cucumber	24
Green pepper	22
Artichokes	22

continues

continued

Protein	Percent of Calories from Protein
Cabbage	22
Celery	21
Eggplant	21
Tomatoes	18
Onions	16
Potatoes, white	11
Sweet potatoes	6

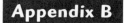

Organizations

To Find a Nutritionally Oriented Health Care Practitioner

American Academy of Anti-Aging Medicine (A4M)
1341 West Fullerton, Suite 111
Chicago, IL 60614
(773) 528-4333
Fax: (773) 528-5390

American Academy of Environmental Medicine
10 East Randolph Street
New Hope, PA 18938
(215) 862-4544

American Association for Naturopathic Physicians
601 Valley Street, Suite 105
Seattle, WA 98109
(206) 298-0126

American Chiropractic Association
Council on Nutrition
1701 Clarendon Boulevard
Arlington, VA 22209
(703) 276-8800

American College for Advancement in Medicine
23121 Verdugo Drive, Suite 204
Laguna Hills, CA 92653
(800) 532-3688
Fax: (949) 455-9679

American Holistic Medical Association
4101 Lake Boone Trail, Suite 201
Raleigh, NC 27607
(919) 787-5146

Foundation for the Advancement of Innovative Medicine (FAIM)
100 Airport Executive Park
Nanuet, NY 10954
(914) 371-3246

International and American Associations of Clinical Nutritionists
5200 Keller Springs Road, Suite 410
Dallas, TX 75248
(972) 250-2829

To Find Help for Medical Problems

Alzheimer's Association
919 North Michigan, Suite 1000
Chicago, IL 60611
(800) 621-0379

American Aging Association
2129 Providence Avenue
Chester, PA 19013
(610) 874-7550
Fax: (610) 876-7715

American Association for Cancer Education
University of Alabama-Birmingham
Vh 700
Birmingham, AL 35294
(205) 934-3054
Fax: (205) 934-3278

American Cancer Society
1599 Clifton Road NE
Atlanta, GA 30329
(800) 227-2345
Fax: (312) 641-6588

American Diabetes Association
1660 Duke Street
Alexandria, VA 22314
(800) 232-3472

American Dietetic Association
216 West Jackson Boulevard
Chicago, IL 60606
(312) 899-0040

American Heart Association
7272 Greenville Avenue
Dallas, TX 75231
(214) 373-6300
(800) 242-8721

American Institute for Cancer Research
1759 R Street, NW
Washington, DC 20009
(800) 843-8114
Fax: (202) 328-7226

National Cholesterol Education Program
NHLBI Information Center
PO Box 30105
Bethesda, MD 20824-0105
(301) 951-3275

National Headache Foundation
5252 North Western Avenue
Chicago, IL 60625
(800) 843-2256

National Osteoporosis Foundation
1150 17th Street, NW, Suite 500
Washington, DC 20036
(202) 223-2226
(800) 223-9994

National Parkinson Foundation
1501 NW 9th Avenue
Miami, FL 33136
(305) 547-8448
(800) 327-4545
(800) 433-7022 (Florida)
(800) 400-8448 (California)
Fax: (305) 548-4403

Federal or Private Agencies for More Information

Academy of Pharmaceutical Research and Science
2215 Constitution Avenue, NW
Washington, DC 20037
(202) 628-4410
Fax: (202) 783-2351

Alliance for Aging Research
2021 K Street, NW, Suite 305
Washington, DC 20006
(202) 293-2856
Fax: (202) 785-8574

American Nutraceutical Association
4647 T Highway 280 East #133
Birmingham, AL 35242
(205) 980-5710
Fax: (205) 991-9302

Council for Responsible Nutrition
1300 19th Street, NW, Suite 310
Washington, DC 20036
(202) 872-1488
Fax: (202) 872-9594

Food and Drug Administration (FDA)
5600 Fishers Lane
Rockville, MD 20857
(301) 443-3170

International Federation on Aging
601 E Street, NW
Washington, DC 20049
(202) 434-2427
Fax: (202) 434-6458

National Council on Aging
409 3rd Street, SW, Suite 200
Washington, DC 20024
(800) 424-9046
Fax: (202) 479-0735

National Foundation for Brain Research
1250 24th Street, NW, Suite 300
Washington, DC 20037
(202) 293-5453

National Institute of Health
9000 Rockville Pike
Building 31, Room 8A06
Bethesda, MD 20892
(301) 496-5751

National Institute of Mental Health
5600 Fishers Lane, Room 7C-02
Rockville, MD 20857
(301) 443-4513

National Institute of Neurological Disorders and Stroke
9000 Rockville Pike
Building 21, Room 8A16
Bethesda, MD 20892
(800) 352-9424

National Institute on Aging
NIA Information Center
Box 8057
Gaithersburg, MD 20898
(800) 222-2225

Office of Alternative Medicine
National Institutes of Health
OAM Clearinghouse
Box 8218
Silver Spring, MD 20907
(888) 644-6226

Index

Symbols

5-HTP (hydroxytryptophan), 109
  depression treatment, 218-219

A

Academy of Pharmaceutical Research and Science contact information, 297
acetyl-L-carnitine, Alzheimer's disease prevention/treatment, 229
additives/preservatives, 32
aerobic activity, 261
  calculating target heart rate, 258-259
  see also exercise
aging, 6-7
  American Academy of Anti-Aging Medicine (A4M) contact information, 295
  American Aging Association contact information, 296
  attitude, 243-244
  horizontal versus vertical disease, 8-9
  International Federation on Aging contact information, 298
  National Council on Aging contact information, 298
  National Institute on Aging contact information, 299
  normal range, 7-8
  statistics, 4
aging gracefully, 243-244
  laughter, 252
  love, 253
  parenting late in life, 251-252
  spirituality, 246-247
    meditation, 250-251
    yoga, 247-249
AIDS treatment, N-acetyl cysteine (NAC), 108
alcohol
  negative effects, 31
    cancer risk, 158
    cataract risk, 235
    osteoporosis risk, 171
  reduced consumption as depression treatment, 215
  wine
    French paradox, 56
    organic wines, 57
    red wine, 56-57
allergies
  food, effect on immune system, 131
  physical examinations, 16
  treatments
    quercetin, 110-111
    stinging nettle, 124
  vitamin C benefits, 89
Alliance for Aging Research contact information, 298
alpha-lipoic acid, 105-106
alternative medicine/practices, 10-11
  Office of Alternative Medicine contact information, 299
aluminum
  Alzheimer's link, 226
  in antacids, 23
Alzheimer's disease, 223-230
  Alzheimer's Association contact information, 296
  cause, 225-226
  diagnosis, 224-225
  dietary prevention/ treatment, 226-229
    acetyl-L-carnitine, 229
    B-vitamins, 227
    ginkgo biloba, 228
    lecithin, 229
    phosphatidyl serine (PS), 229
    vitamin E, 228-229
  discovery of disease, 224
  estrogen treatment, 229-230
  symptoms, 225
American Academy of Anti-Aging Medicine (A4M) contact information, 295
American Academy of Environmental Medicine contact information, 295
American Aging Association contact information, 296
American Association for Cancer Education contact information, 296
American Association for Naturopathic Physicians contact information, 295
American Cancer Society contact information, 296
American College for Advancement in Medicine contact information, 295
American Diabetes Association contact information, 296
American Dietetic Association contact information, 296
American Heart Association contact information, 297
American Holistic Medical Association contact information, 295
American Institute for Cancer Research contact information, 297

American Nutraceutical
  Association contact
  information, 298
American Soybean Association
  contact information, 145
amino acids
  depression treatment, 220
  eye health (taurine), 238
  prostate enlargement
    treatment, 207
andropause (male menopause),
  278
androstenedione, 279-280
angina (angina pectoris), 92,
  140, 147-148
  testosterone level, 277
antacids, aluminum warning,
  23
anthrocyanosides, blueberries,
  58
anti-nutrients, 29-31
antibiotics
  effect on immune system,
    130
  herbal alternatives
    echinacea, 118-119
    urinary tract infections,
      124-125
  over-prescription, 75
  possible adverse effects, 23
antidepressants, 211-213
  see also depression
antioxidants
  alpha-lipoic acid, 105-106
  bilberry extracts, 118
  cancer prevention, 71
  CoQ_{10}, 106-107
  eye health, 238
    cataract prevention,
      233-234
    macular degeneration
      prevention, 236-237
  glutathione, 108-109
  grape seed extract, 111
  green tea, 61
  hawthorn, 120-121
  heart disease prevention/
    treatment, 149
  Kava, 121-122
  lycopene
    prostate health, 207
    tomatoes, 61-62
  supplements, 76-77

wine, 56
zinc, 103
arthritis, 187-196
  osteoarthritis (degenerative
    joint disease, DJD),
    187-188
    benefits of niacinamide
      (vitamin B_3), 84
  prevention/treatment
    anti-inflammatories,
      189-190
    chondroitin sulfate, 194
    curcumin (herb), 193-194
    diet, 190-192
    exercise, 195-196
    fish oils, 194-195
    glucosamine sulfate,
      109, 194
    vitamins, 192-194
  rheumatoid arthritis, 188
  statistics, 188
ascorbic acid, *see* vitamins, C
Atkins diet, 39
attitude, 243
  aging gracefully, 243-244
  exercise, 256-258
  laughter, 252
  love, 253
  optimism, 252
  psychoneuroimmunology,
    288

B

B vitamins, 82-89
  Alzheimer's disease
    prevention/treatment, 227
  B_1 (thiamin), 82
  B_2 (riboflavin), 83
  B_3 (niacin/niacinamide),
    83-84
    see also niacin/
      niacinamide
  B_5 (pantothenic acid), 88
    arthritis prevention/
      treatment, 193
  B_6 (pyridoxine), 86
  B_{12} (cobalamin), 86-87
    normal level, 7-8
  biotin, 88
  choline, 88
  deficiency symptoms, 15-16

depression treatment, 214
folic acid, 87-88
  Alzheimer's disease
    prevention/treatment,
    227
  inositol, 88-89
  lowering homocysteine
    levels, 148
balanced diet, 47-49
  see also diet
beans
  phytochemicals, 62-63
  soy, 52-53
    see also soy
benign prostatic hyperplasia
  (BPH), *see* prostate gland,
  enlargement
beta carotene, 80-82
  CARET (Beta carotene and
    Retinol Efficiency Trial), 82
  eyesight health, 236-237
bilberry, 118
biofeedback, 251
bioflavonoids (flavonoids), 54
  menopausal hormone
    alternatives, 184
biotin, 88
  see also B vitamins
birth control pills, pyridoxine
  (vitamin B_6) depletion, 86
black cohosh, menopausal
  hormone alternative, 185
blindness, *see* eyes
blood pressure
  high, 145-147
    dietary guidelines,
      146-147
    related diseases, 146
    treatment, 146
    white coat syndrome, 14
blood sugar, *see* glucose
blood work
  interpreting results, 18-21
    CBC (complete blood
      count), 20
    cholesterol level, 19-20
  see also lab tests
blueberries, 58
BMI (body mass index), 40
boron, 97
botanicals, *see* herbs
bowels, irritable bowel
  treatment, 122-123

BPH (benign prostatic hyperplasia), *see* prostate gland, enlargement
brain
    Alzheimer's disease, *see* Alzheimer's disease
    biochemistry related to depression, 211
    keeping your mind sharp, 244-246
        educational vacations, 245
        smart drugs, 246
        taking college courses, 245
    memory loss prevention, supplements, 112
bran, oat bran effect on cholesterol, 62
breast cancer
    mammograms, 159
        recommended frequency, 18
    risk factors, 155-157
        menopausal hormone replacement therapy, 180
        storing water in plastic bottles, 156
    see also cancer
broccoli, 57-58
butter, 46
bypass surgery, 141-142

C

caffeine
    consumption prior to physicals, 15
    green tea, 61
    negative effects, 30
    osteoporosis risk, 174
    reduced consumption as depression treatment, 215
calcium, 97-98
    osteoporosis prevention, 170-171, 173
    sources, 170-171
        nondairy, 98
calculating target heart rate, 258-259

calories, 40
    amount burned during exercise
        aerobic activity, 261
        walking, 260
    BMI (body mass index), 40
    calories from protein in common foods, 292-294
    counting, 40
    empty calories, 40
cancer, 153-154
    breast cancer, 155-157
        mammograms, 18, 159
        menopausal hormone replacement therapy risks, 180
    carcinogens, 155
    cell mutation, 154
    CoQ$_{10}$ benefits, 106-107
    detection, 158-159
        hemoccult cards, 158
    organizations contact information
        American Association for Cancer Education, 296
        American Cancer Society, 296
        American Institute for Cancer Research, 297
    prevention, 157-163
        antioxidants, 71, 162-163
        fruits/vegetables, 160
        high-fiber diets, 160
        low-fat diet, 159-160
        macrobiotic diets, 160-161
        phytochemicals, 161-162
        polyphenols, green tea, 60-61
        supplements, 162-163
        vitamin E benefits, 92
        see also miracle foods
    risk factors, 154-155
        breast cancer, 155-157, 180
    statistics, 154
    treatment, 163-165
        tamoxifen, 157
capsaicin cream, arthritis symptom relief, 193
carbohydrates, 43-44
carcinogens, 155

cardiomyopathy, 107
cardiovascular disease, *see* heart disease
CARET (Beta carotene and Retinol Efficiency Trial), 82
carrot cake, nutrition of, 37
cataracts, 233-236
    causes, 233
    prevention
        vitamin C, 91, 234
        vitamin E, 235-236
    statistics, 234
    see also eyes
catheterization (heart), 141
CBC (complete blood count) test, 20
cervical dysplasia, folic acid benefits, 87
cetyl myristoleate (CMO), 112
checkups, *see* physical exams
cheilosis, 83
chelation therapy, heart disease treatment, 150-151
chemicals
    environmental toxins, effect on immune system, 132-133
    pesticides/herbicides/fungicides, 32-33
chemicals in food
    additives/preservatives, 32
    anthrocyanosides, blueberries, 58
    antioxidants, *see* antioxidants
    flavonoids, 54
        wine, 56
    isothiocyanate, 57
    lycopene, tomatoes, 61-62
    pesticides/herbicides/fungicides, 32-33
    phenolic compounds, wine, 56
    phytochemicals, *see* phytochemicals
chewing tobacco, leukoplakia (premalignant cancer), 81
chicken preparation, 46
chiropractic medicine, American Chiropractic Association, 295

cholesterol, 19-20, 45-46
  cholesterol levels in
    common foods, 289-294
  hydrogenated fats, 29
  interpreting lab results,
    19-20
  National Cholesterol
    Education Program, 297
  oatmeal, 45
  reducing, 143-145
    beans, 62-63
    cancer risk of
      cholesterol-lowering
      drugs, 157
    medications, 144
    niacin (vitamin B₃), 83-84
    oat bran, 62
    red wine, 56-57
choline, 88
  see also B vitamins
chondroitin sulfate, arthritis
  prevention/treatment, 194
chromium, 98-99
  food sources, 99
cigarette smoking, 31
  Alzheimer's disease risk, 226
  cancer risk, 157
  cataract risk, 235
  effect on menopause, 179
  osteoporosis risk, 169
  sexual function effects, 273
citrus fruits, *see* vitamins, C
CMO (cetyl myristoleate), 112
cobalamin (vitamin B₁₂), 86-87
  see also B vitamins
coffee, drinking prior to
  physicals, 15
  see also caffeine
cola drinks, sugar content, 28
*Common Form of Joint
  Dysfunction: Its Incidence and
  Treatment, The*, 17
complex carbohydrates, 44
conjunctivitis (eyes), 233
CoQ₁₀, 106-107
  angina treatment, 148
cosmetic surgery, 284-286
  men, 285
  women, 285-286
Council for Responsible
  Nutrition contact
  information, 298

counseling as depression
  treatment, 220
creatine, 112
curcumin (herb), arthritis
  prevention/treatment, 193

D

dairy products
  fat/cholesterol level,
    291-294
  osteoporosis prevention,
    170-171
degenerative joint disease
  (DJD), *see* osteoarthritis
dehydroepiandrosterone
  (DHEA), 269-271
  Alzheimer's disease
    treatment, 230
  benefits, 270
depression, 209-221
  causes (physiological versus
    psychological), 210-211
  heart disease risk factor, 252
  seasonal affective disorder
    (SAD), 216
    statistics, 217
  symptoms, 210
  treatment, 213-216
    5-HTP
      (hydroxytryptophan),
      218-219
    activity, 221
    amino acids, 220
    antidepressants, 211-213
    companionship, 221
    counseling, 220
    diet, 213-215
    exercise, 215
    inositol, 219
    light therapy, 216
    NADH, 219
    St. John's wort, 123-124,
      217-218
DHA (docosahexaenoic acid),
  108
DHEA
  (dehydroepiandrosterone),
  269-271
  Alzheimer's disease
    treatment, 230
  benefits, 270

DHT (dihydro-testosterone),
  202
diabetes
  American Diabetes
    Association contact
    information, 296
  benefits of niacinamide
    (vitamin B₃), 84
  blood sugar test (fasting
    glucose level), 20-21
  insulin, 43
  peripheral neuropathy, 87
diet, 25-35
  Alzheimer's disease
    prevention/treatment,
    226-229
    acetyl-L-carnitine, 229
    B-vitamins, 227
    ginkgo biloba, 228
    lecithin, 229
    phosphatidyl serine (PS),
      229
    vitamin E, 228-229
  angina symptom relief, 147
  arthritis prevention/
    treatment, 190-192
  Atkins diet, 39
  balance, 47-49
  blood pressure-lowering
    dietary guidelines, 146-147
  body mass index (BMI), 40
  calories, *see* calories
  cancer/diet relationship,
    159-163
    antioxidants, 162-163
    effect on cancer risk,
      154-155
    fruits/vegetables, 160
    high-fiber diets, 160
    low-fat diet, 159-160
    macrobiotic diets,
      160-161
    phytochemicals, 161-162
    supplements, 162-163
    treatment, 164
  carbohydrates, 43-44
  cholesterol, *see* cholesterol
  depression treatment,
    213-215
  fat, *see* fat
  fiber, 44-45
  food pyramid, 26-27
  grocery shopping, 35

heart disease risk, reducing, 142
macrobiotic diet, 38-39
  cancer prevention, 160-161
meal recommendations, 47-49
menopausal dietary guidelines, 182-183
  soy, 183
mineral deficiencies, 96-97
Ornish (Pritikin) diet, 39
osteoporosis prevention, 173
prostate health, 204-205
protein, 46-47
RDAs (recommended daily allowances), 33-34
SAD (Standard American Diet), 27-33
  additives/preservatives, 32
  anti-nutrients, 29-31
  pesticides/herbicides/fungicides, 32-33
  sugar, 31-32
  vitamin level, 68
salt, 31
sexual function, 273-274
soft drink sugar content, 28
trans-fatty acids, 30
vegetarian diet, 38
  arthritis prevention/treatment, 191
Zone diet, 39
see also food
digestion, 22-23
  chewing food, 22
  gas, 22-23
dihydro-testosterone (DHT), 202
dimethylglycine (DMG), 112
disease
  Alzheimer's, *see* Alzheimer's disease
  cancer, *see* cancer
  cardiovascular, *see* heart disease
  degenerative joint disease (DJD), *see* osteoarthritis
  heart disease, *see* heart disease
  high blood pressure-related diseases, 146

horizontal versus vertical disease, 8-9
immune system, *see* immune system
peripheral vascular disease, 121
prevention
  nutritional analyses, 77
  nutritional supplements, 69-72
specialized research associations/societies, 296-297
DJD (degenerative joint disease), *see* osteoarthritis
DL phenylalanine (DLPA), depression treatment, 220
DMG (dimethylglycine), 112
docosahexaenoic acid (DHA), 108
doctors
  exams
    mammograms, *see* mammograms
    physicals, *see* physical exams
  finding nutritionally oriented physicians, 287-288
drugs
  5-HTP (hydroxytryptophan), depression treatment, 218-219
  angina symptom relief, 147
  antibiotics, over-prescription, 75
  antidepressants, 211-213
  birth control pills, pyridoxine (vitamin B_6) depletion, 86
  breast cancer risk, 157
  cholesterol lowering-drugs, 144
  Food and Drug Administration (FDA) contact information, 298
  herbs, 115-117
    see also herbs
  micronization, 276
  miracle drugs, 51
  most prescribed drugs, 76
  osteoporosis treatment, 175

Prozac, 211-213
sexual function
  adverse effects of medications, 273
  Viagra, 272-273
  yohimbine, 273
side effects, 74-76
smart drugs, 246

E

eating
  chewing food, 22
  digestion, 22-23
    gas, 22-23
  see also diet; food
echinacea, 118-119
  immune system enhancement, 135
EDTA (ethylene diamine tetra acetic acid), heart disease treatment, 150
eicosapentaenoic acid (EPA), 108
elderly, nutritional deficiencies, 70
electrolytes, 21
empty calories, 40
endorphins, 215
enlarged prostrate, *see* prostate gland, enlargement
EPA (eicosapentaenoic acid), 108
Equal, 32
essential fatty acids, 107-108
  prostate health, 207
estrogen, 275-276
  Alzheimer's disease treatment, 229
  menopausal hormone replacement therapy, 179-180
    natural hormone-replacement, 181-182
ethylene diamine tetra acetic acid (EDTA), heart disease treatment, 150
examinations
  eyes, 232
  mammograms, 18, 159
  physicals, *see* physical exams

exercise, 255-263
 aerobic activity, 261
 angina/chest pain, 147-148
 arthritis prevention/
  treatment, 195-196
 attitude, 256-258
 benefits, 256-258
 consulting physicians prior
  to beginning, 143
 depression treatment, 215
 endorphins, 215
 menopausal hormone
  alternatives, 185
 osteoporosis prevention,
  174-175
 personal program setup,
  262-263
 reducing heart disease risk,
  142-143
 target heart rate, calculating,
  258-259
 walking, 257, 260-261
 warming up, 260
 weightlifting, 261-262
extracts, 117
 bilberry, 118
 buying, 117
 capsaicin cream, arthritis
  symptom relief, 193
 ginkgo biloba, *see* ginkgo
  biloba
 Saw-palmetto (Serenoa
  repens), prostate health,
  205
 standardized extracts, 117
 see also herbs
eyes, 231-239
 cataracts, 233-236
  vitamin C benefits, 91
  zinc benefits, 103
 dry eyes treatment, 236
 examinations, 232
 macular degeneration, 233,
  236-238
 maintaining eye health,
  238-239
  herbs, 239
  sleep, 239
  taurine, 238
 ophthalmologists versus
  optometrists, 232
 sunglasses, 239

F

fasting
 arthritis treatment, 190-191
 fasting glucose level test, 20
fat, 41-43
 butter/margarine, 46
 diet's effect on cancer risk,
  154-155, 159-160
 essential fatty acids, 107-108
  prostate health, 207
 hydrogenation, 29
 levels in common foods,
  289-294
 positive effects, 41
 saturated, 41-42
 trans-fatty acids, 30
 see also oils
FDA (Food and Drug
 Administration) contact
 information, 298
Feverfew, 119
fiber, 44-45
 cancer prevention, 160
finasteride (Proscar), prostate
 gland enlargement treatment,
 202-203
fish/fish oils, 194-195
 arthritis prevention/
  treatment, 191-195
  NSAID drugs
   combination risk, 195
 heavy metals effect on
  immune system, 133
fitness, *see* exercise
flavonoids, 54
 wine, 56
flax seed
 menopausal benefits, 183
 prostate enlargement
  treatment, 207
folic acid, 87-88
 Alzheimer's disease
  prevention/treatment, 227
 food sources, 87
 see also B vitamins
food
 additives/preservatives, 32
 allergies
  effect on immune
   system, 131
  environmental toxins,
   132-133

beans, 62-63
 phytochemicals, 62-63
 soy, 52-53
blood pressure-lowering
 dietary guidelines, 146-147
broccoli, 57-58
butter/margarine, 46
 alternatives, 46
carrot cake, nutrition of, 37
chemicals, *see* chemicals in
 food
chewing, 22
cholesterol-reducing food/
 nutrients, 145
digestion, 22-23
 gas, 22-23
flavonoids, 54
Food and Drug Admin-
 istration (FDA) contact
 information, 298
food pyramid, 26-27
fried food, *see* oils; fat
grocery shopping, 35
hydrogenation, 29
meal recommendations,
 47-49
miracle foods, *see* miracle
 foods
negative effects of, 9
nightshade family, arthritis
 risk, 191
nutritional information
 calories from protein in
  common foods, 292-294
 cholesterol/fat levels in
  common foods, 289-294
 fat, 43
onions, 59
organic, 32-33
 wines, 57
pesticides/herbicides/
 fungicides, 32-33
processed foods, avoiding,
 48
salicylates, 16
salt, 31
soft drinks, sugar content,
 28
soy products, 52-53
spinach, cataract
 prevention, 238
sugar, 31-32
super foods, *see* miracle
 foods

tofu/tempeh, 38
  see also soy foods
tomatoes, 61-62
see also diet
Foundation for the
  Advancement of Innovative
  Medicine (FAIM) contact
  information, 296
free radicals, 76-77
  cancer treatments, 164
  eyesight health
    cataract formation, 233
    macular degeneration,
     236
  see also antioxidants
French paradox, 56
fried foods, *see* oils; fat
fruit
  bilberry, 118
  blueberries, 58
  citrus, *see* vitamins, C
  flavonoids, 54
    wine, 56
  lowering cancer risk, 160
  salicylates, 16
  tomatoes, 61-62
  see also food
fungicides, 32-33

G

gamma-oryzanol, 112
garlic, 59-60
  immune system
    enhancement, 136
gas, 22-23
  possible causes, 22-23
ginger, 58-59
  arthritis prevention/
    treatment, 192
  relieving cancer treatment
    discomfort, 164
ginkgo biloba, 119-120
  Alzheimer's disease
    prevention/treatment, 228
  sex drive, 274
ginseng, 120
  sexual function, 274
glands
  hormone production, 267
  pituitary, human growth
    hormone (HGH), 280-281
  prostate, *see* prostate gland

glaucoma, 233
  see also eyes
glucosamine sulfate, 109
  arthritis prevention/
    treatment, 194
glucose
  fasting glucose level test, 20
  hypoglycemia, 99
  insulin, 43
glutathione, 108-109
golden-seal, immune system
  enhancement, 135-136
grape seed extract, 111
green tea, 60-61
grocery shopping, 35
  herbs, 117
  nutritional information
    calories from protein in
     common foods, 292-294
    cholesterol/fat levels in
     common foods, 289-294
    fat, 43
  supplements, 73-74
  top 10 items purchased, 49
guggul (herb), heart disease
  prevention/treatment, 150

H

hair element analysis, 77
hawthorn, heart disease
  prevention/treatment,
  149-150
HDL (high-density lipoprotein)
  cholesterol, 19-20
headaches
  National Headache
    Foundation contact
    information, 297
  remedies
    Feverfew, 119
    ginger, 58-59
health definition, 69
health care practitioners,
  finding nutritionally oriented
  physicians, 287-288
heart, 139-140
  target heart rate, calculating,
    258-259
heart disease, 140-141
  American Heart Association
    contact information, 297

angina/chest pain (angina
  pectoris), 92, 140, 147-148
cardiomyopathy, 107
high blood pressure,
  145-147
homocysteine levels in
  blood stream, 148
prevention/treatment,
  141-142
  chelation therapy,
    150-151
  CoQ_{10}, 106
  folic acid, 87-88
  hawthorn, 120-121
  supplements, 149-150
  vitamin E, 92-93
reducing risk, 142-143
  controlling cholesterol,
    143-145
  diet, 142
  exercise, 142-143
  relaxation/stress relief,
    143
risk factors, 141
  depression, 252
statistics, 140
surgery, 141-142
testosterone level, 277
heavy metals
  aluminum, Alzheimer's
    disease link, 226
  effect on immune system,
    132-133
hemoccult cards, cancer
  detection, 158
herbicides, 32-33
herbs, 115-125
  bilberry, 118
  buying, 117
  curcumin, arthritis
    prevention/treatment, 193
  echinacea, 118-119
  eye health, 239
  Feverfew, 119
  flax seed
    menopausal benefits, 183
    prostate enlargement
     treatment, 207
  ginger, 58-59
    arthritis prevention/
     treatment, 192
    relieving cancer
     treatment discomfort,
     164

ginkgo biloba, 119-120
  Alzheimer's disease
    prevention/treatment,
    228
  sex drive, 274
ginseng, 120
  sexual function, 274
guggul, heart disease
  prevention/treatment, 150
hawthorn, 120-121
  heart disease prevention/
    treatment, 149-150
healing power, 115-117
heart disease prevention/
  treatment, 149-150
immune system
  enhancement, 135-136
Kava, 121-122
menopausal hormone
  alternatives, 185
milk thistle, 122
muira puama, sex drive, 274
peppermint oil, 122-123
prostate health, 205-206
pygeum africanum, 205
saw palmetto, 123
  prostate health, 205
sex drive enhancement, 274
St. John's wort, 123-124
  depression treatment,
    217-218
stinging nettle, 124
  prostate health, 205-206
tinctures, 117
HGH (human growth
  hormone), 280-281
high blood pressure, 145-147
  dietary guidelines, 146-147
  related diseases, 146
  treatment, 146
Hippocrates, 11
HIV/AIDS treatment, N-acetyl
  cysteine (NAC), 108
homocysteine
  effect of folic acid on, 87-88
  heart disease cause, 148
  osteoporosis risk, 172
horizontal versus vertical
  disease, 8-9
hormones, 265-266
  Alzheimer's disease
    treatment, 229-230
  androstenedione, 279-280

DHEA
  (dehydroepiandrosterone),
  269-271
estrogen, 275-276
glands associated with
  hormones, 267
human growth hormone
  (HGH), 280-281
insulin, 43
melatonin, 268-269
menopausal hormone
  replacement therapy,
  179-180
    natural hormone-
      replacement, 181-182
    risks, 180
    side effects, 180
  natural versus synthetic,
    266-268
  pregnenolone, 279
  progesterone, 276-277
  prostaglandins, 39
  replacement therapy, 266
    risks, 275
  testosterone, 277-279
hot flashes, 178
human growth hormone
  (HGH), 280-281
hydrogenation, 29
hydroxytryptophan (5-HTP),
  depression treatment,
  218-219
hypoglycemia, 99

I

illness, *see* disease; immune
  system
immune system, 129-136
  behaviors affecting
    immunity, 136-137
  causes of dysfunction,
    130-133
    antibiotics, 130
    environmental toxins,
      132-133
    food allergies, 131
    sugar, 130-131
    vitamin/mineral
      deficiencies, 130
  enhancing, 133-136
    herbs, 135-136
    nutrients, 133-135

how it works, 129-130
  signs of weakened system,
    133
impotency treatment
  diet/supplements/lifestyle,
    273-274
  Viagra, 272-273
infections of the eyes, 232
  conjunctivitis, 233
inositol, 88-89
  depression treatment, 219
  see also B vitamins
insoluble fiber, 44
  see also fiber
insulin, 43
International and American
  Associations of Clinical
  Nutritionists contact
  information, 296
International Federation on
  Aging contact information,
  298
iron, 99-100
isoflavones, soy products, 53
isothiocyanate, 57

J-K-L

Kaufman, William, 17
kidneys, effects of protein, 47

L-carnitine, heart disease
  prevention/treatment,
  149-150
lab tests
  cancer detection, 158-159
  hair element analysis, 77
  interpreting lab results,
    18-21
    CBC (complete blood
      count), 20
    cholesterol level, 19-20
  mineral status assessment,
    95-97
  nutritional analyses, 77-78
  osteoporosis detection, 175
  prostate specific antigen
    (PSA), 201
  urinary flow study, prostate
    enlargement diagnosis, 202
laughter, 252
LDL (low-density lipoprotein)
  cholesterol, 19-20

lecithin, Alzheimer's disease prevention/treatment, 229
libido, *see* sex drive
lipoic acid, 105-106
lipoproteins (cholesterol), 19
listening to your body, 21-22
liver health
  liver profile test, 21
  milk thistle herb, 122
love, benefits, 253
lycopene
  prostate health, 207
  tomatoes, 61-62

M

macrobiotic diet, 38-39
  cancer prevention, 160-161
macular degeneration, 233, 236-238
  see also eyes
magnesium, 100-101
  angina treatment, 148
  heart disease prevention/ treatment, 149-150
  osteoporosis prevention, 172
mammograms, 159
  recommended frequency, 18
margarine, 46
meal recommendations, 47-49
  see also diet; food
meat
  alternatives, 38
    soy foods, 52-53
  chicken preparation, 46
  fat/cholesterol level, 289
medication, *see* prescription medication; drugs
meditation, 250-251
  biofeedback, 251
  see also relaxation
melatonin, 268-269
memory
  Alzheimer's, *see* Alzheimer's disease
  loss prevention, supplements, 112
men
  andropause (male menopause), 278
  cosmetic surgery, 285

physicals, 18
prostate health, *see* prostate gland
menopause, 177-185
  alternatives to hormone replacement therapy, 181-185
    diet, 182-183
    exercise, 185
    herbal remedies, 185
    natural hormone-replacement, 181-182
    vitamins, 184
  andropause (men), 278
  average age, 178
  estrogen therapy benefits, 275
  hormone replacement, 179-180
    risks, 180
    side effects, 180
  perimenopause, 178
  symptoms, 178-179
  testosterone benefits, 279
menstrual periods, need for fat intake, 41
metals (heavy metals)
  aluminum
    Alzheimer's disease link, 226
    in antacid, 23
  effect on immune system, 132-133
  minerals, *see* minerals
MethylSulfonyl methane (MSM), 112
micronization, 276
milk
  dairy products
    fat/cholesterol level, 291-294
    osteoporosis prevention, 170-171
  soy milk, osteoporosis prevention, 174
milk thistle, 122
minds, keeping sharp, 244-246
  educational vacations, 245
  smart drugs, 246
  taking college courses, 245
  see also brain
minerals, 95-103
  boron, 97

calcium, 97-98
  nondairy sources, 98
  osteoporosis prevention, 170-171, 173
chromium, 98-99
deficiencies, 72-73, 96-97
  caused by medication, 76
  effect on immune system, 130
diet, 96-97
eye health, cataract prevention, 237
hair element analysis, 77
immune system enhancement, 134
iron, 99-100
magnesium, 100-101
  angina treatment, 148
  heart disease prevention/ treatment, 149-150
  osteoporosis prevention, 172
menopausal hormone alternatives, 184
mineral status assessment, 95-97
phosphorus, osteoporosis risk, 174
prostate enlargement treatment, 206-207
selenium, 101-102
  eyesight health, 237
silicon, osteoporosis prevention, 172
zinc, 102-103
  see also zinc
see also supplements
miracle drugs, 51
miracle foods
  beans, 62-63
  blueberries, 58
  broccoli, 57-58
  flavonoids, 54
    wine, 56
  garlic/onions, 59-60
  ginger, 58-59
  green tea, 60-61
  phytochemicals, 54-56
    increasing content in your diet, 55-56
    phytochemical-containing foods, 55
    see also phytochemicals

red wine, 56-57
soy, 52-53
tomatoes, 61-62
miso, *see* soy foods
monounsaturated fat, 41-42
  see also fat
mouth condition
  leukoplakia (premalignant
    cancer), 81
  physical examinations, 15
MSM (MethylSulfonyl
  methane), 112
muira puama (herb), increased
  sex drive, 274
multivitamins, choosing, 73-74
  see also vitamins
mushroom extracts, 109-110

N

N-acetyl cysteine (NAC), 109
NADH (nicotinamide adenine
  dinucleotide), 110
  depression treatment, 219
nails, physical examinations,
  16
National Cholesterol Education
  Program contact information,
  297
National Council on Aging
  contact information, 298
National Foundation for Brain
  Research contact information,
  298
National Headache Foundation
  contact information, 297
National Institute of Health
  contact information, 298
  Office of Alternative
    Medicine, 299
National Institute of Mental
  Health contact information,
  299
National Institute of
  Neurological Disorders and
  Stroke contact information,
  299
National Institute on Aging
  contact information, 299
National Osteoporosis
  Foundation contact
  information, 297

National Parkinson Foundation
  contact information, 297
neurofibrillary tangles
  (Alzheimer's disease), 224-225
neurotransmitters
  biochemistry related to
    depression, 211
  smart drugs, 246
niacin/niacinamide (vitamin
  B$_3$), 17, 83-84
  arthritis prevention/
    treatment, 192-193
  cautions, 84
  cholesterol reduction, 83-84
    dosage recommenda-
      tions, 144
  food sources, 84
  see also B vitamins
nicotinamide adenine
  dinucleotide (NADH), 110
nightshade food family,
  arthritis risk, 191
nonsteroidal anti-
  inflammatory drugs (NSAIDs),
  189-190
  fish oil combination risk,
    195
  normal range, 7-8
  American diet vitamin
    level, 68
noses
  allergies, *see* allergies
  physical examinations, 16
NSAIDs (nonsteroidal
  anti-inflammatory drugs),
  189-190
  fish oil combination risk,
    195
NutraSweet, 32
nutrients
  5-HTP, 109
  alpha-lipoic acid, 105-106
  Alzheimer's disease
    prevention/treatment,
    227-229
  anti-nutrients, 29-31
  cetyl myristoleate (CMO),
    112
  cholesterol-reducing food/
    nutrients, 145
  CoQ$_{10}$, 106-107
    angina treatment, 148
  creatine, 112

dimethylglycine (DMG), 112
essential fatty acids, 107-108
gamma-oryzanol, 112
glucosamine sulfate, 109
glutathione, 108-109
grape seed extract, 111
heart disease prevention/
  treatment, 149-150
  chelation therapy,
    150-151
immune system
  enhancement, 133-135
MethylSulfonyl methane
  (MSM), 112
mushroom extracts, 109-110
N-acetyl cysteine (NAC), 109
NADH (nicotinamide
  adenine dinucleotide), 110
octacosanol, 112
phosphatidyl serine (PS),
  111-112
prostate enlargement
  treatment, 206-207
pycnogenol, 111
pyruvate, 112
quercetin, 110-111
synergy, 102
see also diet; supplements
nutritional analyses, 77-78
nutritional information
  calories from protein in
    common foods, 292-294
  cholesterol/fat levels in
    common foods, 289-294
  fat, 43
  RDAs (recommended daily
    allowances), 33-34
nutritionally oriented
  physicians, finding, 287-288

O

oat bran, effect on cholesterol,
  45, 62
obesity
  effect on immune system,
    136
  increased cancer risk, 158
  obesity rate in ages 35 to 45,
    256
octacosanol, 112

Office of Alternative Medicine contact information, 299
oils
    essential fatty acids, 107-108
        prostate health, 207
        see also Omega-3 oils
    hydrogenation, 29
    saturated fat, 41-42
    see also fat
Omega 3 oils, 107-108
    arthritis prevention/ treatment, 191-193
        fish oils, 194-195
    flax seed
        menopausal benefits, 183
        prostate enlargement treatment, 207
onions, 59
ophthalmologists, 232
optometrists, 232
organic foods, 32-33
    wines, 57
organizations
    Academy of Pharmaceutical Research and Science, 297
    Alliance for Aging Research, 298
    American Nutraceutical Association, 298
    Council for Responsible Nutrition, 298
    Food and Drug Administration (FDA), 298
    International Federation on Aging, 298
    National Council on Aging, 298
    National Foundation for Brain Research, 298
    National Institute of Health, 298
    National Institute of Mental Health, 299
    National Institute of Neurological Disorders and Stroke, 299
    National Institute on Aging, 299
    nutritionally oriented health care practitioners, 295-296
    Office of Alternative Medicine, 299

specialized research associations/societies, 296-297
Ornish (Pritikin) diet, 39
osteoarthritis (degenerative joint disease, DJD), 187-188
    benefits of niacinamide (vitamin B$_3$), 84
    see also arthritis
osteoporosis, 167
    description, 168
    detection, 175
    National Osteoporosis Foundation contact information, 297
    prevention, 169-170
        calcium, 170-171, 173
        diet, 173
        exercise, 174-175
        magnesium, 172
        protein, 173-174
        silicon, 172
        sodium intake, 172
        vitamin D, 171-173
        vitamin K, 173
    risk factors, 94, 169-170
        surgical menopause, 178
    statistics, 168
    treatment, 175

P

pantothenic acid (vitamin B$_5$), 88
    arthritis prevention/ treatment, 193
    see also B vitamins
parenting late in life, 251-252
Parkinson's disease, National Parkinson Foundation contact information, 297
PCOs (proanthrocyanidins), 111
PEA (phenylethylamine), depression treatment, 220
peppermint oil, 122-123
perimenopause, 178
    see also menopause
peripheral neuropathy, 87
peripheral vascular disease, 121
pesticides, 32-33
    effect on immune system, 132

pharmaceuticals, *see* prescription medication
phenolic compounds, wine, 56
phenylalanine (amino acid), depression treatment, 220
phosphatidyl serine (PS), 111-112
    Alzheimer's disease prevention/treatment, 229
    osteoporosis risk, 174
physical fitness, *see* exercise
physical exams, 13-23
    allergies, 16
    coffee intake prior to, 15
    interpreting lab results, 18-21
        CBC (complete blood count), 20
        cholesterol level, 19-20
    hair element analysis, 77
    listing complaints, 14
    men, 18
    mineral status assessment, 95-97
    mouth condition, 15
    nails condition, 16
    nose condition, 16
    nutritional analyses, 77-78
    pulse rate, 15
    respiratory rate, 15
    scalp condition, 15
    skin condition, 16
    symptoms/treatments, 17
    white coat syndrome, 14
    women, 18
physicians
    finding nutritionally oriented physicians, 287-288
    ophthalmologists, 232
    optometrists, 232
phytochemicals, 54-56
    beans, 62
    broccoli, 57-58
    flavonoids, 54
    increasing content in your diet, 55-56
    phytochemical-containing foods, 55
    sulforaphane, broccoli, 57-58
    supplements, 55

phytoestrogen, 52
  isoflavones in soy foods, 53
pituitary gland, human growth
  hormone (HGH), 280-281
plastic surgery, 284-286
  men, 285
  women, 285-286
polyphenols, green tea, 60-61
polysaccharide K (PSK)
  mushroom extract, 110
polyunsaturated fat, 41-42
  see also fat
pregnancy
  breastfeeding,
    docosahexaenoic acid
    (DHA), 108
  folic acid benefits, 87
  nutritional supplements, 71
  vitamin A warning, 81
pregnenolone, 279
prescription medication
  5-HTP (hydroxytryptophan),
    depression treatment,
    218-219
  angina symptom relief, 147
  antibiotics, over-
    prescription of, 75
  antidepressants, 211-213
  birth control pills,
    pyridoxine (vitamin B₆)
    depletion, 86
  breast cancer risk, 157
  cholesterol lowering-drugs,
    144
  micronization, 276
  most prescribed drugs, 76
  osteoporosis treatment, 175
  Prozac, 211-213
  side effects, 74-76
preservatives/additives, 32
Pritikin (Ornish) diet, 39
proanthrocyanidins (PCOs),
  111
probiotics, 23
processed foods, avoiding, 48
progesterone, 276-277
  menopausal hormone
    replacement therapy,
    179-180
    natural hormone-
      replacement, 181-182

Proscar (finasteride)
  danger to women, 202
  prostate gland enlargement
    treatment, 202-203
prostaglandins, 39
prostate gland, 199-207
  enlargement (benign
    prostatic hyperplasia,
    BPH), 200-202
    causes, 202
    diagnosing, 201-202
    Proscar (finasteride)
      treatment, 202-203
    research dollars, 200
    statistics, 200-201
    surgery/surgery options,
      203-204
    symptoms, 201
  function, 199
  maintaining health, 204-207
    diet, 204-206
    herbs, 205-206
    nutrients, 206-207
    saw palmetto herb, 123
    vitamins/minerals,
      206-207
  PSA (prostate specific
    antigen) test, 18
  size, 200
protein, 46-47
  calories from protein in
    common foods, 292-294
  effect on kidneys, 47
  osteoporosis prevention,
    173-174
  sexual function, 273
Prozac, 211-213
  side effects, 211
PS (phosphatidyl serine),
  111-112
  Alzheimer's disease
    prevention/treatment, 229
  osteoporosis risk, 174
PSA (prostate specific antigen)
  test, 201
PSK (polysaccharide K)
  mushroom extract, 110
psychoneuroimmunology, 288
pulse rate, 15
  target heart rate, 258-259
pycnogenol, 111

pygeum africanum, prostate
  health, 205
pyridoxine (B₆), 86
pyruvate, 112

Q-R

quercetin, 110-111
RDAs (recommended daily
  allowances), 33-34
recipes, spaghetti squash, 48
recommended daily allowances
  (RDAs), 33-34
red wine, 56-57
  French paradox, 56
  see also alcohol
relaxation
  effect of stress on immune
    system, 136
  biofeedback, 251
  meditation, 250-251
  reducing heart disease risk,
    143
  yoga, 247-249
remedies
  garlic/onions, 59-60
  ginger, 58-59
  herbs, *see* herbs
research studies
  CARET (Beta carotene and
    Retinol Efficiency Trial), 82
  nutritional supplements/
    disease prevention, 71-72
  vitamin D deficiencies, 91
  vitamin E benefits, 92
respiratory rate, 15
rheumatoid arthritis, 188
  see also arthritis
riboflavin (vitamin B₂), 83
  see also B vitamins

S

SAD (seasonal affective
  disorder), 216
  statistics, 217
  see also depression
SAD (Standard American Diet),
  27-33
  additives/preservatives, 32

anti-nutrients, 29-31
    pesticides/herbicides/
        fungicides, 32-33
    sugar, 31-32
    vitamin level, 68
salicylates, 16
salt, 31
saturated fat, 41-42
saw palmetto, 123
    prostate health, 205
scalp condition, physical
    examinations, 15
seasonal affective disorder
    (SAD), 216
    statistics, 217
    see also depression
seitan, 38
selenium, 101-102
    eyesight health, 237
    recommended dosage, 102
senile plaques (Alzheimer's
    disease), 224-225
    see also Alzheimer's disease
Serenoa repens, *see* Saw
    palmetto
serotonin, 85
    elevating with 5-HTP, 109
    serotonin reuptake
        inhibitors (SSRIs),
        depression treatment,
        211-213
sex drive, 271-274
    diet/supplements/lifestyle,
        273-274
    Viagra, 272-273
shopping, *see* grocery shopping
sickness, *see* disease; immune
    system
silicon, osteoporosis
    prevention, 172
simple carbohydrates, 43-44
skin
    physical examinations, 16
    preserving skin health, 286
sleep, eye health, 239
smart drugs, 246
smoking, 31
    Alzheimer's disease risk, 226
    cancer risk, 157
    cataract risk, 235
    effect on menopause, 179
    osteoporosis risk, 169
    sexual function effects, 273

social activity, depression
    treatment, 221
sodium, osteoporosis risk, 172
soft drinks
    caffeine, *see* caffeine
    sugar content, 28
soluble fiber, 44-45
    see also fiber
soy foods, 52-53
    American Soybean
        Association contact
        information, 145
    cholesterol reduction, 145
    isoflavones in soy products,
        53
    menopausal dietary
        guidelines, 183
    osteoporosis prevention,
        174
spinach, cataract prevention,
    238
spirituality, 246-247
    meditation, 250-251
    yoga, 247-249
SSRIs (serotonin reuptake
    inhibitors), depression
    treatment, 211-213
St. John's wort, 123-124
    depression treatment,
        217-218
Standard American Diet (SAD),
    27-33
    additives/preservatives, 32
    anti-nutrients, 29-31
    pesticides/herbicides/
        fungicides, 32-33
    sugar, 31-32
standardized extracts, 117
stinging nettle, 124
    prostate health, 205-206
stress
    effect on immune system,
        136
    reducing
        Kava, 121-122
        relaxation, *see* relaxation
substance P, arthritis symptom
    relief, 193
sugar, 31-32
    alternatives, 32
    cravings due to chromium
        deficiency, 99

effect on immune system,
    130-131
glucose
    fasting glucose level test,
        20
    hypoglycemia, 99
    insulin, 43
sulforaphane, broccoli, 57-58
sun-damaged skin, 16
sunglasses, cataract prevention,
    239
super foods, *see* miracle foods
supplements
    5-HTP, 109
    alpha-lipoic acid, 105-106
    Alzheimer's disease
        prevention/treatment,
        227-229
    antioxidants, *see*
        antioxidants
    arthritis prevention/
        treatment, 192-195
        chondroitin sulfate, 194
        curcumin (herb), 193-194
        fish oils, 194-195
        glucosamine sulfate, 194
        vitamins, 192-194
    cancer prevention/
        treatment, 162-164
    cetyl myristoleate (CMO),
        112
    choosing, 73-74
    CoQ$_{10}$, 106-107
        angina treatment, 148
    creatine, 112
    deficiencies, 72-73
        caused by medication, 76
    depression treatment,
        217-220
    dimethylglycine (DMG), 112
    docosahexaenoic acid
        (DHA), 108
    eicosapentaenoic acid (EPA),
        108
    eye health
        cataract prevention,
            233-236
        macular degeneration
            prevention, 236-238
    fatty acids, 107-108
    gamma-oryzanol, 112
    glucosamine sulfate, 109
    glutathione, 108-109
    grape seed extract, 111

heart disease prevention/ treatment, 149-150
herbs, *see* herbs
immune system enhancement
  herbs, 135-136
  vitamins/minerals, 133-135
menopausal hormone alternatives
  herbs, 185
  vitamins/minerals, 184
MethylSulfonyl methane (MSM), 112
minerals, *see* minerals
mushroom extracts, 109-110
need for, 67-72
  disease preventions, 69-72
  pregnancy, 71
nicotinamide adenine dinucleotide (NADH), 110
nutritional analyses, 77-78
octacosanol, 112
osteoporosis prevention, calcium, 170
phosphatidyl serine (PS), 111-112
phytochemicals, 55
probiotics, 23
prostate enlargement treatment, 206-207
pycnogenol, 111
pyruvate, 112
quercetin, 110-111
sexual function, 273-274
taking, 74
vitamins
  A, potential toxicity, 80
  E (tocopherols), 93
  multivitamins, 73-74
  time-release/ sustain-release, 74
  see also vitamins
surgery
  cosmetic, 284-286
    men, 285
    women, 285-286
  heart, 141-142
  prostate gland enlargement, 203-204

surgical menopause, osteoporosis risk, 178
symptoms
  listening to your body, 21-22
  symptoms/treatments table, 17

T

tamoxifen, cancer treatment, 157
target heart rate, calculating, 258-259
taurine, eye health, 238
tea
  ginger tea, arthritis prevention/treatment, 192
  green tea, 60-61
tempeh, 38
testosterone, 277-279
tests
  Alzheimer's disease, 225
  cancer detection, 158-159
  CBC (complete blood count), 20
  cholesterol level, 19-20
  electrolytes, 21
  fasting glucose level (blood sugar), 20
  hair element analysis, 77
  interpreting lab results, 18-21
  liver profile, 21
  mineral status assessment, 95-97
  nutritional analyses, 77-78
  osteoporosis detection, 175
  prostate specific antigen (PSA), 18, 201
  thyroid, 21
  urinalysis, 21
  urinary flow study, prostate enlargement diagnosis, 202
therapy as depression treatment, 220
thiamin (vitamin B$_1$), 82
  see also B vitamins
thyroid tests, 21
time-release/sustain-release supplements, 74

tinctures, 117
tobacco
  arthritis risk, 191
  chewing, leukoplakia (premalignant cancer), 81
  see also smoking
tocopherols (vitamin E), 93
tofu, 38
  see also soy products
tomatoes, 61-62
toxins (environmental), effect on immune system, 132-133
trans-fatty acids, 30
transurethral resection of the prostate (TURP), 203-204
tryptophan, 109
TURP (transurethral resection of the prostate), 203-204
Tyrosine (amino acid), depression treatment, 220

U

urinalysis, 21
urinary flow study, prostate enlargement diagnosis, 202
urinary tract infections, herbal treatment, 124-125

V

vegetables
  flavonoids, 54
  lowering cancer risk, 160
  salicylates, 16
  tomatoes, 61-62
  see also food; diet
vegetarian diets, 38
  arthritis prevention/ treatment, 191
  meat substitutes, 38
vertical versus horizontal disease, 8-9
Viagra, 272-273
vitamins, 79
  A, 80-82
    potential toxicity, 80
  Alzheimer's disease prevention/treatment
    B vitamins, 227
    E, 228-229

arthritis prevention/
  treatment, 191
B, 82-89
  Alzheimer's disease
    prevention/treatment,
    227
  B$_1$ (thiamin), 82
  B$_2$ (riboflavin), 83
  B$_3$, *see* niacin/
    niacinamide
  B$_5$, *see* pantothenic acid
  B$_6$ (pyridoxine), 86
  B$_{12}$ (cobalamin), 86-87
  biotin, 88
  choline, 88
  deficiency symptoms,
    15-16
  folic acid, 87-88
  inositol, 88-89, 219
  lowering homocysteine
    levels, 148
  normal level, 7-8
  pantothenic acid
    (vitamin B$_5$), 88
beta carotene, 80-82
  CARET (Beta carotene
    and Retinol Efficiency
    Trial), 82
  eyesight health, 236-237
C (ascorbic acid), 89-91
  cataract prevention, 91,
    234
  dosage recommenda-
    tions, 90
  macular degeneration
    prevention (eyes),
    236-237
cancer prevention, 162-163
D, 91
  osteoporosis prevention,
    171-173
  sources, 91
deficiencies, 72-73
  B$_6$ (pyridoxine), 85
  caused by medication, 76
  effect on immune system,
    130
  vitamin D, 91
depression treatment, 214
E, 92-93
  Alzheimer's disease

prevention/treatment,
  228-229
cataract prevention,
  235-236
dosage
  recommendations, 93
macular degeneration
  prevention (eyes),
  236-237
tocopherols, 93
eye health, 238
  cataract prevention,
    234-236
  macular degeneration
    prevention, 236-237
heart disease prevention/
  treatment, 149
immune system
  enhancement, 133-135
K, 94
  food sources, 94
  osteoporosis prevention,
    173
menopausal hormone
  alternatives, 184
niacinamide, 17
normal American diet
  level, 68
prostate enlargement
  treatment, 206-207
supplements
  choosing, 73-74
  multivitamins, 73-74
  time-release/
    sustain-release
    vitamins, 74
see also supplements;
  minerals

W

walking, 257, 260-261
warming up before exercise,
  260
water
  cancer risk from storing in
    plastic bottles, 156
  enlarged prostate symptom
    relief, 204
  intake recommendations, 49

weight loss
  BMI (body mass index), 40
  calories
    counting, 40
    empty calories, 40
    aerobic activity, 261
    walking, 260
  fat, 41-43
    need for, 41
  see also diet
weightlifting, 261-262
white coat syndrome, 14
white flour, mineral
  deficiency, 96
wine
  French paradox, 56
  organic wines, 57
  red wine, 56-57
  see also alcohol
women
  birth control pills,
    pyridoxine (vitamin B$_6$)
    depletion, 86
  cancer detection tests,
    158-159
  cervical dysplasia, folic acid
    benefits, 87
  cosmetic surgery, 285-286
  green tea, 61
  menopause, *see* menopause
  menstrual periods, need for
    fat intake, 41
  physicals, 18
  pregnancy, *see* pregnancy
  RDAs (recommended daily
    allowances), 34

X-Y-Z

yoga, 247-249
  health benefits, 248-249
  learning, 249
yohimbine, sexual function
  drug, 273

zinc, 102-103
  deficiency symptoms, 16
  eyesight health, 237
  immune system
    enhancement, 134
  prostate enlargement
    treatment, 206
Zone diet, 39

DR. ALLAN MAGAZINER'S
Life Essentials Nutritional Supplements
Are Now Available to You!

My Pledge of Quality

I designed these products using therapeutic doses of the most efficacious nutrients available. After I selected the core ingredients for each product, I added a base of additional nutrients to provide important synergistic benefits. These formulas are unique because I carefully formulated each product using the latest scientific evidence *and* the principles of Natural Medicine.

I selected the ingredients from the world's leading suppliers. Many of these ingredients are patented and trademarked, which ensures consistent quality from batch to batch. The Standardized herbal extracts are purchased from Europe's leading phyto-pharmaceutical companies where each product is meticulously extracted to achieve the optimum levels of biologically active compounds. Also, each product features nutrient types that are easily absorbed and utilized by the human body.

My products are rigorously tested by independent laboratories with particular expertise in the analysis of nutritional supplements.

During the manufacturing process Quality Assurance procedures are meticulously followed to ensure high quality finished products.

I take great pride in featuring products with the finest ingredients in the world. I am proud that my products are carefully manufactured, scientifically formulated and laboratory tested. I believe these products can be important tools in your quest for optimal health.

Dr. Allan Magaziner

BRAIN ESSENTIALS contains herbs and nutrients that have been traditionally associated with a healthy mind including Standardized Ginkgo Biloba Extract, Phosphatidyl Serine, Acetyl L-Carnitine and many other nutrients.

CARDIO ESSENTIALS utilizes Coenzyme Q10, Standardized Hawthorn Extract, L-Carnitine and other nutrients to help promote optimal health during the mature years of life.

FEM ESSENTIALS provides herbs and nutrients such as Standardized Black Cohosh Extract, Standardized Soy Isoflavones and many other nutrients that may help ease the symptoms during a woman's normal mid-life transition.

IMMUNE ESSENTIALS is a full spectrum formulation of herbs and nutrients such as Standardized Echinacea, Astragalus Extract, Zinc and Vitamin C that may help to maintain optimum health.

JOINT ESSENTIALS features Glucosamine Sulfate and Chondroitin Sulfate and many other nutrients that may help maintain optimal flexibility during the mature years.

MOOD ESSENTIALS is a blend of herbs and nutrients that are commonly associated with a healthy state of mind such as Standardized St. John's Wort Extract, L-5-HTP and Standardized Kava Root Extract.

OSTEO ESSENTIALS features Calcium, which helps prevent osteoporosis, and many other important nutrients such as Soy Isoflavones and Vitamin K.

PROSTATE ESSENTIALS contains Standardized Saw Palmetto Extract, Standardized Pygeum Extract and Opti-Zinc, which may help mature men maintain optimal health.

VISION ESSENTIALS helps promote optimal health with Standardized Bilberry Extract, Lutein, Vitamin C, Zinc and other important nutrients.

To order call: 1-800-LIFE-595

Many other products are available such as Vitamin E, Antioxidants, B-Complex, Multivitamins and Ester-C.

For more information, please write to:

Life Essentials Nutritional Supplements
P.O. Box 426
Whitehouse, NJ 08888

These statements have not been evaluated by the Food and Drug Administration. These statements are not intended to diagnose, treat, cure, or prevent any disease.